Reason and Medicine

Reason and Medicine: Art and Science of Healing from Antiquity to Modern Times

The author Daya R Varma, MD, PhD is Professor Emeritus, Department of Pharmacology and Therapeutics, McGill University, Montreal, QC, Canada.

This is an abridged and updated version of the book *The Art and Science of Healing Since Antiquity* (Xlibris, Bloomington, 2011).

Reason and Medicine

Art and Science of Healing from Antiquity to Modern Times

Daya Ram Varma MD, PhD

Three Essays
COLLECTIVE

First Edition February 2013

ISBN 978-81-88789-83-2

Three Essays
COLLECTIVE

B-957 Palam Vihar, GURGAON (Haryana) 122 017 India
Phone: 91-124 2369023, +91 98681 26587, +91 98683 44843
info@threeessays.com Website: www.threeessays.com
Printed and bound by Glorious Printers, New Delhi

In memory of my mother Sampati and father Matabadal, of the Village Narion in the Eastern Uttar Pradesh (UP) district of Azamgarh, who, like most parents, dedicated their lives to my well-being.

Young men should prove theorems, old men should write books.

Godfrey Harold Hardy[1]

1 Hardy (1877-1947) was a distinguished British mathematician on number theory; the quote is from *Selected Papers of Freeman Dyson* (publisher, American Mathematical Society, 1996, page 43). When Dyson was in Cambridge in 1942, he asked Hardy "why he had spent so much of his time writing books, such as the elementary textbook *An Introduction to the Theory of Numbers* instead of doing mathematical research." Hardy answered without any pathos in his voice, "Young men should prove theorems, old men should write books." Hardy was responsible for getting the Indian Mathematician Srinivasa Ramanujan (1887-1920) to Cambridge and ensuring that he was elected to the prestigious Fellow of Royal Society (FRS) despite Ramanujan having no formal academic degree.

Contents

Acknowledgments

The original version of the book contained 413 pages. It received many compliments from historians, political scientists, philosophers, reviewers and readers. At the same time, I inferred from reviews by Mridula Ramanna in *Economic and Political Weekly* (July 30, 2011) and William Dere in *Frontier* (December, 2011) and from personal comments by my friend Professor Iqbal Niazi that the book could be shortened. Original book had abstracts preceding the text of each Chapter. Professor Nalini Taneja suggested that abstracts are not necessary in a book. I value these remarks and this abridged version is a response to their suggestions.

I wish to thank Asad Zaidi of the Three Essays Collective for producing this abridged version in India.

Note on Abridgement

The original version of the book had abstracts preceding each chapter; these have been deleted in this abridged version. Appendix 1 (Medical Historiography) and Appendix 3 (The 1978 declaration of Alma-Ata on primary health care) have been deleted. The book was written for a broad readership. However, some portions in Chapter 13 (Therapeutics Since Antiquity) and Chapter 14 (Modern Medicine Comes of Age) are of greater interest to medical professionals than to the general public; both these chapters have been greatly modified. As well, I have attempted to avoid repetition in this version of the book.

Preface

There is an old Chinese expression about 'the Rivers going to pay court to the Sea', and indeed one can well consider the older streams of science in the different civilisations like rivers flowing into the ocean of modern science. Modern science is indeed composed of contributions from all the peoples of the Old World, and each contribution has flowed continuously into it, whether from Greek or Roman antiquity, or from the Islamic world or from the cultures of China and India.

Joseph Needham[1]

Notwithstanding the views of Joseph Needham (1900-1995) quoted above, there is something unique about medical science. Here too, rivers pay court, but also continue to behave as if each rivulet was a sea. Consequently, there is the modern medicine as well as other schools of medicine like Ayurveda, Chinese medicine, homeopathy, naturopathy, chiropractic, and so on. The journal *Nature* even talks of "Asian medicine" (*Correspondence*, 2012).

Medical historians have dealt with this issue, but their emphasis has been on modern medicine rather than a comparative exposure of different schools of medicine. There are not many narratives of medical history that can help a lay person gain insight into the different schools of medicine and assist them in making a rational choice.

Modern medicine, like all schools of medicine, is a child of spiritual medicine, commonly known as witchcraft. It has made gigantic advances, but not enough to remain unchallenged by other streams of witchcraft. This book is an attempt to analyze how witchcraft unfolded into its different variants and why modern medicine is its most rational expression.

When I was a medical student at King George's Medical College, Lucknow, India, during the years 1950-1955, I often visited one Dr. Narendra Gupta, a professor of pathology but no fan of Ayurveda, who, nevertheless, on one occasion remarked that Ayurveda had made a great contribution to medicine by ushering a departure from spiritualistic to materialistic medicine. Since then I have pondered over the significance of Dr. Gupta's remarks, and over what socio-political or philosophic factors could have contributed to this switch from one to another phase of medicine. It occurred to me then that, someday, I would make it a complete story. However, this idea remained dormant for over fifty years and would never have materialized into this book had some bizarre developments not taken place in India.

In 2006, the followers of Yoga Guru Ramdev attacked the office of the Communist Party of India (Marxist), for criticising certain practices of his Ayurvedic Divya Yog Pharmacy. This episode received much publicity in the Indian media and provoked me to write an article 'The Uninterrupted Journey of Medical Science from Witchcraft to Allopathy' (Varma, 2006); there I used the term allopathy a bit loosely because the expected readership is more familiar with this term than with any other definition of modern medicine. In this book, the terms "medicine" and "modern medicine" are used for what commonly and erroneously is called allopathy. This book is an expanded version of that article in the Indian journal.

Here I endeavour to show that witchcraft, or spiritual medicine, is the medical expression of a gathering and hunting society, Ayurveda, Chinese and Greek medicine of an agricultural society and modern medicine of a capitalist society.

January 2013
St. John's, Newfoundland, Canada

Notes

1. Joseph Needham (1900-1995) in *Science and Civilisation in China, V. 7* (Cambridge: Cambridge University Press, 2004), 25.

References

Correspondence. "Asian Medicine..." *Nature 35* (2012) 35.

Varma, D. R. "From Witchcraft to Allopathy: Uninterrupted Journey of Medical Science," *Economic and Political Weekly* (Mumbai) 41 (2006) 3,605-3,611.

CHAPTER 1

Introduction

Biology is certainly not applied physics or chemistry but an independent science, not only with its own domain but also with laws of its own; the latter may be characterized, in contrast to the general laws of matter treated in physics, as laws of specific complications (M. Hartmann). A striking testimony is the chromosome theory of inheritance, which accounts for a vast array of facts. But the great progress in biology since the turn of the century has been achieved by the same methods of generalizing, induction, of comparison and experiment, which also govern physics.

Hermann Weyl[1]

Historians and sociologists of medicine have engaged during the past two decades in a thoroughgoing re-evaluation of the historical relationship between scientific knowledge and medical practice.... What they found suggested that physicians took up science as an ideal before it offered much to help them allay the ills of the sick. The American medical profession chose to march under the banner of science for a variety of reasons that had little to do with its clinical application.

John Harley Warner[2]

Why Multiple Schools of Medicine?

Science has developed on the foundations of keen observation, appropriate experimentation and induction, and by discarding what has been proven false. While the natural sciences, as a rule, abide by these general principles, the case with medicine is not the same. There is no such thing as Chinese or Indian, Hindu or Islamic physics or chemistry, but all these societies possess their own medicines. Why is this so? Why are there distinct schools of medicine (Ayurvedic, Chinese, Homeopathic, etc.)? We find the answer in the differing tasks which natural and medical sciences perform.

Social Domain of Medical Science

A medical practitioner derives material benefit, reasonable or otherwise, from each and every interaction with the patient. Money can be made by good as well as bad medicine; and patients find out only later, if at all, which kind it was. Accordingly, in no other area are myth and reality, rationality and irrationality, science and spiritualism as intertwined, each claiming superiority over the other, as in medicine. People expect from medicine both the possible and the impossible, and consequently there is always a stream of patients with real or imaginary sicknesses, all ready to be preyed upon. Naturally, we encounter different kinds of healers.

Not only do we have practitioners of Ayurveda, homeopathy, acupuncture, and naturopathy, we also have gurus, some of whom claim to calm the mind and soul like Sri Sri Ravi Shankar of the Art of Living, Maharishi Mahesh Yogi (1917-2008) and Sathya Sai Baba (1926-2011). Fuelling the erroneous but popular perception that the West is materialistic and the East, particularly India, is spiritualistic, most "god" men and women happen to be of Indian origin; but for some reason, they prefer to operate in the United States of America, where they promise to solve problems of health as well as wealth. This environment is favoured by the limits of medical science itself, which is further compounded by unsatisfactory institutions of medical care, including medical professional bodies, public health care systems, and affordability.

Popular Expectations from Medicine

People expect cures from medicine but are unaware of the limitations that science faces; the sick would go to anyone in the hope of finding a cure. Usually, the practitioners of alternate medicine are more reassuring than the physicians of modern medicine. The culture of spiritualism, especially the more recent culture of godless spiritualism among a large section of intelligentsia who tenaciously uphold the superiority of natural over artificial, affects the attitude of people toward health and disease – all these allow the survival of different schools of medicine.

For better or worse, people's lives are affected by science, independent of their will. However, the relationships of physicians and of natural scientists with society are not identical. Mathematicians, physicists and chemists do not interact with individuals through their professions while medical practitioners very much do. The discoveries of natural scientists are transformed into gadgets for general use at a designated price and are operated according to the instructions provided by the supplier. On the other hand, a patient receives assistance directly from the physician, often in the context of a hospital setting, through a complex system that could include diagnostic, supportive, and nursing facilities. The expertise and temperament of the physicians are not uniform. Dissatisfaction with any aspect of the interaction with the physician persuades the patient to seek alternative approaches. It is not uncommon for a patient suffering from an incurable disease, such as cancer, to move from a modern hospital to a homeopath to a naturopath and eventually to the church, mosque, synagogue, or temple.

The Complexity of Biological System

There is yet another limitation faced by medical science. Biological systems are far too complex to achieve the same precision, at least for the time being, as is the case for the natural sciences. On the other hand, biology itself may be considered to be the most complex expression of physics and chemistry. In the final analysis, the elements of the periodic table, in some complex combination and interaction with each other, create living organisms, which can be as tiny as a virus or as big as an elephant.

Herbert Spencer (1820-1903) was perhaps the first to comment on the evolution of life; he wrote (Spencer, 1875), "Life is the definite combination of heterogeneous changes, both simultaneous and successive." Physics Nobel laureate Erwin Schrödinger (1887-1961) argues (Schrödinger, 1958), "How can the events *in space and time* which take place within the spatial boundary of a living organism be accounted for by physics and chemistry? The obvious inability of present-day physics and chemistry to account for such events is no reason at all for doubting that they can be accounted for by those sciences." John Desmond Bernal

(1901-1971) makes an identical point when he writes (Bernal, 1967), "*Life is a partial, continuous, progressive, multiform and conditionally interactive, self-realisation of the potentialities of atomic electron states* [italics in the original] ...all life has some material structure in common, in the form of enzymes, nucleic acids and essentially reproducing organs or molecules."

Natural Sciences Versus Medical Science

The commonality between natural and biological sciences, as pointed out above, is reflected in their history as well; the difference, however, is that erroneous assumptions in both chemistry and physics are abandoned in the light of contrary evidence while they often persist in medicine. Here I present one example from chemistry and one from physics to illustrate this point.

Until 1845, chemists believed that organic compounds were produced under the influence of a vital force and could not be made artificially. Even the synthesis of urea (an organic compound) by Friedrich Wohler (1800-1882) in 1828 could not dispel the vital force theory because he used ammonium cyanate, which was, until then, only obtained from animals. Only when Hermann Kolbe (1818-1884) synthesized acetic acid in 1845 from its elements could the vital force theory be discarded. But this was discarded for good. This was soon followed by the synthesis of many organic compounds like ethanol, methane, benzene, and acetylene by Pierre Berthelot (1827-1907). There is no chemistry now that is based on the existence of a vital force as a mediator of change from inorganic to organic substances. Had the vital force theory not been discarded, we would have no synthetic drugs, and the possibility of synthesizing a protein molecule in a test tube would be unthinkable.

Many ancient philosophers and a good many physicists believed that the speed of light is infinite and that ether is essential for the motion of light (or elecromagnetic waves). Philosopher René Descartes (1596-1650) felt that if the speed of light were finite, his whole philosophy would crack (Mackay and Oldford, 2000).

However, in 1676, the astronomer Olaf Roemer (1644-1710) suggested on the basis of experiments that the speed of light was finite, incredibly fast, but finite. This assertion was confirmed in 1728 by the astronomer James Bradley (1692-1762), who estimated the speed of light to be approximately 298,000 kilometres per second, not very far off from the present estimate of 299,792,458 meters per second or approximately 300,000 kilometres per second. This became the basis of one of the greatest advances of the twentieth century when Albert Einstein used the transformation equation of Mendrik Lorentz (1853-1928) to present his theory of special relativity ($E = mc^2$), where *c* served as a universal constant, to demonstrate the equivalence of mass *m* and energy *E*.

Simultaneously, the experiments by Albert Michelson (1852-1931) and Edward Morley (1838-1923) in 1887, together with Einstein's corpuscular theory of light for which he was awarded the Nobel Prize in 1922, demolished the erroneous notion of ether as a medium for the motion of waves (Einstein and Infeld, 1942). Descartes would never know that the speed of light is finite, but his philosophy still reigns supreme. There are comparable stories in medicine as well, but here, the old and the new continue to coexist.

The Origin of Medicine

All knowledge is based on first conjecturing the causes of an event and then applying the most modern tools available to verify the conjecture. Medical science is no exception. Most probably, disease is as ancient as humankind. However, given the habitat of our aboriginal ancestors in caves and jungles, it is very likely that pain was the first recognized disease symptom and that the "first cry of pain through the primitive jungle was the first call for a physician" (Robinson, 1931a). There was the belief that the "stoppage of physical life was due to supernatural causes – to the wrath of the dead, the uncanny powers of human enemies, the revenge of offended spirits" (Robinson, 1931b).

So our earliest ancestors came up with an explanation for the cause of diseases. In a way, this was a revolutionary development because it offered an explanation for the disease. The treatment naturally was to appease the evil spirit. Thus, the origin of spiritual medicine or witchcraft was meant to heal. In its own way, this is a complete system linking theory with practice. The approach is scientific even if its foundations are faulty.

As the hunting and gathering society yielded to agricultural society, which introduced the system of producing things for consumption as distinct from depending upon natural sources, a materialistic outlook superseded the belief in offending spirits. By its very nature, agriculture and domestication of animals requires experimentation and a keen sense of observation. Just take the case of smallpox. Women involved in dairy farming knew long before Edward Jenner (1749-1823) conquered smallpox (Winkelstein, 1992) that cowpox was prophylactic against smallpox.

It is thus not surprising that the transition from a gathering to an agricultural society led to the realization that disease has a physical as opposed to a supernatural basis. *This was a revolutionary departure and ushered in the phase of medicine that we witness today.* In the thousands of years that followed, there has merely been a refinement of this concept and an attempt to reach a precision, through experimentation and conjectures, as to the physical factors underlying a disease state.

It is also not surprising that this breakthrough from spiritual to materialistic medicine came from the oldest civilizations, India, China, and Greece approximately between 700 BC and 400 BC. Sir William Osler (1849-1919) was wrong when he pronounced in 1913 that by the middle of the seventeenth century "What disease really was, where it was, how it was caused, had not even begun to be discussed intelligently" (Osler, 1921).

Indian scientists of that time came up with a new theory of disease termed *Tridoshas* (imbalance between three elements, see Chapter 6 on Ayurveda). China came up with the theory of interaction between two opposites – *yang* and *yin* (see Chapter 7 on Chinese medicine) and in Greece, Hippocrates (468-377 BC) advanced his theory of four humours (see Chapter 8 on Greek medicine). These were milestones in the progress of medical science. The first Ayurvedic text, *Agnivesha Samhita* was written in the sixth-seventh century BC. The Chinese *yang* and *yin* concept might have been formulated between 700 and 500 BC. Hippocrates' four humours theory arrived a bit later than Chinese and Indian medicine, and perhaps for this very reason, it is a bit more materialistic than the latter two. Essentially, hewever, these three concepts are contemporary.

Just as the spiritual basis of disease led to witchcraft, the theory of the physical basis of disease led to the exploration of physical means for the alleviation of diseases. Thus began the search for remedies from plants, animals, minerals, and soil, and from the twentieth century on, in the laboratory as well.

The Sources of Medicaments

Humans, animals, and vegetation evolve in constant interaction with the environment and, in turn, are changing the environment. In many instances, chemicals that are endogenous to the body produce their biological effects by stimulating or inhibiting specific receptors on the surface of, or inside, the cells. It is easy to comprehend why the body has receptors for endogenous molecules. But human and animal bodies also contain receptors for foreign substances like for atropine (from *Atropa belladonna*, which dilates the pupil, morphine (from the poppy plant, *Papaver somniferum*), the most effective analgesic, cannabinoids (the active ingredient of marijuana or *ganja*), which elevates mood, and for many other chemicals. Furthermore, the liver contains a highly developed enzyme system, which can destroy almost any substance foreign to the body.

These facts simply denote a common origin and hence interaction between humans and the rest of living and nonliving matter during evolution; hence there is always a probability that plants, animals, and minerals in nature can cure or kill. Therefore, the claim that natural products can cure is very much justified, and the scorn for herbal products reflects as much prejudice on the part of scientists as the fear of synthetic products does to worshippers of god-given remedies.

The culture of faith in natural as opposed to synthetic drugs is universal. The environmental movement, justifiable on some grounds, has also its spiritual side. There are books on herbal medicine and natural products (Culpeper [1814], 1944; Murray and Pizzorno, 1991; Johnson et al., 2012).

Toward Modern Medicine

There is a lot of bias, naturally in favour of the West, in assigning landmarks in history. Modern medicine has been named as Hippocratic medicine. While Hippocrates' medical postulates could be considered a continuation of the philosophical conjectures of Thales of Miletus (620-c.540 BC) and essentially materialistic, it would still be appropriate to consider modern medicine as an extension of Indian, Chinese and Greek medicine.

No science is the product of the work of a single individual although there have been august figures in each of the schools. Pythagoras (580-490 BC) and Isaac Newton (1642-1727) in mathematics, Galilei Galileo (1564-1642) and Albert Einstein in physics, Charles Darwin (1809-1882) and Gregor Johann Mendel (1822-1884) in biology are household names. However, Einstein and Darwin do not spring from a vacuum; rather, they reflect a gigantic jump in the socially contributed knowledge up to that time; that is precisely why they are the products of nineteenth and twentieth centuries and not of the first and second centuries. At the same time, none of them have written the final chapter in the field of their expertise. In contrast, ossification is the dominant theme of all other branches of medicine with the exception of modern medicine. For example, proponents of Ayurveda or homeopathy feel that, by and large, the final answer was already provided by Charaka of Ayurveda or Hahnemann of homeopathy. Could there have been a genius three thousand years ago (Ayurveda) or even three hundred years ago (homeopathy) who could have supplied the correct and final answer to all ailments, specially when some of the modern diseases did not exist at that time?

Medical science, like any other branch of science, needs continuous revision and experimentation, and each new advance poses new questions requiring new tools for solutions. Likewise, advances in any branch of the sciences and humanities cannot take place unless society as a whole advances economically, politically, socially, and culturally.

That might be the single most important factor that caused modern medicine to advance slowly from the time of Hippocrates until about the seventeenth century and, then rather rapidly, in the nineteenth and twentieth centuries, which the historian Eric Hobsbawm (1997) describes in the series *The Age of Revolution* (1789-1848), *The Age of Capital* (1848-1875), *The Age of Empire* (1875-1914), and *The Age of Extremes* (1914-1991). That may also be the reason why major advances were witnessed in England, Germany, and France. In contrast, the sciences either stagnated or regressed in Egypt, Persia, India, and China because these societies lagged behind, in the modern period primarily due to colonialism. I return to this subject in Chapter 16 titled "The Sun Rises in the West."

Modern medicine is not a conceptual advance over Ayurveda, nor was Hippocrates' theory of four humors; it incorporates all systems of medicine, is in continuum with and an advance over all of them to the most rational stage possible. Either the causes of disease have been established beyond doubt through a series of observations and experimentation as is the case for tuberculosis, malaria, and many other infective diseases, or they are the subject of intensive investigation like essential hypertension, Alzheimer, and diabetes.

How then does modern medicine differ from all other schools of medicine? It suffices to say that modern medicine, like all other branches of science, is based on constant inquiry and renewal determined by careful experimentation and observation. Take, for example, the case of tuberculosis. Modern medicine considered tuberculosis to be a constitutional disease, giving rise to the term *consumption* about one hundred years ago, and the only treatment was to go to sanatoria. As soon as it was recognized that the disease is caused by *Mycobacterirum tubercule* the old theory was discarded.

The essence of medical science is to discard what cannot be proved to be beneficial for whatever it has been used or prescribed for; this is done from laboratory study using animals or tissues to clinical trials and epidemiological re-evaluations once the drug is in general use.

This is not to say that modern medicine evolved without going through episodes of prejudice and scepticism. Some of them are as horrendous as the church's indignation against Galileo.

Sterilization during surgery and childbirth is, perhaps, the second greatest advance in medical science after the discovery of the anti-smallpox vaccine. Nothing has saved more lives and decreased puerperal sepsis and neonatal mortality as much as washing hands and boiling surgical instruments prior to use. Even to this date, with the emergence of multidrug resistant bacteria and virulent viral infections, washing hands is considered the most effective prophylaxis. And yet, when the physician Ignaz Semmelweis (1818-1865) proposed in 1846 that surgeons should wash their hands before handling wounds or births, surgeons argued that this practice would waste precious time. A great scientist was thus driven to death in an insane asylum for telling the truth because traditions were much more convenient to surgeons (see Szasz, 1974).

Louis Pasteur (1822-1895) suggested in 1865 that organisms in the air might cause sepsis. This led the surgeon Joseph Lister to start using antiseptics, and he announced the marvellous outcome in 1867; this contribution too was greeted with some scepticism. However, once the value of sterilization became recognized, it became the norm.

The essence of medical science is not that it uses synthetic as opposed to natural drugs. Indeed, almost all medications used by physicians of all schools of medicine until the end of nineteenth century were derived from plants or minerals (Flückiger and Hanbury, 1879) and many remained popular until quite late; many are still used today, and many are being added.

One of the pioneers of medicine, Thomas Sydenham (1624-1689), whom the English philosopher John Locke (1632-1704) placed alongside Sir Isaac Newton, said in 1680, "Among the remedies which it has pleased Almighty God to give to man to relieve his sufferings, none is so universal and so efficacious as opium." Andean natives chewed coca (*Erythoxylon coca*) leaves (the source of cocaine) for stimulatory action as did Sigmund Freud (1856-1939) in the late nineteenth century and it is in competition with heroin in the twenty-first century. Vitamins, which are essential for life but generally cannot be made by the human body, are solely derived from foods or the environment (like the action of sunlight on skin producing vitamin D). Many naturally occurring drugs such as emetine for amebiasis, digitalis for heart failure, quinidine for heart irregularities, ergot for migraine, caffeine and ephedrine for asthma, vinca alkaloids for cancer, atropine for reducing secretions and intestinal spasm, colchicines for gout, and so on are still in use. Lithium, the lightest of the alkali metals, which cannot be synthesized, proved invaluable in the treatment of manic-depressive illness. Arsenic was the only treatment for syphilis until the discovery of penicillin in the mid 1940s. Most antibiotics, including penicillin, are derived from micro-organisms themselves; and the source of insulin, until very recently, was the pancreas of beef and pork, albeit used by people of all religions.

In short, the sources of drugs (herbs, plants, metal, living organism) are not and cannot be the basis of different branches of medicine. I have listed in Appendix I many of the natural drugs still in use in modern medicine.

Indeed, the major contributions of modern medical science until the mid-twentieth century were not in the area of drug discovery but rather in the area of physiology, biochemistry, genetics, diagnostics, and pathology. However, neither of these developments in basic medical science is a solace to the patient who needs a cure more than a diagnosis and often detests the prognosis. More patients are saved in hospitals by supportive therapy, which could involve maintaining the fluid balance, giving blood transfusion if necessary, maintaining respiration and blood pressure, than by spectacular drugs. With the exception of a few poisons (cyanide, morphine, methanol, and war gases), the treatment of drug overdose or poisoning does not require an antidote – even if antidotes exist – but rather supportive therapy. Indeed, the WHO list of essential drugs is very small and can easily be made much smaller.

In terms of applied medicine, gigantic advances have been made in surgery, but that is another matter, concerned more with technology than medical science.

Since John Desmond Bernal introduced the field of molecular biology, gigantic advances have been made, and yet no useful drug of any significance has come out of this line of investigation.

It should be recognised that medical research pays greater attention to diseases of the rich and of the developed countries than to diseases that afflict the majority in developing countries.

Factors Contributing to the Popularity of Alternative Schools of Medicine

The reasons for the survival of Ayurveda, homeopathy, Chinese medicine, chiropractic, and naturopathy are not the same as the reasons for the persistence of man-drawn rickshaws in the age of automobiles; the former is by choice, the latter by necessity. There are still too many who would opt for homeopathy (first choice) or Ayurveda (second choice). The rickshaw puller would opt for a taxi anytime if he could.

The foremost of factors contributing to the survival of alternate medical practices is the limitation of medical science. Modern medicine cannot cure all existing diseases or even relieve all unpleasant symptoms; also, it is neither readily available nor always affordable. Moreover, diseases are a part of biology, some treatable, some not, at least for the time being. However, the limitation of medical science is not easily acceptable to patients, who will, naturally and justifiably, search for a cure. They are ready to try anything, and there will always be available a practitioner of alternate schools of medicine who will promise good results.

Unlike many consumer goods, which arrive from major industrial centres, medical treatment must be available in the proximity of the sick, especially during acute illnesses. In a place like India, where public health care is very poor while fancy private profit-making modern hospitals do exist in major cities, the marginalized population has little to choose from. An Ayurvedic practitioner is always available at a lower cost than the modern physician.

Biological systems have an inbuilt method of correcting abnormal episodes. Mechanisms do exist for combating infections, correcting changes in blood pressure, suppressing cancer, etc. Indeed, one of the practitioners of hygiene in the late nineteenth century, Dr. Russell T. Trall (1812-1877),[3] advocated that drugs should never be used to treat a disease because disease is a part of health (Trall, 1880).

It is common knowledge that people recover from episodes of fever without taking medication and often without even knowing the cause of the fever. India's current population is over one billion. I am not aware of any studies to determine what percentage of population seeks medical help from any kind of healer; there is a good chance that more than 50 percent of Indians (500 million) never see a doctor or a dentist in their lifetime. There are drugs to relieve asthma, but there are no cures available to modern medicine; yet many asthmatic children recover completely as they grow older. Given this situation, a great majority of common diseases can be cured by any drug, provided the drug itself is not too toxic to make the patient worse off than he or she would be due to the disease.

Given the natural inbuilt mechanism of healing, the physician of any branch of medicine has a good chance of satisfying a good percentage of her or his patients. That is a part of the reason why a number of practitioners, without training in any type of medicine, can carry on with their business in India and other countries where strict regulations do not exist. Indeed, almost all the great physicians of the distant past, including Hippocrates and Paracelsus, were essentially self-trained. Moreover, all drugs produce a placebo effect (Wolf, 1959), which may be all that is needed in the majority of cases.

Moreover, biology and medicine are placed in greater conflict with religion than are the natural sciences. A 768-page glossy *Atlas of Creation* by Harun Yaha (pen name for Adnam Oktar),[4] the head of the Foundation of Scientific Research in Ankara, is widely distributed to counter Darwin. Revivalists take advantage of weaknesses of medical science to boost the mystic merit of Ayurveda, homeopathy, or Chinese medicine. The emergence of personalities like Dr. Deepak Chopra of America, who champions a fusion of the old and new, Dr. Hari Sharma (1993) who attributes even modern medical concepts as originating from Ayurveda, or Baba Gurudev of India, who claims to combine Ayurveda with Yoga to cure cancer and AIDS, are recent sophisticated examples of this revivalist trend.

Conclusions and Outline of the Book

In summary, living organisms and the diseases they harbour are the most complex expression of the interactions between fundamental particles; an understanding of this complex relationship is beginning to unfold. Medical science started as spiritualism and still carries its birth pangs. The limits that this situation places on rational therapy allow the survival of the unfit and the fit in medicine. The primary aim of this book is to address why there are many kinds of medical schools and why they are likely to continue for a long time. In order to do this, I will discuss the evolution of medicine in the socio-political context throughout the ages.

Notes

1. Harmann Weyl (1885-1955). *Philosophy of Mathematics and Natural Science* (Princeton: Princeton University Press, 1949), 214-215. Hermann Weyl is regarded as one of the greatest mathematicians of the twentieth century. He was born in Germany and taught at the Institute for Advanced Study in Princeton, New Jersey.

2. John Harley Warner is a noted science historian and the quote is from his article "Ideals of Science and Their Discontents in Late Nineteenth-Century American Medicine," *ISIS* 82 (1991): 454.

3. Dr. Trall was the Director of the Hygiene Institute in New York. He shunned both allopathic and homeopathic medicine. One of the early historians of medicine, Dr. David Allyn Gorton (1832-1916), the author of the book *The History of Medicine, Philosophical and Critical: From Its Origin to the Twentieth Century* (New York: G. P. Putnam's Sons, 1910), worked in the clinic of Dr. Trall before drifting to homeopathy.

4. Yaha, H. *Atlas of Creation*. Istanbul: Global Publishing (available free on Internet: *www.harunyaha.com*). It is lavishly illustrated with the appearance of a well-researched book.

References

Bernal, J. D. *The Origin of Life* (London: Weidenfeld & Nicolson, 1967) xv.

Culpeper, N. *Culpeper's Complete Herbal & English Physician Enlarged*([1814] (Reprinted Glenwood, IL: Meyerbooks, 1944).

Einstein A. and Infeld L. *The Evolution of Physics: The Growth of Ideas from Early Concepts to Relativity and Quanta* (New York: Simon and Schuster, 1942).

Flückiger, F. A. and Hanbury, D. *A History of the Principal Drugs of Vegetable Origin* (London: Macmillan, 1879).

Hobsbawm, E. *On History* (London: Weidenfield & Nicolson, 1997).

Johnson, R.L., Foster, S., Dog, T.L. and Kiefer, D. *National Geographic Guide to Medicinal Herbs* (Washington National Geographic, 2012).

Mackay, RJ and Oldford, RW. "Scientific Method, Statistical Method and the Speed of Light," *Statistical Science* 15 (2000): 254-278.

Murray, M. and Pizzorno, J. *Encyclopedia of Natural Medicine* (Rocklin, CA: Prima Publishing, 1991).

Osler, W. *The Evolution of Modern Medicine* (New Haven: Yale University Press, 1921), 183.

Robinson, V. *The Story of Medicine* (New York: Tudor Publishing, 1931a), 1.

Ibid., 1931b. 3.

Schrodinger, E. *What is Life? With Mind and Matter and Autobiographical Sketches* (1944) (Cambridge: Cambridge University Press, 1958), 3-4.

Sharma, H. *Freedom From Disease: How to Control Free Radicals, a Major Cause of Aging and Disease.* (Toronto: Veda Publishing, 1991).

Spencer, H. *The Principles of Biology, V. 1* (New York: D. Appleton and Company, 1875), 69.

Szasz, T. S. *The Myth of Mental Illness* (New York: Harper-Perennial, 1974), xvii-xviii.

Trall, R. T. *True Healing Art or Hygienic VS Drug Medication (1880)* (Kessinger Publishing: *www.Kessinger.net*; ISBN 1-5645-9808-X).

Winkelstein, W. "Not Just a Country Doctor: Edward Jenner, Scientist," *Epidemiologic Reviews* 14 (1992): 1-15.

Wolf, S. "The Pharmacology of Placebos," *Pharmacological Reviews* 11: (1959): 689-704.

CHAPTER 2

The Art and Science of Medicine

The 'real' mathematics of the 'real' mathematicians, the mathematics of Fermat and Euler and Gauss and Abel and Riemann, is almost wholly 'useless' (and this is as true of 'applied' as of 'pure' mathematics). It is not possible to justify the life of any genuine professional mathematician on the ground of the 'utility' of his work.

G. H. Hardy[1]

There has always been a close interaction between the development of science and that of material techniques. Neither would be possible without the other, for without the advance of science techniques would fossilize into traditional crafts, and without the stimulus of techniques science would return again to pure pedantry. It does not follow, however, that this association is either conscious or efficient; in fact, the application of science to practical life has always been faced with the greatest difficulties and is even now, when its value is beginning to be recognized, carried on in the most haphazard and ineffective way.

J. D. Bernal[2]

Introduction

The medical discipline includes a scientific aspect like the natural sciences and a social aspect like the humanities. Both are important; when the applied medicine falters, the science gets discredited. Medical science does not control the nature or the time frame of its application. While physics and chemistry, and even other biological sciences, get due recognition for unraveling the mysteries of nature, medical science is primarily judged for its healing capacity; that might be why so often surgery gets more recognition than medical science.

The applied aspect of medical science takes the form of therapeutics, which could be treated as the art of medicine (Warner, 1995).

Broadly speaking, advances in civilization are first reflected in philosophical discourses, which become the forerunner of scientific advances, and the latter can go through a short or a very long period of incubation before being put to application. This is true for physics, for chemistry, as well as for medicine, but perhaps more so for medicine. Astrophysicist Stephen Hawking and Mlodinow (2010) contend that, "philosophy is dead. Philosophy has not kept up with modern developments in science, particularly physics." This might be a harsh conclusion. The world has changed over the years, and we cannot hope for the philosophy of Plato and Aristotle, but there is and would remain a place for philosophy as the forerunner of changes, notably in biology, more particularly in the area of the most complex question of biology – the origin of life, cognition, and the ethics of science.

There is an important distinction between therapeutics and all other human achievements. For example, there are less and more efficient methods of fetching water, cutting trees, building houses and providing transportation, and endless other activities. A tent serves the purpose of a mansion and an hoe does the job of a tractor; the difference is not fundamental. However, only the right kind of medicine can heal; alternatives are either useless or harmful. Many current diseases are the same as they existed thousands of years ago; but because they date from antiquity does not mean that the remedies of Galen (AD 129-c.216), Avicenna (980-1037), and Paracelsus (1493-1541), jotted down in the earlier textbooks (Wood, 1874), were effective.

From Science to Its Application

Science rarely leads to instant application. For example, in one of the greatest achievements in physics, Galilei Galileo proved that the theory of Nicolaus Copernicus (1473-1543) about planets circling around the sun was correct; this milestone in physics got him in trouble with the Church, but no one else was harmed by it and no one else benefited from it. Almost six decades later, Isaac Newton took Galileo's physics to new heights with his three laws of motion, the first of which was merely an extension of Galileo's discoveries. These were gigantic advances in science, but neither Galileo's nor Newton's physics found any use until much later. The same could be said about Einstein's theory of relativity.

What is true of physics is also true of chemistry. Because drugs are central to the discipline of medicine, advances in therapeutics depend much more on advances in chemistry than in physics. However, advances in chemistry are generally slower than in physics because the former is less theoretical than the latter. It was not until 1869 that Dimitri Mendeleev (1834-1907) could place elements in chemical families, in what is known as the periodic chart or table. This, no doubt, was a big step forward but happened more than three hundred years after Galileo.

Almost six hundred years elapsed from the discovery of ether in 1275 by Raymundus Lullus (1232-1316) and its synthesis in 1540 by Valerius Cordus (1515-1544) to its application on October 16, 1846, by William T. Morton (1819-1868) to anaesthetize the patient Edward Gilbert Abbott at the Massachusetts General Hospital in Boston.

The tale of nitrous oxide (laughing gas) is similar. Joseph Priestley (1733-1804) discovered it around 1772. Its potential as an anaesthetic was also demonstrated by Humphrey Davy (1778-1829) in 1799. And yet seventy-four years had to elapse before it was tested as an anaesthetic at the same operation theatre in Boston where ether was first tested.

Ether is flammable, an irritant, and unpleasant to the patient during induction as well as recovery. For these reasons, it was soon replaced by chloroform, which is not flammable but is more toxic. As it happens far too often, when the lead is given by one drug, many and better ones follow, of which many examples are provided in Chapter 13. Ether and chloroform are no longer used and have been replaced by halothane, enflurane, isoflurane, and so on; although none fulfil all the criteria of an ideal anaesthetic, their inadequacies are compensated for by the simultaneous use of other drugs, like very fast and very short-acting barbiturates for induction, morphine-like drugs for analgesia, and curare-like drugs for relaxation of muscles. Paradoxically, the laughing gas nitrous oxide (N_2O) – very different from similar-sounding nitric oxide (NO) – that failed the first test is still used, mainly by dental surgeons.

Gigantic advances were made by medical science during the 2,500 years from the time of the Indian surgeon Susruta (sixth century BC) and the Greek Hippocrates to the first quarter of twentieth century in our understanding of human physiology and the pathology of diseases. Yet in terms of therapy, there was minimal progress until the beginning of the twentieth century. In other words, developments in basic medical science could not be translated into therapeutics for thousands of years.

The Distinct Nature of Surgery and Dentistry

Both surgery and dentistry are primarily applied arts. The answer to what should be done if there is a fracture or a rotten tooth is obvious. That is why both surgery and dentistry had made considerable progress even without effective anaesthetics while therapeutics lagged behind. The Indian surgeon Susruta, most likely the first surgeon of repute and the originator of dentistry, describes techniques of different surgical procedures including plastic surgery for the repair of a severed nose.[3] All ancient civilizations had devised methods of treating toothache, cosmetic tooth surgery, and tooth extraction.

The 320-page atlas by Malvin E. Ring (1985) is an excellent text on the evolution of dentistry over three thousand years in the context of the specific characteristics of evolving civilizations in Peru, Mexico, Egypt, Greece, India, China, and elsewhere. Interestingly, Ring (1985) writes, "It is interesting that such a variety of people, who have had no contact with each other and whose cultures are in other respects very different have developed such similar customs." This analysis is similar to what Edward Augustus Freeman (1823-1892) expounded in his book *Comparative Politics* (Freeman, 1896).

The Essence of Medical Science

Medical science involves the understanding of human physiology, biochemistry, and genetics, discovering the causes of diseases and specific remedies to treat them, finding out how a drug works, and why do living organisms age, and why do they die or should they die at all? In short, the science of medicine is whatever can eliminate the difference between biology, physics, and chemistry, the possibility of which is real and was anticipated by Schrodinger (1944; see Chapter 1). Applied medicine is the reason we go to the physician or hospital.

Use and Misuse of Medical Science

"The practice of science cannot be, nor should it be, entirely apolitical," editorialises the journal *Nature* (Editorial, 2012). Science is not neutral and unfolds its true social impact in application. Just as an understanding of the anatomy of the atom has been put to good and bad use, so also advances in medical science can be put to good and bad use. The unravelling of the mysteries of the human body is the science of medicine, and implanting a pacemaker to make the heart beat with regularity is its good application while prescribing diethylstilbestrol (DES) to prevent miscarriage is its bad application.

Sometimes, scientific intervention fails to benefit the patient. This leads to renewed investigation and new approaches, which, in reality, is the essence of any science.

Take, for example, the case of barbiturate poisoning. Until the discovery of benzodiazepines (e.g., diazepam or Valium) in the early 1960s, barbiturates were the most commonly used sedatives. There are many differences between benzodiazepines and barbiturates, but the most important difference is that an overdose of barbiturates can kill by depressing respiration, among other effects, while death is rare with benzodiazepines. Self-administration of a barbiturate used to be a common method of suicide, the incidence of which was quite high in the Scandinavian countries. A group of drugs known as analeptics or central nervous system stimulants such as picrotoxin, metrazol (pentylenetetrazol), nikethamide, and even strychnine (rat poison) were recommended to treat barbiturate poisoning; the rationale was that these drugs would stimulate the respiratory centre and, hence, would overcome the depressant effects of barbiturates.

However, the treatment of barbiturate poisoning by administering these stimulants yielded disappointing results. There are complex reasons for this, but the most important is that the time course of action of these stimulants and of barbiturates is not identical; moreover, barbiturates do more than just depress respiration, and the stimulation of the brain itself is followed by a depression as is often noted after an epileptic seizure. Somewhat similar phenomena, but more frequent than barbiturate poisoning, are encountered at social gatherings. When someone is too drunk to drive, a strong coffee is offered to reduce the effects of alcohol; all that the coffee does is give a false sense of sobriety and, of course, greater chances of an accident.

In view of the poor results with this stimulant approach to treat barbiturate overdose, the Scandinavian physicians (Nilsson, 1951; Clemmesen and Nilsson, 1961) advocated an approach that did not include any analeptic, and for that reason, they were ridiculed as nihilists (Koppanyi and Fazekas, 1952). Despite this criticism, they went ahead with their new approach developed at the poison centre of the Bispebjerg Hospital in Copenhagen. A physician and accessory staff remained in waiting for a victim of barbiturate poisoning at the hospital centre with no other responsibility. As soon as the ambulance brought a case of barbiturate poisoning, the medical staff at once resorted to supportive therapy, which comprised of maintaining fluid balance, preventing acid/base disturbance, and maintaining respiration mechanically if necessary and not by drugs. The result was stunning. Fatalities from barbiturate poisoning were dramatically reduced. Now this approach, known as the Scandinavian method, is used to treat not only barbiturate poisoning but also poisoning by a diverse group of toxic substances; this is so because, in the final analysis, most poisons kill by depressing respiratory and cardiovascular systems or causing kidney failure.

The acquisition of knowledge of the osmolarity of the blood, its pH and its composition and its critical role in all functions of the body is science. The recognition that natural recovery is possible if the patient can be kept alive by supporting vital functions is also science. Treating victims of overdose of barbiturate by this approach is a rational application. Central nervous system stimulants were used to treat barbiturate poisoning on the basis of a faulty understanding of the cause of death and the pharmacology of stimulants.

Very few poisons such as cyanide, morphine and methanol can be treated by antidotes, based on the knowledge of the mechanism of action of the poison and the antidotes, which is illustrated below in the case of cyanides such as hydrogen cyanide and methanol.

Hydrogen Cyanide

Hydrogen cyanide (HCN) is present in the atmosphere of the earth and other planets; it is even speculated that polymerization of HCN might have contributed to the origin of life. HCN normally exists in gaseous form and is the most toxic of all cyanides, followed by potassium cyanide, which is a powder and, for that reason, is preferred for suicidal and homicidal purposes. Poisoning is caused by the cyanide ion, and the toxic potency of a cyanide depends upon the rate at which the cyanide ion is liberated from the parent molecule, which is faster in the case of HCN than in the case of potassium cyanide (KCN), and the latter, in turn, is faster than in the case of sodium cyanide. The cyanide ion possesses a very high affinity for ferric iron – an essential constituent of many enzymes including the enzyme cytochrome oxidase, which is responsible for the ultimate utilization of oxygen in the body. Once the cyanide ion combines with cytochrome oxidase, oxygen cannot be utilized and death ensues. In short, death by the ingestion of cyanide is like execution by hanging. But there is another side to it. Because of the association of the living organism with cyanide during evolution, there has also evolved a mechanism of neutralizing cyanide by another enzyme called rhodanase (thiosulfate sulfurtransferase).

Contrary to popular belief, cyanide is not a very potent poison, but it is a very fast-acting poison if ingested in sufficient dosages. Indeed, if in suicidal or homicidal cases the amount of cyanide is insufficient and the victim does not die within a few hours, death is extremely unlikely because the cyanide is metabolized into innocuous thiocyanate. One of the antidotes against cyanide poisoning is sodium thiosulfate, which can bind to cyanide and not let the cyanide ion act on the vital body enzyme cytochrome oxidase. So, if sodium thiosulfate is administered early enough in sufficient dosage, cyanide will not be able to kill; inhalation of oxygen adds to its efficacy. So here is an example of an effective antidote based on scientific knowledge of the mechanism of action of a poison.

Methanol

Methanol is methyl alcohol (CH_3OH). What we drink at parties or at leisure is ethyl alcohol (C_2H_5OH) or ethanol, simply known as alcohol.

Ethanol is the product of fermentation of carbohydrate and therefore exists in nature. It has been used from time immemorial for inebriation. Alcohol inhibits the normal inhibitory activities of the brain, and so it leads to boisterous behaviour and sexual aggressiveness, but it really does not contribute to sexual prowess. William Shakespeare (1564-1616) knew it so he could write in act 2, scene 3 of *Macbeth* when the porter, while narrating the effect of alcohol to Macduff, says, "Lechery, sir, *it provokes, and unprovokes; it provokes the desire, but it takes away the performance* [emphasis added]."

In the body, ethanol is converted into acetaldehyde by the enzyme alcohol dehydrogenase; the resulting acetaldehyde is then broken down by aldehyde dehydrogenase into acetic acid, which breaks down further and becomes part of the carbon pool of the body.

Methanol is miscible with ethanol; it is much cheaper than ethanol because it does not carry the usual duty. From time to time, one hears that a number of poor workers in India suddenly went blind in the morning after a night of drinking. What had happened is that the liquor shops had adulterated ethanol with methanol. Methanol undergoes the same kind of metabolism as ethanol except that it is reduced to formic acid and not to acetic acid, which is the case with ethanol. This is because methanol is *methyl* and not *ethyl* alcohol. The blindness is caused by the toxic effects of formic acid on the retina. Because of this knowledge, achieved through biochemical research, an effective treatment against methanol poisoning has been devised. It involves the administration of ethanol (alcohol). Ethanol offers itself to the enzyme alcohol dehydrogenase so that the enzyme is busy acting on ethanol and not available to convert methanol into formic acid; methanol gets excreted in its native form.

Bhopal Disaster

On the other hand, most poisons are quite nonspecific in their action. A case in point is the Bhopal disaster of December 2-3, 1984, in India. The disaster was caused by the release of a toxic chemical methyl isocyanate, which is a very potent irritant of lung tissue and much more potent as a toxic agent than hydrogen cyanide. There was a public outcry for an antidote, but there is no antidote, nor can there be, against general respiratory irritants, which maim or kill by producing pulmonary oedema resulting in reduced oxygen intake. In the absence of an antidote against such poisons, only supportive therapy can help. Unfortunately, supportive therapy in the case of pulmonary oedema, just as in cases of SARS (severe acute respiratory syndrome) outbreak of 2003 in Toronto that was caused by a viral infection, required positive pressure respiration and other supportive therapy (see Varma and Mulay, 2009). It is difficult to assemble these devices on a large scale during an unexpected mass poisoning.

Science and Scientists

Most modern researchers in medicine are concerned with unravelling the mysteries of life rather than applied research. The discovery of the three dimensional structure of DNA in the mid 1950s was not aimed at finding therapeutics for any disease but at getting the precise structure of one of the key molecules in evolution. More than fifty years have passed but no specific therapy has yet come out of the knowledge of the structure of DNA. On the other hand, the discovery of the chemical bond by Linus Pauling (1901-1994) resulted in significant advances in therapeutics.

Sometimes, scientists consciously combine basic research and its application. There are many examples of this and I am citing here one of the earliest achievements. The story concerns the menace of carbon monoxide (CO), the silent painless killer, which the late celebrated actress Audrey Hepburn (1929-1993) was shown as using to kill herself by turning on the ignition keys of a luxury car in a closed garage in the film *Sabrina*.

Carbon monoxide (CO) is the product of any combustion. So, where there is smoke, there is not only fire but also CO. Fire fighters die of CO poisoning more often than of burns. The Industrial Revolution and the discovery of the New World introduced coal for domestic heating and cooking. Procuring coal needed mining and mines contained CO, a hazard that was often the cause of death of miners. This menace was quite common in the fast-industrializing Britain. The physiologist John Scott

Haldane (1860-1936), much concerned with the well-being of workers, undertook the task of finding out why miners died in the pit and what could be done to protect them.

Doing experiments upon himself (this is important in view of the fact that the first subject on whom Jenner tested his anti-smallpox vaccine was not himself but a small boy) and on mice, Haldane established that death was caused by CO, which binds to haemoglobin-generating carboxyhaemoglobin (COHb); he established that the affinity of CO for haemoglobin is about three times greater than that of oxygen so that when normal oxyhaemoglobin is replaced by carboxyhaemoglobin, oxygen is not available to body tissues. Haldane made the most ingenious observation that mice were more sensitive to the poisonous effect of CO than humans. From then on, miners carried mice in cages as they descended into the pit and would get out if their mice died. Mice were later replaced with canaries and canaries by modern detectors. Haldane also showed that CO poisoning could be treated by oxygen inhalation, preferably at high pressure (see Varma et al., 2009). There are many examples of need-based research. The increased public pressure is forcing governments to find solutions speedily for new health hazards, be it pollution or the swine flu.

Sometimes, a therapy is based on false understanding of diseases or physiology. Such is the case with excessive use of purgatives, cathartics, emetics, tonics, and astringents, and above all bloodletting to treat a wide variety of diseases, including fever (Wood, 1874).

Singh and Ernst (2008) present a detailed description of how the first President of the United States, George Washington (1732-1799), was subjected to bloodletting to treat a bad attack of the common cold by a team of three of the top physicians of the country, Dr. James Craik (1730-1814), Dr. Gustavus Richard Brown (1747-1804), and Dr. Elisha Cullen Dick (1762-1825). The enthusiastic bloodletting led to his death on December 14, 1799.[4] Even by the late eighteenth century, when the most important citizen of a country died of quackery, enough was known about the physiology of circulation; it was known that, ultimately, everything from essential nutrients to oxygen are distributed throughout the body by the blood. It was known that people die of wounds that cause excessive bleeding. There was nothing to suggest that difficulty in breathing, the major complaint of President Washington, can be relieved by bloodletting. So why did the top physicians of the newly independent United States of America resort to bleeding their President until his blood colour changed? This can only be explained by the astounding lack of existing knowledge of medical science and, of course, the lack of common sense on the part of the attending physicians, who were all taught by the famous Dr. Benjamin Rush (1745-1813), America's most vociferous and famous advocate of bloodletting.

Bloodletting is an outcome of Hippocrates' theory of four humours, taken to absurdity by Galen. Whatever be the case, bloodletting to treat the sore throat of George Washington or yellow fever during the same time frame by Dr. Rush is an irrational application of rational medical science. It is still used by Unani-tibb even for such conditions as a peptic ulcer.

If George Washington had been the emperor of India and his wife, Martha, had consulted her Indian maid, she would have advised her to give the President salt gargles in warm water and he would probably have recovered. The drawing out of blood, preferably by leeches because it is slower, is advised in the case of stroke. They tried it to save the life of Joseph Stalin (1879-1953)[5] but Stalin died just the same. Currently it has been found useful in plastic surgery because slow removal of blood from the site of incision leads to good cosmetic results.

Do Harm!

A famous Hippocratic principle *Do No Harm* is the title of the book by Belkin (1993). But physicians can do harm. Like everyone else, physicians too are subject to societal prejudices and have unlimited opportunities to apply them. This is a big area and a subject of many books. Here I only raise the issue of how gender prejudices are reflected in the application of medical science or pseudoscience from the cradle to the grave.

The horrendous practices of female foeticide and genital mutilation are not universal; the former is basically limited to India and the latter to Africa. However, some gender biases are universal.

The life cycle of a woman is punctuated with major physiological changes from menstruation through pregnancy and childbirth. The clinical implications of these changes in a woman's life are described by Baxter and Prior (2009). Naturally, perimenopause is followed by menopause, which too alters the physiology of the body; this may be no different from what happens to males, but there is a significant difference – it is obviously recognizable in women. For each and every one of these physiological changes in the life of a female, some method of intervention has been devised. In each of the examples I am about to present, medical science has been applied rather unscientifically, to say the least.

Major contributions by physicists and chemists have been made in the field of diagnostics and therapeutics; the use and misuse of these developments have been the privilege of physicians and surgeons. One of these techniques is ultrasound.

In the past, some women with considerable experience of observing the gait of a pregnant woman, at least in India, claimed that they could predict the sex of the unborn baby. Whether or not their forecast was true could only be confirmed once the baby was born. Now, however, the unborn baby hiding in the safest abode possible cannot escape eavesdropping by doctors. They are monitored by the ultrasound machine, which makes almost no mistake.

There is a long story of how this gadget came into being. Briefly, it started with the publication of the treatise *The Theory of Sound* in 1877 by the 1904 physics Nobel laureate Lord Rayleigh (John William Strutt [1842-1919]). The generation of sound waves of frequencies higher than human auditory sensitivity was accomplished in 1876 by Sir Francis Galton (1822-1911), a cousin of Charles Darwin. The demonstration of the interrelationship between electrical potential and mechanical pressure in 1880 was done by the 1903 physics Nobel Prize winner, Pierre Curie (1859-1906), husband of the other Nobel Prize winner Marie Curie.

The use of ultrasound in obstetrics was introduced by Professor Ian Donald (1910-1987) in 1959 (Donald, 1962). While describing the history of ultrasound, Joseph Woo (1998) writes, "Within the next few years it became possible to study pregnancy from beginning to end and diagnosis of complications like multiple pregnancy, fetal abnormality and placenta previa (which causes life-threatening haemorrhage) became possible."

However, sex detection emerged as the most popular use of ultrasound, especially in India, not to satisfy the curiosity of the mother but to cater to the vengeance of the father and the family against girls. Millions of girls have perished even before they could have their first cry (Jha et al., 2006), and that happened and is happening in India, the country acclaimed to be of high spirituality.

In front of most medical establishments hangs a signboard "Ultrasound for sex detection is against the law"; however, unscrupulous doctors, of whom there are plenty, reveal the sex of the child to the father without formally using the word *male* or *female* – by using thumbs up, a smile, suggesting distribution of sweets, and many other ways. They have devised portable ultrasound gadgets so that the doctor could predict the sex of the unborn even in remote villages.

This is not the end of the saga of women. The human species has survived for 200,000 years or more precisely because women give birth to new members. The increase in the means of sustenance has led to an increase in population. But the Reverend Thomas Robert Malthus (1766-1834), an admirer of the famous economist Adam Smith (1723-1790), conjectured (Malthus, 1798) that population grows geometrically while the means of sustenance grow arithmetically; this implied that sooner than later there would be more people than there would be food to feed them. However, even till the time of Malthus, the population of Europe had not grown geometrically. Indeed the population of Europe increased from 27.5 million in 500 AD to a mere 50 million 900 years later in 1450 AD (Russell, 1972). There is more food available in 2009 than is needed for nearly seven billion people although not all of them get their share of resources. Notwithstanding the gross errors in the formulation of Malthus, fanatic efforts have been made to curb population since the 1950s, especially in China, India, and other developing countries.

China introduced the one-child policy (expected to change soon since they are suddenly short of labour power). India started all kinds of programs to curb population growth. Men felt that vasectomy might interfere with virility, so fallopian tubes became the main target. Gregory

Goodwin Pincus (1903-1967) introduced high-dose oral contraceptives; the search for new oral contraceptives started. For some reason, a less complex reproductive biology of males still remains untouched. Not satisfied with all these steps, funds were made available to test the efficacy of introducing quinacrine (a twin of quinine) pellets into the uterus to produce scar tissue through inflammation, which would block the fallopian tubes. Surgery without scalpel that can be performed by anyone after minimal training (Mulay, 1997)!

The reverse is also true. If pregnancy is evading women, most often due to the inadequacies of the semen or sperm, she is subjected to in vitro fertilization (IVF). Not much is done to men who would become the father. The pioneer of IVF is the British scientist Dr. Robert G. Edward, who, with the assistance of gynaecologist Dr. Patrick Steptoe (1913-1998), succeeded in the first IVF birth of Louise Brown and, for this technique, was awarded the Nobel Prize in physiology and medicine in 2010.

Most pregnancies are normal and proceed smoothly from conception to the birth of the child. However, in some cases, something goes wrong and there is a miscarriage. Some women have experienced more than one miscarriage, which may require some therapeutic intervention. But there has never been an epidemic of miscarriages warranting mass prophylaxis. The USA has the most restrictive laws governing introduction of drugs, so that thalidomide, which caused malformations in nearly ten thousand babies in Europe, was not approved in the United States, and the total number of affected babies was only seventeen. However, this was not the case with diethylstilbestrol (DES).

The story of DES is a vivid illustration of the convergence of the enthusiasm of the medical profession for novelty, the natural inclination of pharmaceutical industries to create a need for what they can sell, and the force of advertising, which can make a whole population succumb to drugs for prophylaxis when none is needed.

Oestrogen and progesterone are the principal female hormones. Until 1938, the world supply of oestrogen was limited because its main source was pregnant mare urine (hence the name Premarin was used by Ayerst pharmaceutical). Synthesis of diethylstilbestrol (DES) by Dodds et al. (1938) was a major scientific breakthrough. Suddenly, there was big-enough supply of oestrogen even to inject them into chicken, lambs, sheep, and cattle to expedite growth. According to Marcus (1994):

> The discovery of stilbestrol, as well as the drug's regulatory approval and application in feedlots, involved a partnership between state and federal government, industries, universities, producers, and consumers. Science, and by extension scientists linked these diverse groups; each partner depended on science – seen as objective and nonpartisan, and personified in scientists – to ensure continued well-being.

But sheep and cattle were not the only beneficiaries of this enthusiasm for the use of DES. More than five million women were prescribed DES as a prophylaxis against miscarriage without any evidence whatsoever that oestrogen indeed prevented miscarriage; the practice continued even when its efficacy was questioned (Dieckmann et al., 1953). Years later, many had to pay the price with vaginal cancer. It is only when the influential *New England Journal of Medicine* (Herbst et al., 1971) reported unusual types of vaginal cancer in women treated with DES that the practice was stopped. In the meantime, these effects were transferred to the second generation as well; soon, we might know what happened to the third generation.

The story of DES is not very different from the story of hormone (oestrogen) replacement therapy (HRT) to overcome the effects of menopause. At any given time, approximately 15 percent of the women in the world are in menopause, that is, about 750 million women. Naturally millions of women could be a potential target of HRT, which was advocated to stop hot flushes, decrease the risk of cardiovascular complications, decrease or delay osteoporosis and bone fractures, elevate mood, prevent vaginal dryness, and much more. The possibility of increase in uterine cancer was not raised until quite recently. Pharmaceutical companies exist to promote the sale of drugs, and it is easy to infer that the sales would be significantly higher if a drug is pushed for prophylaxis than for cure because everyone is a potential customer in the first case.

Once synthetic oestrogens became available, gynaecologist Robert Wilson (1966) assured women with his book *Feminine Forever* that age is not a problem. How reassuring! Wilson declared that menopause was not only preventable but also curable. Many women were placed on hormone replacement therapy on the assurance of alleviating every consequence of menopause from hot flushes to bone fractures – this too without conclusive evidence. Despite the fact that the serious adverse effects of DES on the daughters, mothers, and sons became obvious, no lessons were learned, and the risk of widespread use of HRT, which had been pointed out earlier by many, became too difficult to deny by the beginning of the twenty-first century. The story of DES and HRT is too important to be passed over in a paragraph even if it is being presented here only as an example of the divorce of science from practice. The subject has been well dealt with in books. Readers are encouraged to read the beautifully written books on the not so beautiful subject by Baxter and Prior (2009), Seaman and Seaman (1977), and Holmes et al. (1981).

In summary, because the very purpose of medicine is to cure the sick and alleviate suffering as much possible when there is no cure, the applied aspect of medicine, and therefore the governmental attitude toward health-care and doctors' compliance with the Hippocratic Oath, are more important to society than medical science in the strict sense.

Notes

1. Hardy, G. H. (1877-1947). *A Mathematician's Apology*, 1940. Calgary: *http://www.math.ualberta.ca/mss/* 32-33.
2. Bernal, J. D. (1901-1971). *The Social Function of Science* (London: George Routledge, 1939), 126.
3. It would seem that severing the nose as a punishment, especially of women suspected of adultery, still prevalent in many cultures, started in antiquity; why else should there be a very detailed description of nose repair by Susruta?
4. According to two scientific publications, one by M. P. Gross and J. Apesos (*Aesthetics Plastic Surgery* 1992[16] : 343-348) and the other by L. Abel (*Journal of American Medical Association* 1970 [214]: 900-901), the bloodletting of President Washington was done by Dr. Benjamin Rush (1745-1813).
5. Giacometti, L. *American Journal of Cardiology*, 1987 (60): 1128-1131. There are anecdotal reports that Stalin was poisoned.

References

Baxter, S. M. and Prior, J. *The Estrogen Error: Why Progesterone Is Better for Women's Health* (Westport CT: Greenwood Publishing, 2009).

Belkin, L. *First, Do No Harm*. (New York: Random House, 1993).

Clemmesen, C. and Nilsson, E. "Therapeutic Trends in the Treatment of Barbiturate Poisoning," *Clinical Pharmacology and Therapeutics* 2 (1961): 220-229.

Dieckmann, W. J., Davis, M. E., Rynkiewicz, L. M, and Pottinger, R. E. "Does the Administration of Diethylstilbestrol During Pregnancy Have Therapeutic Value?" *American Journal of Obstetrics and Gynecology* 66 (1953): 1062-81.

Dodds, E. C., Goldberg, L., Lawson, W., and Robinson, R. "Oestrogenic Activity of Alkylated Stilboesterols," *Nature* 142 (1938): 34.

Donald, I. "Clinical Applications of Ultrasonic Techniques in Obstetrical and Gynaecological Diagnosis," *British Journal of Obstetrics and Gynaecology* 69 (1962):1036.

Editorial. "Political Science", *Nature* 483 (2012). 123.

Freeman, E. A. *Comparative Politics* (Danvers, MA: General Books, [1896], 2009), 120.

Hawking, S. and Mlodinow, L. *The Grand Design* (New York: Bantam Books, 2010), 5.

Herbst, A. L., Ulfelder, H., and Poskanzer, D. C. "Adenocarcinoma of the Vagina. Association of Maternal Stilbestrol Therapy with Tumor Appearance in Young Women," *New England Journal of Medicine* 284 (1971): 878-81.

Holmes, H. B., Hoskins, B. B. and Gross, M. *The Custom-Made Child: Women-Centered Perspectives*. (Clifton, NJ: Humana Press, 1981).

Jha P., Kumar R., Vasa P., Dhingra N., Thiruchelvam D., Moineddin R. "Low Male-to-Female Sex Ratio in Children Born in India: National Survey of 1.1 Million Households," *Lancet* 367 (2006): 211-218.

Koppanyi, T. and Fazekas, J. F. "Pharmacotherapeutic Nihilism in the Treatment of Acute Barbiturate Poisoning," *American Journal of Medical Science* 224 (1952): 577-585.

Malthus T. R. *An Essay on the Principle of Population*. (Oxford: Oxford World Classics reprint, 1798), Chapter 1, 13.

Marcus, A. I. *Cancer from Beef: DES, Federal Food Regulation and Consumer Confidence* (Baltimore: The Johns Hopkins University Press, 1994), 11.

Mulay, S. "Quinacrine Sterilization: Unethical Trials," *Economic and Political Weekly*, Mumbai, India 32 (1997): 877-879.

Nilsson, E. "On the Treatment of Barbiturate Poisoning: a Modified Clinical Aspect," *Acta Medica Scandinavia 139* (supplement 253, 1951), 127.

Ring, M. E. *Dentistry: An Illustrated History* (Baltimore: Mosby, 1985), 25.

Russell, J. C. *Population in Europe*: in Carlo M. Cipolla, ed., *The Fontana Economic History of Europe*, Vol. I: The Middle Ages (Glasgow: Collins/Fontana, 1972), 25-71, posted on the *Internet Medieval Source Book.* The sourcebook is a collection of public domain and copyright-permitted texts related to medieval and Byzantine history. (c)Paul Halsall Jan 1996, halsall@murray.fordham.edu.

Schrödinger, E. *What Is Life?* (Cambridge: Cambridge University Press, 1944).

Seaman, B. and Seaman, G. *Women and the Crisis in Sex Hormones* (New York: Rawson Associates, 1977).

Singh, S. and Ernst, E. *Trick or Treatment?: Alternative Medicine on Trial* (London: Transworld Publishers, 2008).

Varma, D. R. and Mulay, S. "Methyl Isocyanate: The Bhopal Gas," in *Handbook of the Toxicology of Chemical Warfare Agents*, ed. Ramesh C. Gupta (San Diego: Elsevier, 2009), 293-312.

Varma, D. R., Mulay, S., and Chemtob, S. "Carbon Monoxide: Public Health Risk to Painless Killer," in *Handbook of the Toxicology of Chemical Warfare Agents*, ed. Ramesh C. Gupta (San Diego: Elsevier, 2009), 271-292.

Warner, J. H. "The History of Science and the Sciences of Medicine," *Osiris* 10 (second series, 1995):164-193.

Wilson, R. A. *Feminine Forever* (New York: M. Evans, 1966).

Woo, J. A Short History of the Development of Ultrasound in Obstetrics and Gynecology. Part I. This website is listed in the Humbul Humanities Hub, Resource Discovery Network, University of Oxford, the Wellcome Library for the History of Medicine and Science Links website of the United States National Science Teachers Association. Copyright 1998-2002.

Wood, H. C. *Treatise on Therapeutics, Comprising Materia Medica and Toxicology* (Philadelphia: J. B. Lippincott, 1874).

CHAPTER 3

Socio-political Determinants of Medical Science

The abstract concept "society" means to the individual human being the sum total of his direct and indirect relations to his contemporaries and to all the people of earlier generations. The individual is able to think, feel, strive, and work by himself; but he depends so much upon society – in his physical, intellectual, and emotional existence – that it is impossible to think of him, or to understand him, outside the framework of society. It is "society" which provides man with food, clothing, and most of the content of thought; his life is made possible through the labor and the accomplishments of the many millions past and present who are all hidden behind the small word "society."

Albert Einstein[1]

Science, like other productive activities, like the state, the family, sport, is a social institution completely integrated into and influenced by the structure of all our other social institutions ...Scientists do not begin life as scientists, after all, but as social beings ...they view nature through a lens that has been molded by their social experience.

R. C. Lewontin[2]

Introduction

Our planet Earth was born some 4.6 billion years ago. What happened since then and how it happened has been extensively investigated by archaeologists, anthropologists, biologists, and historians.

The pace of change was much slower in the earlier stages of history than it is now. Almost twenty thousand years separate the Old Stone Age and the Middle Stone Age. It is very likely that the Stone Age was preceded by the Wood Age since wood was more abundant and more pliable than the stone (Day, 1967). Given this slow pace at which civilization moved until a few hundred years ago, it is hard to establish when and how the science of medicine in the form and shape of spiritual medicine came into being and what political factors influenced its evolution to modern medicine. Even if we examine different aspects of medicine in the last one hundred years, it is not always obvious what factors led to certain developments and what factors prevented the universal application of advances in medical science.

Role of Individuals in History

The McGill University icon Sir William Osler says (1908):

> History is simply the biography of the mind of man; and our interest in history, and its educational value to us, is directly proportional to the completeness of our study of the individuals through whom this mind has been manifested.

If I agreed with Osler, the context of this chapter, indeed of the whole book, would have been different. But I think this statement of Osler is based on an erroneous understanding of the history of medicine and, by implication, of history in general. Individuals do play a role in history, but not in the way Osler perceives. I am more inclined to agree with the analysis of Karl Marx (1818-1883) made in his treatise *The Eighteenth Brumaire of Louis Bonaparte*:

> *Men make their own history, but they do not make it as they please; they do not make it under self-selected circumstances, but under circumstances existing already, given and transmitted from the past.*

In a similar vein, Bertrand Russell (1872-1970) writes (1945a):

> The rise of liberalism, in politics and philosophy, provides material for the study of a very general and very important question, namely: What has been the influence of political and social circumstances upon the thoughts of eminent and original thinkers, and, consequently, what has been the influence of these men upon subsequent political and social developments?

Osler's statement is made in the context of his essay on William Harvey (1578-1657), the discoverer of blood circulation. However, the search for the circulation and source of blood started thousands of years before Harvey, at least since Galen. Moreover, Harvey did not answer how blood from the arteries enters the veins, a puzzle that was solved soon after Harvey's 1628 publication, by Marcello Malpighi (1628-1694). Malpighi had access to the microscope and was able to demonstrate the link between arteries and veins through a web of tiny capillaries.

While socio-political determinants of applied medicine are more obvious than those of basic medical science, they operate at all levels. Arnold Toynbee (1946) writes as follows:

> Forces in action are not national but proceed from wider causes, which operate upon each of the parts and are not intelligible in their partial operation unless a comprehensive view is taken of their operation throughout the society.... Throughout, it is impossible to grasp the significance of any particular member's behaviour under a particular ordeal without taking some account of the similar or dissimilar behaviour of its fellows and without the successive ordeals of a series of events in the life of the whole society.

Is Modern Medicine Hippocratic Medicine?

If Toynbee, as quoted above, is correct and I think he is, the question arises why modern medicine is considered Hippocratic medicine and not Egyptian medicine or Charak medicine or just medicine, as is the case with physics and chemistry. Is it because Hippocrates placed medicine on a scientific footing, which Egyptians, Hindus, and Chinese did not? Or is it because modern (often called Western) medicine is the only form in which Hippocratic medicine exists while Hindu and Chinese medicines continue to exist as separate entities? Or is it because the economic and political dominance of the West propels it to relate better to what is Christian and Western than to 'alien' civilizations like the Egyptian, Indian and Chinese?

In my opinion, the acclaimed lineage of modern medicine to Hippocrates is an assertion of Western supremacy rather than a genuine scientific derivation, which, in general terms, has been pointed out by others (Frank, 1998; Toynbee, 1946; Needham, 1954; Said, 1978; Conner, 2005); Bhishagratna (1963) has pointed to Western bias in historiography specifically with relation to Hindu and Greek medicine. As far as the science of medicine is concerned, Hippocrates would rate poorly relative to both the Hindu and Chinese theories of health and disease. I will return to this subject again in Chapter 8 devoted to Greek medicine.

Determinants of Medical Progress

The story of almost all advances in medical science would support the generalization that social, political, and economic factors exert profound effects on the progress of all branches of science, technology, and humanities, including the medical profession as a whole and medical science in its strictest sense.

Here I present five examples relating to highly significant events in the evolution of medical science to substantiate the above assertion. The first example relates to what would be considered basic research, namely the discovery of the structure of DNA. The second example concerns the discovery and treatment of a major disease, namely malaria. The third example concerns public health measures and cholera. The fourth example concerns China, Britain, and the Opium Wars. The fifth example illustrates how an appropriate political climate is a prerequisite for advances in medicine – it concerns the discovery of anaesthesia.

The Discovery of the Double Helical Structure of DNA (Deoxyribonucleic Acid)

Deciphering of the structure of DNA in 1958 is, undoubtedly, a landmark in biology. The belief that everything about human beings is contained in the sequence of their DNA has culminated in the Human Genome Project in the United States and its international analogue, the Human Genome Organization (HUGO). This program aims at deciphering a complete ordered sequence of As (adenine), Ts (thymine), Cs (cytosine) and Gs (guanine), which make up all the genes in the human genome, a string of letters that will be three billion elements long (Lewontin, 1991).

A perusal of scientific papers of the last fifty years would reveal how all advanced laboratories have been focusing on researches linked to the discovery of the structure of DNA, ostensibly because the suppression or expression of genes and the identification of specific genes responsible for physiological and pathological state would solve the problems of health and disease more conclusively than has been accomplished so far. Nobel Prizes to Watson, Wilkins and Cricks, and more recently to Venkatraman Ramakrishnan, Thomas A. Steitz, Carol Greider, Elizabeth Blackburn, and Jack Szostak are on grounds of DNA-related researches.

However, the principal reason for using DNA as an example in this book is not so much to detail the significance of DNA as it is to show how numerous socio-political factors played a role in deciphering the structure of DNA (Maddox, 2002).

The unraveling of the structure of DNA would not have been possible without the availability of crystallography as a tool. However, John Desmond Bernal, who is the acclaimed pioneer of crystallography, was not the one who applied his technique to study DNA. Moreover, even Bernal, a physicist himself, could not have developed the technique of crystallography without overall advances in physics in the first half of the twentieth century. Rosalind Franklin (1920-1958), who spent her last years in Bernal's laboratory at Birkbeck College in London and whose historic x-ray photograph no. 51 was the starting point that formally culminated in the identification of the double helix structure of DNA, was not credited for her role during her life time. Only Wilkins mentioned her name in his Nobel lectures; Watson and Crick, the other sharers of the Nobel Prize, do not.

It is not presumptuous to suggest that the resurgence of the feminist movement, especially after the publication of *Le Deuxième Sexe* (*The Second Sex*) by Simone de Beauvoir (1908-1986) in 1949 created the conditions for the posthumous recognition of the role of Rosalind Franklin; during her life, she was just Rosy, with an unpredictable and undesirable temperament – a charge never laid against Watson. How a young Jewish woman in Britain of the 1950s was sidelined until she moved to Bernal's laboratory is not a pleasant episode. Franklin neither received the Nobel Prize in medicine nor in chemistry.

Moreover, sufficient technical and scientific advances had taken place by the 1950s so that many more people were struggling to unravel the structure of DNA, including the Nobel laureate Linus Pauling, who too conjectured a helical structure for DNA. Maddox (2002) passionately describes the complex and not-so-clean world of science and scientists and of society at large in the context of the discovery of the double helix and the neglected role of Rosalind Franklin.

The message contained in the x-ray photographs was identified using the Patterson function, developed by Arthur Lindo Patterson (1902-1966), who had received his PhD in physics from McGill University. Patterson was studying other chemicals and not DNA. None of the three Nobel laureates connected with DNA acknowledge Patterson in their Nobel lectures.

Malaria

The second example concerns the identification of the cause and cure of malaria. Malaria is a disease of the tropics and sub-tropics and, even in the twenty-first century, afflicts 300-500 million people annually and kills one million of them, mostly children of poor countries. The sub-Saharan region of Africa registers the most deaths. Malaria is perhaps the biggest killer, except for wars of aggression or genocide. Why should a disease as ancient as malaria still cause havoc? Given the political and medical significance of malaria, it is a subject of numerous books. The description in this book is mainly based on these books: *The Malaria Capers* by Robert S. Desowitz (1991), *Epidemics and History* by Sheldon Watts (1997), *A People's History of Science* by Clifford D Conner (2005), and *The Fever* by Sonia Shah (2010).

Malaria is an ancient disease. Chinese literature refers to malaria (*Nei Ching*) 4,700 years ago. Almost 4,000 years ago, Sumerian and Egyptian texts describe a fever associated with the enlargement of the spleen (caused by the accumulation of destroyed blood cells) and pale nails (due to anaemia resulting from the destruction of red blood cells preceding the chill). The Vedic scriptures of India (1500-500 BC) make reference to a fever which most likely was malaria because the text describes its association with time of the year, the onset of the rainy season, and with the bite of mosquitos. In all probability, the terms *jungle fever*, *marsh fever*, and *swamp fever* refer to malaria since they link the disease with a rich habitat for mosquitos. Village folks in India always diagnosed malaria as something distinct from other fevers because of its cyclic nature and characteristic chill. However, not a Chinese, not an

Indian but the Greek Hippocrates is often described as the first malarialogist though he had nothing to do with it except the use of the word *quartan fever*.

Malaria is transmitted by *Anopheles* mosquitos; it is caused by the parasites *Plasmodium* (*P.*) *falciparum*, *P. vivax*, *P. ovale*, *P. malariae* – each producing fever, chill, enlargement of the spleen, pale nails, and conjunctiva; however, the interval between episodes of fever and virulence of different *Plasmodium* are not identical.

The discovery of the mode of transmission of malaria corresponds to the discovery of the new world by Europeans, the colonization of India by Britain, and of Algeria by France. The British recognition of immense rewards from the 'jewel in the crown' that was India triggered a massive transformation of the country, including the introduction of the English language, railways, roads, a number of modern engineering marvels, elaborate administrative machinery, educational institutions, and modern scientific research. Calcutta (now Kolkata) in Bengal was the first British colonial capital and, hence, the first to start English education, thanks to the much-praised and equally much-maligned Lord Thomas Babington Macaulay (1800-1859). It is no wonder that the two Indian scientists mentioned in this book, Satyen Nath Bose (1894-1974), in whose honour is named the fundamental particle Boson, and Jagdish Chandra Bose (1858-1937), were from the Bengal region of India and the products of this English-science education.

Once settled in the newly found country, Britain had to deal with malaria and with other parasitic infections such as *kala-azar*. In 1897, Ronald Ross (1857-1932), born in Almora, India, got interested in malaria. His interest must have been provoked by the frequent sickness and death of British nationals and the soldiers in the British Indian army. It is clear from the many writings of Ross (later Sir Ronald Ross) that, unlike Robert Koch (1843-1910), the founder of the germ theory of disease and a humanist, Ross was concerned with the well-being of only white settlers rather than with the health of 'natives'. For example, after his trip to West Africa, he authored a set of instructions for the Liverpool School of Tropical Medicine titled "Malaria and Mosquitos" in which he writes (Ross, 1900), "In a community in which natives form the great bulk of the population, it is obvious that intelligent cooperation on large scale can hardly be looked for." These instructions concern white settlements in Africa; although the name Ross does not appear on the note in the journal, it is clearly indicated that the author is Ronald Ross.

Ross began his research on malaria in Madras (now Chennai) and then in Sikanderabad, the twin city of the better-known Hyderabad. Ross discovered the presence of the malarial parasite in *Anopheles* mosquito while in Osmania University. He had fed the mosquito on a malaria patient named Hussain Khan. Ross later proved the key role of mosquitos in the transmission of malaria by his experiments on birds; he ascertained the entire life cycle of the *malarial parasite*, including its presence in the mosquitos' salivary glands. This clearly implied that mosquitos could inject parasites through their bite.

Alphonse Laveran (1845-1922) in the French colony of Algeria earlier hypothesized the possibility that mosquitos acted as vectors in transmitting the disease. Ross was aware of Laveran's hypothesis. Laveran had observed black particles in the red blood cells of malaria patients and became the first to prove that malaria is caused by a parasite.

Italian scientists (Ottaviani et al., 1998) contend, and rightly so, that the Italian zoologist Grovanni Battista Grassi (1854-1925) was the first to establish the life cycle of the malarial parasite and its migration between mosquitos and humans. However, Italy was not a colonial power while both Britain and France were. In the controversy that followed over who was the first, Ronald Ross won. Grassi's name hardly appears in textbooks. Ross of Britain was awarded the Nobel Prize in medicine in 1902 and Alphonse Laveran of France in 1907.

Two other Nobel prizes recognized research on malaria – one went to the neurologist Julius Wagner-Jauregg (1857-1940) in 1927 and the other to the chemist Paul Müller (1899-1965) in 1948. Neither actually worked on the cause and cure of malaria, but what they did do had something to do with malaria. Dr. Julius Wagner-Jauregg, a professor of neurology at the University of Vienna, injected malarial parasites into demented syphilitic patients to produce fever. The reason for his doing so is as follows.

Syphilis is a sexually transmitted infection by the bacteria *Treponema pallidum*. For that reason, syphilis had humbled kings and commoners, generals and soldiers, poets and painters, good people and bad people. There are three stages of syphilis. In the primary stage, a painless chancre appears at the point of sexual contact (in males at the tip of the penis) with a syphilitic subject; the chancre heals, only to haunt again after months with what is called the secondary stage, during which tiny ulcers may appear anywhere or all over the body; other symptoms like fever, malaise, pain, etc., may accompany. These ulcers are loaded with the bacteria and can easily be transmitted. They also disappear even in the absence of therapy. Syphilis then enters into the third stage – tertiary syphilis – which leads to various complications, prominently vascular and neurological. While during the primary stage, syphilis can now be eradicated with penicillin, arsenic and mercury were used in the past, including during the time of Napoleon Bonaparte (1769-1821). The treatment of tertiary syphilis is highly problematic. It is the tertiary stage of syphilis, which Wagner-Jauregg attempted to treat by producing malaria. The rationale was that because the bacteria *Treponema pallidum* are very susceptible to heat, the fever produced by the malarial parasite would kill the bacteria and arrest further deterioration in the mental state of patients with tertiary syphilis.

Müller also did not do research on malaria; he rediscovered *DDT* (dichlorodiphenyltrichloroethane) and got a Swiss patent in 1940 although the chemical had been originally made in 1873 by an Austrian student who never received any particular attention.

DDT could kill a host of insects including mosquitos. Soon after its discovery, it was being sprayed all over the world, often by personnel without gloves on their hands or masks on their faces. Indeed, DDT dramatically reduced the incidence of malaria, and it appeared that malaria would disappear like the bubonic plague. During my student days (1950-1955) at the King George's Medical College, Lucknow, a malaria-prone region, finding blood smear slides with *Plasmodium* was easier than finding one without it. Soon after 1955, however, whenever the pathology department encountered a patient of malaria, hundreds of slides would be made to demonstrate to future doctors what the malaria parasite looked like. Everybody thought that malaria was a disease of the past.

· Once it was known that mosquitos transmitted malaria, entrepreneurs made full use of this knowledge. The American Army Surgeon William C. Gorgas (1854-1920) cleared Panama and Cuba of mosquitos, and the Panama Canal was built. In 1939-1940, Fred Soper (1893-1977) of the Rockefeller Foundation cleared Brazil of *Anopheles gambiae* by Paris green and *pyrethrum* to be followed by Müller's DDT.

However, as is the case with bacteria, parasites too acquire methods of safeguarding themselves from unwelcome intruders. The tiny bacteria invisible to the naked eye can find ways and means of negating the effects of penicillin. Indeed, there seems more camaraderie among bacteria than among humans. A recent study found that antibiotic-resistant bacteria find a way of protecting their non-resistant fellow beings (Lee et al., 2010). The emergence of multidrug resistant microbes is not the subject of this chapter, but the emergence of resistance of mosquitos to DDT and of *Plasmodium* to chloroquine and other anti-malarial drugs is.

Not too long after Paul Müller was awarded the Nobel Prize for worldwide use of DDT, Rachel Carson (1907-1964) released her book *Silent Spring* (Carson, 1962). Rarely has a book had so much impact as did *Silent Spring*. As expected, the industry pounced on her. Also as expected, the public fell for her. *Silent Spring* initiated the environment movement of which, ultimately, former Vice-President of the United States, Al Gore, became the beneficiary and won a Nobel Prize for peace. Governments, weak or strong, are now forced to deal with the issue of the environment. In any event, Carson's *Silent Spring* led to a ban on the use of DDT in the USA in 1972 and, soon after, elsewhere. What happened to thousands of technicians who sprayed DDT and people who live on DDT-contaminated lands in Asia, Africa, and Latin America is a matter of conjecture. All we know is that DDT can no more kill a mosquito, but it is going to remain in the soil for a very long time, and its target would be human beings. Malaria is back and DDT is gone.

Until World War II, quinine, a constituent of the Peruvian (cinchona) bark, was the only drug therapy for malaria. Peruvian Indians used the powdered bark of the cinchona tree to treat the symptoms of malaria in the seventeenth century; this powder got named as Jesuit powder after having been brought to Europe by Brother Augostino Salumbrino (1561-1642), an apothecary by training who lived in Lima. It was first used to treat malaria in Rome in 1631 and was available in London in 1649 to treat *agues*, a term used by William Shakespeare in several of his plays as a synonym for malaria. However, Shakespeare's conjecture in the *Tempest* (act II, scene II) in which the slave Caliban tries to treat his master Stephano's trembling with alcohol is misplaced because alcohol is of no value in malaria.

Quinine was isolated in 1817 by the French researchers Pierre Joseph Pelletier (1788-1842) and Joseph Bienaimé Caventou (1795-1877). The name was derived from the original *Quechua*, the Inca word for cinchona tree bark. As was the case with the knowledge of the role of mosquitos in the transmission of malaria, the knowledge of the anti-malarial properties of quinine was put to good and bad uses. With the blessings of quinine, Africa ceased to be the white man's grave; "it was quinine's efficacy that gave colonists fresh opportunities to swarm into the Gold Coast, Nigeria and other parts of West Africa" (Conner 2005a).

There is also another side to quinine. Quinine was so much in demand that to maintain their monopoly on cinchona bark, Peru and the surrounding countries began outlawing the export of cinchona seeds and saplings in the early nineteenth century. However, the Dutch government smuggled the seeds out, and by the 1930s, its colony, Java, was producing 22 million pounds of cinchona bark or 97 percent of the world's quinine production. Then came World War II. Japan occupied Southeast Asia after having caused devastation in China. The supply of quinine to the Allied powers was cut off, which triggered a number of steps. The United States started cinchona plantations in Costa Rica. Britain started cinchona plantations in India. British and American researchers embarked on a project to find a substitute for quinine; and they did succeed. Quinine was synthesized in the laboratory, but the process was less economical than extracting it from natural sources. The anti-malarial property of chloroquine, first synthesized in Germany in 1934, was discovered by British researchers; chloroquine became the most important drug in the prophylaxis and treatment of malarial thanks to

World War II. Not only that, but a team of American scientists, which included George H. Hitchings (1905-1998) and Gertrude B. Elion, both winners of the 1988 Nobel Prize in medicine for discovering antileukaemia drug, synthesized the antimalarial drug pyrimethamine. These discoveries ended the nearly three-hundred-year dominance of quinine. Although quinine is still used in selected cases of malaria, other uses for it have been found; it is added to certain drinks because of its bitter taste.

Cholera

The third example deals with a scientific aspect of public health measures. It is the story of the discovery of the mode of transmission of cholera. Between 1817 and 1831, at least fifty million people perished due to global cholera epidemics (*Quarterly Review*, 1831).

We know now that cholera is caused by the bacterium *Vibrio cholerae* and spread by ingestion of contaminated foods. Before we came to know this simple fact a lot happened. The disease is now rare in the Western world but quite frequent in other parts, especially in India, where, on certain religious occasions such as the Kumbh Mela (Kumbh congregation), almost seventy million people assemble in the relatively small city of Allahabad, the birthplace of Jawaharlal Nehru (1889-1964), to take a dip in the already dirty holy river Ganges. Every precaution is taken by the Indian government to prevent cholera epidemics during the Kumbh Mela, but it never completely succeeds.

What is cholera? The nineteenth-century big cities such as London were like many big cities of India today. Here is the story of a little girl described in the medical journal *Lancet* of November 11, 1837.

> Ellen Green, aged seven years, of Irish extraction, living with her parents, in a miserable apartment, on the second floor of a small house ...Altogether, the inmates of that single apartment amounted to eight individuals. The remaining rooms of the house were also tenanted by several other families, whilst immediately opposite the door was a heap of manure and filth, the joint produce of the house, and of a pigstye, which abutted upon the wall.
>
> On the evening of 26th October (1837), this girl was first attacked with vomiting and purging, attended with cramps of the legs and thighs, which continued all night ...the next day ...Her features were remarkable ...eyes sunk deep into the orbits; the conjunctiva effused; lips quite blue; tongue

quite white and cold; skin on the hands, fingers, and feet corrugated; the extremities very cold, and of a leaden hue; which was more particularly apparent in the hands, feet, and nails. Her pulse was occasionally perceptible ...*She had passed no urine* [emphasis added] from the time she was first attacked ...Brandy and port wine were also occasionally administered, but she gradually became worse, and expired about six the next morning, having been ill altogether about twenty-four hours.

Soon after,

Thomas Green (father of the child Ellen Green), aged 38, an Irish labourer in the West India Docks ...Daniel M'Carthy, aged 30, an Irish labourer, living, with his wife and child, in the same room with Green and his family ... Daniel Green, aged 3 years, another child of the man Green died one after another.

The above description in the *Lancet* is as typical of cholera now as it was in 1837. And yet, writes Wilson (2003a):

A society's attitude towards disease reveals more than the state of its medical knowledge. Victorian England, destined to become so densely populous, so politically powerful throughout the world, so dirty and so rich, poured much of its paranoia and its ambivalence concerning mammon-worship into its feeling about cholera. The disease came from India, source of so much British wealth and guilt ...We have witnessed in our days the birth of a new pestilence which in the short space of fourteen years (1817-1831), has desolated the fairest portions of the globe, and swept off at least fifty million of our race.

The narration above tells what happens when afflicted by cholera; it is like death by heat stroke with the added agony of diarrhea and vomiting before almost all water is expelled out of the body.

Wilson (2003a) says that in 1858 the Thames was so dirty that when Queen Victoria (1819-1901) and Prince Albert (1819-1861) attempted a short pleasure cruise, they were forced to return after a few minutes because of the terrible odour. Parliament had to rise early because of unbearable odour. People were obliged to drink the dirty water.

Edwin Chadwick (1800-1890) drew public attention to the filthy conditions in the manufacturing towns. However, the great scientific demonstration that cholera was waterborne was made by Dr. John Snow (1813-1858) against fierce opposition. The false conjectures regarding where cholera came from and how it spread in certain quarters of London is a vivid illustration of the prejudices of science and society against the poor in London's heartland and, of course, against the colonies – in this case India.

We now know that the ingestion of any substance already contaminated by *Vibrio cholerae,* invariably present in the excreta of a cholera patient, can produce cholera, which is why congregations as in the Kumbh Mela, or the drinking of contaminated water, are associated with outbreaks of cholera.

However, in 1849, Dr. John Snow, the son of an unskilled labourer raised in one of poorest residential area of York, had to fight hard against anticontagionists to prove this fact through his pamphlet *On the Mode of Communication of Cholera.*

Dr Snow's pamphlet (Snow, 1849b, 1851) provides different lines of evidence to support the thesis that cholera is "propagated by human intercourse".

In a specific case in Albion Terrace, South London, Dr. Snow followed the water supply and the drainage in the houses numbered 11-17. Summarizing Dr. Snow's pamphlet, Wilson (2003b) writes:

> Cholera extended to all the houses in which the water was tainted. However, Dr. Milroy, an advocate of the miasmas theory and an anticontagionist, attributed the mortality in Albion Terrace to three causes – an open sewer ... odour from the sinks ...and an accumulation of rubbish.
>
> Dr. Snow's other feat was to deliver the eighth child of Queen Victoria on April 7, 1853, under chloroform anesthesia. Chloroform is quite toxic, and Dr. Snow must have known it quite well since none of his patients died due to chloroform. He would administer just enough chloroform to produce analgesia and light anesthesia, which, aside from being safe, also allowed the woman to respond to his instructions.

Wilson goes on to add (2003b):

> The majority of the medical profession refused to accept Snow's findings. It was not until the cholera microbe was isolated and identified in 1883 by Robert Koch (1843-1910) that Snow's brilliant hunch – turning to circumstantial deduction – was proven. Snow and Chadwick did everything to promote cleanliness as a safeguard against waterborne diseases especially in area housed by coal miners who suffered from cholera more than any

> other group of people. Snow urged that their work conditions be divided into four hour shifts so that they did not need to use the coal pits as privies. But, of course, such measures could not be introduced without control, and – as in the case of the Irish famine – the true laissez-faire liberal would, quite literally, prefer death to state interference.

Dr. Snow was absolutely right in saying that cholera is caused by bacteria and that bacteria are transmitted through contaminated water or foods. And yet, cholera is a disease of poverty. No rich person now dies of cholera.

Opium

My penultimate example concerns exploiting drug addiction for profit and conquest. More than 150 years before the Talibans of Afghanistan discovered the commercial benefits of the poppy, one of the powers engaged since 2002 in defeating them, namely England, had discovered the benefits of selling opium as a legitimate business.

Early in the nineteenth century, traders of the British East India Company were exporting opium from India to China. They knew as well as everyone else that opium is addictive; indeed, that is why it was being exported to China. There were areas of China where almost 70 percent of the population had become addicted to opium. When the Chinese government attempted to stop the opium trade, the first Opium War (1839-1842) broke out. The Chinese lost the war and the Treaty of Nanjing was signed in which China had to pay a huge indemnity and give Britain the right to have access to five ports.

Not content with this gain, the British engineered the Second Opium War (1856-1860); the French also joined in. As expected, China was defeated again and had to sign the Treaty of Tianjin in 1858. This had much bigger implications. It allowed for residential status to foreign powers in Beijing, the opening of several new ports to Western trade and residence, the right of foreign travel in the interior of China and, more importantly, the freedom of movement for Christian missionaries. The settlements further detached Hong Kong from China and introduced the principle of extraterritoriality whereby foreigners could not be tried under Chinese law on the assumption that the Chinese were barbarians. The opium trade was legalized.

It is to the credit of Chinese resilience that its people and the country limped along to survive not only this ordeal but also the loss of nearly thirty million people during the Taiping rebellion (1850-1864) and the savage attack by Japan (1937-1945) to finally achieve liberation in 1949. In the twenty-first century, the West had to reckon with a new China, politically, economically and socially strong.

The question, however, still remains – are drugs still being pushed for profit? For a good answer to this question, read the book *The Push to Prescribe* edited by Ford and Saibil (2009).

Anaesthesia

Socio-political factors play a role in the discovery of drugs. Many examples can be cited to support this contention, but I wish to narrate a story that is of universal relevance. It is about the discovery of anaesthetics. In Chapter 2 I mentioned how hundreds of years passed between the discovery of ether and the discovery that it can be used as an anaesthetic. Here I intend to tell what the anaesthesiologist Nicholas M. Greene (1922-2004) thought about the factors delaying the discovery of anaesthesia. I quote relevant parts of the article by Greene (1971):

> The richness of the history of anesthesia unfolds when one considers the factors which determined why anesthesia was introduced when it was … In the absence of humanitarianism, political freedom could not develop, child labor would continue, penology would remain medieval, the care of the insane would remain cruel and inhumane, and also, in the absence of humanitarianism, anesthesia could not be discovered. Control of pain required the simultaneous development of a desire on the part of the society to correct all the ailments which affect man.
>
> So long as witches were being burned in Salem, anesthesia could not be discovered 20 miles away in Boston.
>
> In 1591, a woman by the name of Eufame MacAlyane was burned alive on Castle Hill in Edinburgh because she sought relief of pain during delivery of her two sons.

Greene (1971) also elaborates why it was a dentist and not a physician who discovered anaesthesia; it was because the former encountered pain on a daily basis in his practice while the latter did surgery rather rarely. He refers to the Salem witch-hunt as a deterrent to the discovery of anaesthesia; I think the festivity of witch-hunt, which was more widespread in Europe than in the USA (see Chapter 11) was perhaps also a factor why anaesthesia could not be discovered in England, Germany and France.

Medicine and Humanities

The progress or stagnation of intellectual contribution can be traced to the progress or stagnation of societies as a whole. Moreover, the progress in any one field of science cannot happen without concurrent advances in all other branches of science as well as humanities, notably philosophy. Many examples of the interrelationship between different branches of science can be quoted; indeed, this can constitute a book in its own right and some such books may exist like the *Great Transformation: The Political and Economic Origins of Our Time* by Karl Polanyi [1886-1964] (1944, 1957, 2001) with a foreword by Joseph E. Stiglitz (1957 edition), winner of the 2001 Nobel Prize in economics.

The role of philosophy in the advancement of the natural sciences is not as obvious as it should be. Biologists, and especially medical scientists, seem particularly reluctant to admit any role of philosophy in advancing the sciences. This is partly because reductionism in science simultaneously leads to a narrow outlook about science and, in many cases, to unjustified arrogance on the part of the scientists.

The reductionist approach in science has its own culture; it can be pursued with detailed knowledge of the subspecialty concurrent with a minimum familiarity with other branches of science and perhaps no familiarity with the social sciences; as a result the research might lose its relevance.

At the same time a number of sociologist critics of reductionism in science have a microscopic vision of science and society; for example, Nettleton (2006) absurdly chooses the "Germ theory"[3] of disease as an example of reductionism. Medical science is more aware than Nettleton type sociologists that bacteria are by themselves not sufficient to cause diseases like cholera, tuberculosis, typhoid etcetera; nonetheless these diseases can never be contracted in the absence of germs, and when they do occur, the treatment is directed against specific micro-organisms.

Russell (1946b) stresses the role of philosophy in the advancement of science as follows:

> Like theology, it (philosophy) consists of speculation on matters as to which definite knowledge has, so far, been unascertainable; but like science, it appeals to human reason rather than to authority, whether that of tradition or that of revelation. All definite knowledge – so I should contend – belongs to science; all dogmas as to what surpasses definite knowledge belongs to theology. But between theology and science there is a No Man's Land, exposed to attack from both sides; this No Man's Land is philosophy.

Indeed in most, if not all, scientific pursuits, the investigator starts with a hypothesis, which might be called the philosophical aspect of the inquiry and then goes on to test it by appropriate experimentation.

Advances in modern surgery and diagnostics which far surpasses advances in therapeutics best illustrates the interdependence of different branches of science as they impact on medicine. Laser surgery is less an advance in the skill of the surgeons than of the physicists who made laser possible. Likewise, the quantification of tiny amounts of chemicals and hormones in the body by RIA (radioimmunoassay), the visualization of inaccessible parts of the body by x-rays, NMR (nuclear magnetic resonance), CAT (computer assisted tomography), and PET (positron emission tomography) scan were contributed to the medical profession by discoveries made by scientists in other fields. Indeed, of the 195 Nobel Prize winners in medicine from 1901 to 2010, only 87 (45 percent) were medical persons; and of these 87, a majority were researchers in the laboratory like other biologists. Of the nine Nobel laureates in medicine since 2007, only one holds a medical degree.

Gender Bias in Medicine

The relative silence on the role of women in medicine reflects many things. It is very likely that women gave birth to the science of medicine during the era, which got characterized as witchcraft. But the progress of medicine, like that of all other sciences, goes hand in hand with development of arguments to sideline women under various pretexts, the most common being that, relative to men, they are less fit for the rigor of science and more fit for household chores.

The admission of women to medical schools was so restrictive that history was made in the nineteenth century of the United States when Elizabeth Blackwell (1821-1910) became the first female graduate of a medical institution in 1849. Even Rita Levi-Montalcini (1910-2011), the 1986 Nobel laureate in medicine, whose one hundredth birthday celebration was reported in no lesser a journal than *Nature* (Abbott, 2009), had to displease her loving father to enter the medical school in Turin, Italy. This was a pleasant interlude compared with what she faced when she graduated. Mussolini (1883-1945) came to power. World War II broke out. Being a Jew, she had to hide from the reach of the Nazis and Fascists and set up her laboratory in her bedroom and later had to move from one place to another to pursue her research. Despite these hard times, Levi-Montalcini discovered the nerve growth factor (NGF), a molecule of great significance, which could prove of potential benefit in alzheimer's disease.

The medical historian Robinson wrote his book in 1931; Sigerist's second volume, which appeared posthumously in 1961, is limited to early Greek, Hindu, and Persian medicine. Robinson does talk about Marie Curie (1867-1934), who was awarded exceptionally two Nobel Prizes, one in physics (1903) and one in chemistry (1911), and whose discoveries on radiation proved of immense importance in medicine. So Robinson and Sigerist cannot be blamed for not referring to what happened after their deaths.

Roy Porter (1997-2002) mentions Nobel laureate Marie Curie and highlights the medical significance of her discovery; however, he too does not mention any other, except Rosalyn Yalow (1921-2011), and then falsely credits her for the discovery of the pituitary hormone, which was indeed a contribution of the Nobel Prize co-winner Roger Guillemin and not Yalow (Porter, 1997), who discovered the technique of radioimmunoassay, which is to date the most sensitive tool to measure chemicals in the body.

There have been ten women Nobel laureates in physiology and medicine up to 2009; if we add the names of Marie Curie, whose Nobel Prize-winning discovery of radiation opened important progress in medicine, and Dorothy Hodgkin (1910-1994), whose work is directly relevant to medicine but whose Nobel Prize is in chemistry, we have at least twelve women of the highest accomplishment in science. Rosalind Franklin died at the age of thirty-eight of ovarian cancer; she is justly recognized by many to be deserving of a Nobel Prize for her work on the structure of DNA; that makes a list of at least thirteen outstanding women. These distinguished women Nobel laureates highlight the role of women researchers.

The ten winners of the Nobel Prize, specifically in physiology and medicine, are the following: (1947) Gerti Cori (1896-1957), a medical doctor from Prague for her work on carbohydrate metabolism; (1977) Rosalyn Yalow, a physicist who combined her physics with biology to develop the technique of radioimmunoassay (RIA); (1983) Barbara McClintock, a botanist, who, while working on the mutations of maize, discovered transposable genes, like the currently known jumping genes; (1986) Rita Levi-Montalcini, mentioned above; (1988) Gertrude B. Elion (1918-1999), a chemist who exemplifies need-based research and who synthesized the first effective drugs against leukaemia (mercaptopurine, thioguanine) and against transplant rejection (azathioprine); (1995) Christiane Nüsslein-Volhard, a molecular biologist who made significant contribution to our understanding of the genetic control of embryonic development; (2004) Linda B. Buck, an immunologist who, through a tortuous course, started examining the mechanism whereby different odours are sensed by the brain; (2008) Françose Barré-Sinoussi, a virologist and co-discoverer of the role of human papilloma virus in cervical cancer, which led to the development of the prophylactic vaccine already in use; (2009) Elizabeth Blackburn and Carol W. Greider who discovered how telomeres are protected and thus the integrity of chromosomes.

In addition to gender bias, there is also a racial bias in historiography. There are books, theatrical portrayal, and movies on the life of Florence Nightingale (1820-1910), but one cannot make out if this honour is bestowed upon her because she was an ideal nurse or because she served in the British army during the bloody Crimean war (1853-1856); her companion nurse at the same battlefield, Mary Seacole (1805-1881) of Jamaica, perhaps more ingenious than Nightingale and equally sacrificing but black, is naturally less well-known.

Science and the Mode of Production

One fundamental difference between feudal and capitalist orders of production, which has the maximum impact on scientific advances, is that the latter requires continuous renovations in the means of production and interdependence in different branches of production.

It is thus not surprising that the capitalist order of production was necessarily accompanied by major advances in medical science and also in the fields of natural sciences, economics, sociology, philosophy, literature, and the methods of governance. It follows that the major impetus for advances in medicine, as in natural sciences, occurred in England, France, and Germany and in America and not in Egypt, India, and China. I dwell on this subject in Chapter 16.

It should be noted that while the capitalist order created conditions for major advances in science and technology, it also puts constraints because the medical profession simultaneously entails scientific discoveries on one hand and the monetary interests of the pharmaceutical industry as well as of doctors on the other hand. In the process, the promotion of doubtfully necessary drugs and concerns of the rich countries and rich people take undue priority.

In Chapter 2 I discussed how a market was created for stilbestrol against miscarriage and for hormone replacement therapy to prevent physiological changes of menopause. Women's bodies are subjected to other uncalled-for interventions due to the creation of a market. For example, 364,000 breast implants were done in the United States in 2005 alone. In the past, caesarean section was reserved for special situations like baby distress or breech presentation (feet first). However, 29 percent of all births in the United States in 2004 occurred by caesarean section. Women past fifty years of age can bear children, thanks to *in vitro* fertilization techniques, and the subject of 2010 Nobel Prize. In Chapter 15, in dealing with medical ethics, I discuss the rationale or lack of rationale for the use of lipid-lowering drugs.

Political considerations also affect the training of medical professionals. In most countries, medical training is need-based and not as a system of imparting the best possible knowledge of medical science. This, by itself, might not be a bad thing because training of medical professionals as doctors, nurses, and technologists is to meet health-care needs rather than advance medical science, which has no national identity. So that barefoot doctors of China may be what China needed (Connel and Gover, 1974).[4] But a barefoot doctor is not obliged to know basic aspects of the totality of medical science. Likewise, a doctor from premium medical institutions in the West may have little idea of diseases of the South, like parasitic infections. In contrast, the programs in natural sciences might differ between the developed and developing countries in terms of excellence of professors, but they do not substantially differ in content. This bias is also reflected in textbooks of medical science.

Notes

1. Einstein, A. "Why Socialism?" *Monthly Review*, New York, May 1949. In *Ideas and Opinions*, A. Einstein (New York: Crown Publishing, 1954), 153-154.

2. Lewontin, R. C. *Biology as Ideology: The Doctrine of DNA* (New York: Harper Perennial, 1991), 3.

3. The 1905 Nobel Laureate Heinrich Hermann Robert Koch (1843-1910) identified anthrax, tuberculosis and cholera bacteria. From his research it was conclusively established that, for example, tuberculosis cannot be produced in the absence of tuberculosis bacillus but he never conjectured that infection with the bacteria was sufficient condition for getting tuberculosis. Treatment of tuberculosis is directed against the bacteria; fresh air and good nutrition cannot cure tuberculosis. He and other eminent bacteriologists like Louis Pasteur (1822-1895), the founders of the "Germ Theory" were fully cognizant of the domain of diseases caused by bacteria. Sociologists would be on firmer footing if they dug deeper into finding out what is really reductionism in science.

4 The delegation of the Science for the People, which visited China in 1974, comprised of the following American scientists: Mary Altendorf, David Aronow, John Dove, Ginger Goldner, Judy Greenberg, Marvin Kalkstein, Frank Mirer, Geri Steiner, and Vinton Thompson.

References

Abbott, A. "Neuroscience: One Hundred Years of Rita," *Nature* 458 (2009): 564.

Bhishagratna, K.L. *Sushruta Samhita (English translation) Vol. 1* (Chowkhamba Sanskrit Series, Varanasi, 1963), vii-x.

Carson, R. *Silent Spring* (New York: Houghton Mifflin, 1962).

Connel, D. and Gover, D. Ed. *China: Science Walks on Two Legs: A Report from Science For The People* (New York: Avon Books, 1974).

Conner, Clifford D. *A People's History of Science: Miners, Midwives, and 'Low Mechanicks'*, (New York: Nation Books, 2005).

Ibid., 2005a. 96.

Day, C. S. *Quipus and Witches' Knots* (Lawrence: University of Kansas Press, 1967), 80.

De Beauvoir, S. *Deuxième Sexe* (Paris: Gallimard, 1949).

Desowitz, R. S. *The Malaria Capers: More Tales of Parasites and People, Research and Reality* (New York: W. W. Norton & Company, 1991).

Ford, A. R. and Saibil, D. (Ed.). *The Push to Prescribe: Women & Canadian Drug Policy* (Toronto: Women's Press, 2009).

Frank, A. G. *ReOrient* (Berkley: University of California Press, 1998).

Greene, N. M. "A Consideration of Factors in the Discovery of Anesthesia and Their Effects on Its Development." *Anesthesiology* 35 (1971): 515-522.

Lee, H. H., Molla, M. N., Cantor, C. R. and Collins, J. J. "Bacterial Charity Work Leads to Population-Wide Resistance," *Nature* 467 (2010): 82-85.

Lewontin, R. *Biology as Ideology: The Doctrine of DNA* (New York: HarperPerennial, 1991), 61-62.

Maddox, B. *Rosalind Franklin: The Dark Lady of DNA* (New York: Harper Collins, 2002).

Marx, K. *The Eighteenth Brumaire of Louis Bonaparte* (1852) (*www.ReadHowYouWant.com*), 2006),1.

Needham, J. *Science and Civilisation in China: Biology and Biological Technology* (Cambridge: Cambridge University Press [1954], 2000).

Nettleton, S. *The Sociology of Health and Illness*, 2nd ed. (Cambridge: Polity Press, 2006), 2.

Osler, W. *An Alabama Student and Other Biographical Essays* (London: Henry Frowde, 1908), 296.

Ottaviani, R., Vanni, D. and Vanni, P. "The Centenary of G. B. Grassi's Discovery," *International Journal of Anthropology* 13 (1998): 177-179.

Polanyi, K. *The Great Transformation: The Political and Economic Origins of Our Times* (Boston: Beacon Press, 1957 (1944, 2001).

Porter, R. *The Greatest Benefit to Mankind* (New York: Norton, 1997).

Ross, R. "Malaria and Mosquitos," *British Medical Journal*, February 10, 1900, 329.

Russell, B. *The History of Western Philosophy* (New York: Simon & Schuster, 1945a), 596.

Ibid., 1945b. xiii.

Said, E. W. *Orientalism* (New York: Vintage Books, 1978).

Shah, S. *The Fever: How Malaria Has Ruled Humankind for 500,000 Years* (New York: Sarah Crichton Books, 2010).

Snow, J. "On the Mode of Communication of Cholera," *London: Pamphlet August/September* 1849a.

——, "On the Pathology and Mode of Communication of Cholera," *London Medical Gazette* 44 (1849b) :745-752, 923-929. First delivered on October 13, 1849.

——, "On the Mode of Propagation of Cholera," *Medical Times (London)* 3, 29 *November* 1851: 559-562.

Toynbee, A. R. *A Study of History,* Abridgement of Volume I by DC Somervell (Oxford: Oxford University Press, 1946), 3-4.

Watts, S. *Epidemics and History: Disease, Power and Imperialism* (New Haven: Yale University Press, 1997).

Wilson, A. N. *The Victorian* (London: W. W. Norton 2003a), 34.

Ibid., 2003b. 156-157.

CHAPTER 4

The Age of Spiritual Medicine

The human spirit craves for scientific knowledge, and if the right kind is not available, men's desire may easily overcome their prudence. Nowhere are those desires stronger and wilder than in the medical field, for is not health the greatest blessing, and the lack or loss of it, the greatest misfortune? This explains also why medical quackery has always flourished and will continue to do so as long as there are distressing and incurable diseases.

George Sarton[1]

Mystery, magic, and medicine: In the beginning they were one and the same. And the healing methods that thousands of years ago sprang up and were developed by one group of primitive savage people were the same type as those developed by all others.

H. W. Haggard[2]

Introduction

In this book, the term *witchcraft* refers to "primitive spiritual medicine" and is not intended to carry any of the negative connotations of the *Oxford Dictionary*, which defines *witch* as a "woman practicing sorcery" and *witchcraft* as "sorcery, use of magic."

I had suggested earlier that witchcraft and magic are the forerunners of medicine and natural sciences (Varma, 2006), which is almost identical to what was postulated by Sir James George Frazer (1854-1941) in his classic *The Golden Bough* (Frazer, 1922a):

> From the earliest times man has been engaged in a search for general rules whereby to turn the order of natural phenomena to his own advantage ... The true or golden rules constitute the body of applied science which we call the arts; the false are magic.

In this sense, magic is like scientific hypotheses, except that it might persist despite evidence to the contrary. If magic fails, it is not science but becomes a kin of religion, which, according to Frazer (1922b), "consists of two elements, a theoretical and a practical, namely, a belief in powers higher than man and an attempt to propitiate or please them."

The medical historian Victor Robinson (1886-1947) wrote (1931a) that out of primitive man's need "arose the first professional class – antedating even prostitution and older than any religion – the profession of magician or mystery man, the Medicine Man." Witchcraft has been considered "the common heritage of humanity ...not chargeable to any particular time, or race or form of religion" (Kittredge, 1929).

Witchcraft, magic and sorcery evolved into modern medicine and other sciences. This chapter attempts to situate witchcraft in the long journey of medicine from antiquity to modern times. The vulgarised form of witchcraft is practiced by all kinds of healers even today.

Witchcraft as the Earliest Medicine and the Role of Women

Although the designation of primitive medicine as witchcraft and not wizardcraft (a word not in the dictionary) reflects traditional patriarchy, the term does reflect, even if unintended, the true origin of medicine.

The knowledge of the relationship between coitus and conception must have come thousands of years after a sufficient number of *Homo sapiens* inhabited the earth. However, there is no mistaking the relationship of the newborn to the mother. The mother was the sole caretaker of the newborn; it had no chance of survival without this care. Caring for the infant extended to the care of the community. Therefore we must conclude that women were the harbingers of the rudimentary medical science thousands of years ago, much before the birth of any discipline of medicine as we know it today.

Only with the emergence of a hierarchy in the medical profession and the power that could be exercised through medicine came the sorcerers, the magicians, the medicine men as suggested by Ehrenreich and English (1973).

The Science of Witchcraft

In antiquity, witchcraft did not have the need to invent God, but it did want to understand causes of all events, especially harmful events, and find a method of dealing with them. In a way, it is the earliest science insofar as it makes inferences from the existing possibilities. There is no fixed expression of witchcraft; rather, it too has evolved, occasionally getting vulgarized and finally taking one of the following two forms: in one form, it represents the transition to modern medicine, biology, physics, chemistry, and technology; in another form, it retains links with the old and persists as rituals sanctioned by society and religion.

Robinson (1931b) opens his book *The Story of Medicine* with the sentence: "The first cry of pain through the primitive jungles was the first call for a physician." If so, then witchcraft must have originated at the same time as the birth of *Homo sapiens*. It is hard to imagine life without encountering pain, which is an important prerequisite for the survival of a living creature. The rare instance of absolute resistance to pain because of some genetic abnormality is life-threatening. It is, therefore, reasonable to conclude that experiencing pain and the response to it is the first encounter with disease, and the *cry* is the first appropriate method of dealing with it.

Perhaps Robinson would have been even more correct if he wrote that the "first cry of pain through primitive jungles" elevated the status of the patient to the status of the first physician, for pain would not only be the first recognizable ailment but also the one to which the patient responds by doing something about it, that is, playing the role of a physician. Maybe the cry itself acts as an analgesic. My inquiries from eminent pain researchers failed to provide an answer; some said the cry is intended to solicit help. If so, why should victims of torture in the unfortunate company of only torturers cry?

Almost three hundred years ago, Daniel Le Clerc (1816-1893) wrote in his *Histoire de la Médecine*, considered to be the first book on the history of medicine, that "the first man was the first physician" (Le Clerc,

1723). Even today, when the institution of training medical professionals through university education has become the norm and even practitioners of other schools of medicine go through some form of training, each and every individual continues to act as a physician.

Every ailment needs some attention. However, not for every ailment, one runs to the doctor; were it so, we would be spending a great deal of our lives in doctors' offices. Either the patient establishes prognosis, for example, of the common cold, and decides to suffer until the common cold has passed through its normal course, or applies some form of home remedy. Another common occurrence is minor injury causing some bleeding; practically everyone knows how to stop it without the assistance of a physician. Likewise, every individual does something in the event of minor burns. Even animals have some method of dealing with injuries and fractures; they stop using the broken leg; this is equivalent to immobilization, which is what the orthopaedic surgeons do by means of splints or plasters. Dogs eat grass to induce vomiting and lick the wound to expedite healing. Elephants help sister elephants during birthing and so on. All animals protect their young ones from predators.

If we proceed with the above logic, we could divide the advances of medicine from the birth of humans to the beginning of the materialistic medicine around 700 BC into three phases. The first phase might be called Intuitive Medicine, the second Observational Medicine, and the third Spiritual Medicine. This last phase was followed by the evolution of modern materialistic medicine starting with Ayurveda, Chinese medicine, and Hippocrates.

An example of Intuitive Medicine would be applying some form of tourniquet to stop bleeding, or responding in some way when the baby cried, or immobilizing a fractured limb, or even applying saliva to an injured part. The second, or Observational Medicine, must have developed alongside the discovery of edible or poisonous natural products. This second stage could have consisted of the search for herbs to soothe pain or to treat fever. In the course of these experimentations, and the development of language and formation of communities, theories must have begun to emerge to explain why certain things happen and what can be done to prevent undesired effects on individuals and communities.

Robinson (1931c) writes, "Aboriginal man could not grasp the conception of natural death. Disturbance or stoppage of physical life was due to supernatural causes – to the wrath of the dead, the uncanny powers of human enemies, the revenge of offended spirits." That being so, the primitive human would go to any extent to prevent death. When we talk about the history of naturally occurring drugs like opium, quinine, cocaïne, atropine, et cetera, we document recorded history. But recorded history implies that the drug was already known to certain communities. Also, some physical manoeuvres like the use of knots against headache were known for a very long time, most likely during the second stage of witchcraft – the phase of Observational Medicine.

The third phase of medicine that is witchcraft or Spiritual Medicine, required the emergence of a certain level of hierarchical system, the need to explain the relationship between the cause and the event, and the human desire to control nature. Most historians start with this third stage of medicine, spiritual medicine, and hence detail magic, witchcraft, sorcery, and divination.

Frazer (1922) documents different forms of magic, their intended objectives and their relationship with science as well as religion. Although he does not provide a time frame for the origin of different forms of magic in various countries, and neither does the book *The Origin of Things* by Julius E. Lips (1895-1950) (Lips, 1949), it would seem that magic and sorcery emerged during the last five thousand years.

According to Frazer (1922c), all magic belongs to one of the two categories: homeopathic magic is based on the law of similarity, which assumes that like produces like, while contagious magic assumes that "things which have been in contact with each other continue to act on each other at a distance after physical contact has been severed." In practice, the two forms are often practiced side by side. According to homeopathic magic, hurting the image of an enemy will hurt the enemy. Contagious magic assumes a relationship between a person and any severed portion of his/her person, for example hair or nails, so that through this hair or nails, an effect can be produced at a distance on the person to whom they belonged. Frazer (1922d) takes a balanced view of the institution of magicians. He writes:

> Thus, however justly we may reject the extravagant perceptions of magicians and condemn the deceptions which they have practiced on mankind, the original institution of this class of men has, take it all in all, been productive of incalculable good to humanity. They were the direct predecessors, not merely of our physicians and surgeons, but of our investigators and discoverers in every branch of natural science. They began the work which has since been carried to such glorious and beneficent issues by their successors in after ages; and if the beginning was poor and feeble, this is to be imputed to the inevitable difficulties which beset the path of knowledge rather than to the natural incapacity or wilful fraud of the men themselves.

Frazer, like Robinson, emphasizes an important point, namely that primitive humans believed that they could prevail upon nature. Frazer writes (1922e):

> The conception of gods as superhuman beings endowed with powers to which man possesses nothing comparable in degree and hardly even in kind, has been slowly evolved in the course of history. By primitive peoples the supernatural agents are not regarded as greatly, if at all, superior to man; for they may be frightened and coerced by him into doing his will.

Karl Marx (1863-1883) wrote: "socialized man, the associated producers, govern the human metabolism with nature in a rational way, bringing it under their collective instead of being dominated by it as a blind power" (Marx 1894).

Transformation of the Role of Witchcraft

As civilization progressed, the function of witchcraft changed from the human endeavour to deal with nature to the human lust for belief in myths and obscurantism. Witchcraft ceased to be a method of dealing with the wraths of the elements of nature – sun and moon, wind and water, mountains and waterfalls, and so on. Rather, witchcraft assumed a different function, as Sigmund Freud (1922) opines in the context of the early twentieth century:

> A group, further, is subject to the truly magical power of words; they can evoke the most formidable tempests in the group mind, and are also capable of stilling them. Reasons and arguments are incapable of combating certain words and formulas.[3] And, finally, communities have never thirsted after truth. They demand illusion, and cannot do without them.

Modern witchcraft has many expressions and is practiced not by sorcerers alone, but by a variety of professionals, including physicians (Verrips, 2003). Likewise, its clients are not innocent hapless people, but often enough the elite. The most common expression of this is faith in astrology.

I have designated the third stage of witchcraft as Spiritual Medicine not because of any connection with God, but because diseases were not attributed to physical factors but rather to unknown spiritual factors. Because the cause of disease was assumed to be spiritual, the treatment was, in one form or another, intended to appease the spirit. While the theoretical basis of primitive medicine was, to a great extent, similar all over the world, the methods of appeasing the devil differed from society to society depending on other prevailing social practices and available natural products (Varma, 2006).

All in all, the first stage of medicine should be characterized as the science of witchcraft or spiritualism.

At any given stage of social development, even in far distant places, myths and inventions were very similar because they were the product of material needs of the time at that particular place (Freeman, 1896). Trepanation, for example, was practiced across continents and each continent had independently discovered how to do it in the erroneous hope of curing everything from headache to madness. It might be worth noting that headache and migraine are felt in the head so that associating it with structures inside the skull is somewhat natural. On the other hand, madness and epileptic seizures are manifested through other organs of the body, not the head; associating these with some abnormality of brain function is an advanced intellectual activity, perhaps the beginning of neurology.

Witchcraft and Drug Discovery

Various books, periodicals, and movies portray witchcraft, magic, and sorcery as symbols of evil or acts of bloodthirsty savages, not as harbingers of science. The prime example of this is the film *Dr. Jekyll and Mr. Hyde*, with Frederic March (1897-1975) in the key role, or the *Dracula* series. I am presenting here a few examples of witchcraft where its healing effects appear realistic and can be explained on the basis of known facts. Even in *Dr. Jekyll and Mr. Hyde*, the transformation from good to evil occurs after taking some potion; it may be assumed that the author Robert Louis Stevenson (1850-1894) was either aware of or had heard of hallucinogenic herbs and the ability of these drugs to transform personality. Erratic behaviour due to ingestion of weeds containing hallucinogens – such as *Mandragora officinarum* (mandrake), the source of scopolamine and hyoscyamine, *Hyoscyamus niger*, and *Datura stamonium*, the source of scopolamine, atropine, and hyoscyamine – has been described (Hansen, 1978) and discussed in the Ebers Papyrus from the period 1700-1600 BC.

Witchcraft is also used to explain unusual phenomena in holy texts of practically every religion. Interestingly, *Atharvaveda*, the parent text of the Hindu Ayurveda, is loaded with descriptions of a multitude of wrongs as acts of witches; it says, "Wickedness in a woman could cause her to slay her own husband or bear him no offspring" (Saletore, 1981). Hinduism is replete with sacrifice rituals for practically every human need (Saletore, 1981); these rituals can easily be traced to primitive human's attempts to deal with natural or unnatural disasters.

However absurd a magical ritual might have been in antiquity, in general, it addressed important questions. Water is perhaps the most important matter in the evolution and survival of species. The most obvious and universal source of water is rain. Perhaps for that reason, in each country there is some mysterious method of bringing rain. Frazer (1922) devotes eighteen pages (72-89) of his book to different forms of magic intended to bring rainfall. In the event of drought in India, a team of children generally takes on the task of bringing rainfall. They go from house to house; women come out and sprinkle water in the front of the house and children roll over, asking frogs to bring rain. The association between frogs and water, which Frazer would term *homeopathic magic*, is revealing. Indeed, in all countries, incantations intended to bring rainfall have some form of relationship with water.

Witchcraft also includes medical practices, which involve either the administration of herbs to the patient or subjecting him to certain manoeuvres. The discovery of medicinal herbs in antiquity must have been a gigantic exercise. Take the example of just one drug, the anti-malarial quinine. How does a community living in the Amazon discover the anti-malarial property of cinchona from among thousands of trees in the rain forest? Did Amazonians try all trees and all parts of all trees to find out if any helped a patient of malaria? This is highly unlikely. It is more likely that the discovery of anti-malarial activity of cinchona bark was a result of certain observations like the association of malaria to rain, the bitterness of the cinchona bark to medicinal effect, and obviously much more.

The most common method of applying drugs, even to this date, was either by oral ingestion or by topical application. Both are ancient practices. Ingestion by mouth of a natural product necessarily requires some form of emulsification and extraction. This gave rise to alchemy, the philosophers' stone, and finally, to the science of chemistry on the one hand, and to the *Harry Potter* series of J. K. Rowling on the other hand.

The topical application of an emulsion or paste to treat ulcers, bruises, and cuts is, by far, the easiest technique of drug use, and this approach must have yielded useful therapeutic information. This could be how the people of India had worked out the antiseptic efficacy of *Neem* (*Azadiracta indica*) and turmeric (*Curcuma longa*). It is easier to comprehend how the effectiveness of lime (calcium oxide) paste to stop bleeding was discovered. These are significant discoveries considering how difficult it is even today to discover a new class of drugs despite so many advances in pathophysiology of diseases and chemistry.

There are also many examples since antiquity of how physical manoeuvring of the body served medical purposes. Some methods such as trepanation or immobilization of fractured limbs or extraction of rotting teeth can be easily linked to the evolution of surgery. There are other techniques as well. For example, in villages in India, colic pains among children are common due to the ingestion of leftover foods in hot climate and an abundance of intestinal parasites. When a child complained of abdominal pain, the mother or grandmother would make the child lie down on its back, put an ignited clay lamp on the top of the belly button, and cover it with a small pan. The pain would disappear or, at the very least, decrease. How this method of relieving pain came to be discovered is mind-boggling. This example illustrates at least two points. The first is the ingenuity inherent in this discovery. The second is that the mother or the grandmother did not think it necessary to know how the clay-lap therapy against abdominal pain worked. This shows that knowledge of the mechanism of action of a drug or treatment is not an essential element in its effectiveness. In the case of the lighted-lamp therapy for abdominal pain, perhaps the flame consumed the oxygen creating a vacuum; the suction probably triggered a set of neuronal impulses obscuring the one carried through the spinal cord by pain fibres. The discovery of acupuncture may have a similar history. Clearly, empirical approaches can be effective against pain without the slightest awareness of the gate theory of pain proposed by Melzack and Wall (1965).

This inference is further supported by the experience of the two most important drugs for the relief of pain, namely opium and aspirin (its natural predecessor, salicin); these two drugs still remain the cornerstone of analgesia, and they were discovered a long time ago by practitioners of witchcraft, who neither knew how these drugs acted nor how pain was produced. Like aspirin, opium (source of morphine) too has been known for more than two thousand years. It is only in the 1970s that the natural presence of opium-like chemicals in the brain and the binding targets of morphine were discovered; how exactly pain is relieved by opium is still not known (see Gutstein and Akil, 2006). Sir John Vane (1927-2004) announced the mechanism of the analgesic effect of aspirin-like drugs early in the 1970s.

Perhaps many discoveries were made in antiquity by trial and error. It was possible because, practically, the entire population was involved in discoveries in the ancient times, which is now the task of only specialized experts. Even the last one hundred years can be divided into two periods. Practically all pharmacology departments were involved in drug discovery in the first half of the twentieth century; now this activity is almost entirely in the domain of the giant pharmaceuticals.

Other Medical Interventions

What is true of medicine is also true of other technical devices discovered in antiquity. We all know how the use of knots is central to our modern existence, be it for tightening shoelaces or erecting a building.

But knots have served and continue to serve much more important functions. Knots were used to cure all kinds of ills in every age and in all parts of the world. Hage (2008) discusses the importance of knots in surgical suturing. Thompson (1904) elaborates on the efficacy of knots against pain.

Early humans practically everywhere in the world used Mnemonic knots (by varying their numbers or using different colour strings) long before writing was invented. It is highly probable that the word "abacus" is derived from the Hebrew word "Abaq," the root of which was "knot." The problem with the knot method was that it was very time-consuming, and this might have given birth to Peruvian quipus. Even the Inca Empire of pre-Spanish Peru had inherited them from pre-Inca past (Spence, 1994). According to Day (1967a), "the textile of remarkable artistic and technical excellence, for example, had been produced in Peru since as early as 3000 B.C." Locke (1912) opines that knots on the Peruvian quipu abide by the decimal system of notation. Przytycki (1998), in discussing the classical roots of knot theory, refers to the relevance of knots in the works of mathematics and physics greats like Gottfried Wilhelm Leibniz (1646-1716), Leonard Euler (1707-1783), Carl Friedrich Gauss (1777-1855), James Clerk Maxwell, Gustav Robert Kirchhoff (1824-1887), Hermann Von Helmholtz (1821-1894), William Thomson (Lord Kelvin) (1824-1907), Peter Guthrie Tait (1831-1901), and many others.

It is difficult to imagine that in social interaction, everyone is a friend. A physically stronger man, or one from a different location, may be or may appear to be an enemy. So the tools of healing must also give rise to tools of protection from the enemy. The art and science of witchcraft therefore divides into two branches – one to protect oneself and friends and the other to harm or, better still, to demolish the enemy.

Knowledge of the very early evolution of medicine, say one hundred thousand years ago or even twenty thousand years ago, is, at best, an intelligent guess. At least two physical factors must have affected medical discoveries of antiquity. One is the prevalence of diseases and the other is the relatively short life span. The extremely low density of population must have been a critical factor in restricting the emergence of many of the diseases that we know of today. Injuries, pain, and fever are likely to have dominated human illnesses. *The Cambridge World History of Human Disease* (Kiple, 1993) does not go earlier than three millennium BC; it does say, however, "Hunter-gatherers and early agriculturalists of the Old World, although hardly disease-free, are generally held to have been free of epidemic diseases as well as of many other illnesses now regarded as 'diseases of civilization.'"

Life span is another important determinant of diseases; it must have been extremely short in the earliest times. An estimate of the short life span of our earliest ancestors can be speculated by taking some later reference point. England of the mid-seventeenth century was perhaps the most developed country of the world. Yet approximately 80 percent of the population died before reaching the age of twenty-five, and less than 10 percent lived beyond the age of forty. Even by 1861, when more than 60 percent of the population in England and Wales lived to sixty-five years of age, approximately 25 percent continued to die before reaching the age of ten, suggesting very high infant and child mortality (Wills, 1996). Of course, many diseases, including epidemics, had become prevalent by the seventeenth century in England, which did not exist, say, one hundred thousand years ago. Despite this, it is apparent that the life span of our earliest ancestors must have been very short, but not short enough to avoid encounters with pain or bleeding.

Theory of Disease

The human mind is very inquisitive and the first thing it demands is to know the cause of an event. Some inquiries are directly need-based, some are pure curiosity, and some attain significance a short time or over a very long period after initial curiosity. Questions are almost always correct when driven by real curiosity. The early humans must have come out with answers to all such queries. There is an explanation for stroke in the villages of North India. The explanation is as follows: Serpents develop wings when they get very old, then they fly. If one comes under the shadow of such flying reptiles, one gets a stroke. There is obviously no substance to these explanations, but ordinary village folks felt the need for explanations just as most modern medical scientists feel them now. It is also possible that they died of heat stroke, and their mental confusion gave them the impression of some flying object in the sky. In any case, the significance of this story is that each abnormal event is followed by a definite inquiry into its cause, and the entire history of medical science has been to search for the cause until an unequivocal answer is found.

Questions related to physical well-being must be answered with certain immediacy. Our very early ancestors did it by something, which, as we got more civilized, is called witchcraft. They invented remedies, some of which are obsolete. Witchcraft must have arisen as a genuine inquiry into the cause of an unusual event; the cause could have been a curse by nature as punishment for some wrongdoing; the cure might have been to satiate the angry nature. There is nothing vicious about these questions and answers.

I end this chapter with a quote from Day (1967b):

> The Sun and the Moon, for primitive man, were deities; disease and death were the work of devils; and he took it for granted that a mysterious spiritual power which anthropologists call mana (a Polynesian word) animates things both material and immaterial. Primitive man, reasoning from such premises, may be pardoned for believing in what he would have called, perhaps – if he had been given to conscious metaphysical analysis – the self-evident laws of extra-natural cause and effect.

Notes

1. Sarton, G. (1884-1956). *Introduction to the History of Science.* V. II, *Part I. From Rabbi Ben Ezra to Roger Bacon* (Robert E. Krieger Publishing Co., New York, 1931), 92.

2. Haggard, H. W. (1891-1859). *Mystery, Magic, and Medicine* (Garden City, NY: Doubleday, Doran & Co., 1933), 9.

3. Freud quotes from the book *Psyhologie des foules* (*The Crowd: A Study of the Popular Mind*, New York: Macmillan,1899) by Gustave Le Bon (1841-1931).

References

Day, C. L. *Quipus and Witches' Knots* (Lawrence: University of Kansas Press, 1967).

Ibid., 1967a. 2-3.

Ibid., 1967b. 41-42.

Ehrenreich, B. and English, D. *Witches, Midwives, and Nurses: A History of Women Healers* (Old Westbury, NY: The Feminist Press, 1973): 1.

Frazer, J. G. *The Golden Bough* (1922) (New York: Simon & Schuster, 1996).

Ibid., 1922a. 57.

Ibid., 1922b. 58.

Ibid., 1922c. 12.

Ibid., 1922d. 71-72.

Ibid., 1922e. 105.

Freeman, E. A. *Comparative Politics* (Danvers: General Books [1896], 2009), 12.

Freud, S. *Group Psychology and the Analysis of Ego* (1921). Trans. James Strachey (1922). (London: W. W. Norton & Company, 1959): 16.

Gutstein, H. B. and Akil, H. "Opioid Analgesics," In *The Pharmacological Basis of Therapeutics* (11th ed.), edited by L. L. Brunton, J. S. Lazo and K. L.Parker (New York: McGraw-Hill, 2006): 547-590.

Hage, J. J. "Heraklas on Knots: Sixteen Surgical Nooses and Knots from the First Century," *World Journal of Surgery* 32 (2008): 648-655.

Hansen, H. A. *The Witches Garden* (Santa Cruz: United Press, 1978).

Kiple, K. F. *The Cambridge World History of Human Disease* (Cambridge: Cambridge University Press, 1993): 3.

Kittredge, G. L. *Witchcraft in Old and New England* (Cambridge: Harvard University Press, 1929): 372.

Le Clerc, D. *Histoire de la médecine* (Amsterdam: Aux depens de la Compagnie, 1723).

Lips, J. E. *The Origin of Things* (London: Harper& Co., 1949).

Locke, L. L. D. "The Ancient Quipu, a Peruvian Knot Record," *American Anthropolgist, New Series* 14 (1912): 325-332.

Marx, K. *Capital Volume 3* (London: Penguin, 1981). 959 [Capital V 3 was written between 1863-1883, and first published in 1894 by Frederick Engels in 1894).

Melzack, R. and Wall, P. D. "Pain Mechanism: A New Theory," *Science* 150 (1965): 171-179.

Przytycki, J. H. "Classical Roots of Knot Theory," *Chaos, Solutions & Fractals* 9 (1998):

531-545.

Robinson, V. *The Story of Medicine* (New York: Tudor Publishing Co., 1931a)

Ibid., 1931b. 1.

Ibid., 1931c. 3.

Saletore, R. N. *Indian Witchcraft* (New Delhi. Abhinav Publications, 1981): 55.

Sigerist, H. E. *A History of Medicine: Primitive and Archaic Medicine* (Oxford: Oxford University Press, 1951).

Spence, L. *Mexico and Peru: Myths and Legends* (1920) (London: Senate, 1994)

Thompson, R. C. *The Devil and Evil Spirits of Babylonia*. II. (BiblioLife, 1904)

Varma, D. R. "From Witchcraft to Allopathy: Uninterrupted Journey of Medical Science," *Economic and Political Weekly* (Mumbai) 41 (2006): 3605-3611.

Verrips, J. "Dr. Jekyll and Mr. Hyde: Modern Medicine Between Magic and Science," In Meyer, B. and Pels, P. Ed. *Magic and Modernity: Interfaces of Revelation and Concealment* (Stanford: Stanford University Press, 2003): 223-240.

Wills, C. *Yellow Fever-Black Goddess: The Evolution of People and Plagues* (London: Harper Collins Publishers, 1996).

CHAPTER 5

Empirical Medicine: Egypt

The impetus it [Egyptian culture] had given in the arts and crafts, in literature, medicine, and sciences, was carried into the younger civilizations of the neighboring countries where it proved to be a strong stimulus. And the day came when the genius of Champollion and the spade of archeologist lifted the veil and we stood looking in deep reverence at the great and manifold achievements of Egyptian culture.

H.E. Sigerist[1]

The Egyptians could not eliminate magic from their medicine, or divorce their sacred and secular knowledge. The ibis-headed Thoth, the hawk-headed Horus, the lion-headed Sekhmet, the cat-headed Pacht, the asp-headed Rannu, overwhelmed the laws of science. Never were demons more prolific than on the Nile, and they attacked not only mortals but the healing divinities ... The Egyptians say the workings of nature in the annual inundation of the river which created their nation, cast out nature with occult formulas.

V. Robinson[2]

Introduction: Ode to Egyptian Civilization!

Egyptian medicine originated between 3000-2000 BC, more than a thousand years before the birth of Indian, Chinese, and Greek medicine. Various medical papyri such as Edwin Smith Ebers, Kahun and others are the earliest medical texts. Despite abundance of gods and magic, Egyptian medicine is basically empirical and materialistic. The lifeline of Egypt was the river Nile; it affected all aspects of Egyptian civilization, including medicine, which flourished when central authority prevailed and declined during the era of multiple local rulers and numerous invasions, The medical papyri which possibly could not account for everything, nonetheless lead us to conclude that ancient Egypt had physicians of different specialties, veterinarians, dentists, surgeons and a host of medicaments mainly of animal and chemical origin. The principal weakness of Egyptian medicine was its silence on a general theory of health and disease, and hence, it became a history, like the Egyptian civilization.

The two quotes cited above from two eminent historians of medicine give contradictory messages. Yet both are true; they reflect the ups and downs of Egyptian science and culture, which is simultaneously both beautiful and admirable as well as sad and depressing. What Egyptians did in 3,000 BC or even earlier, no other civilization, not India, not even China, let alone Greece, would accomplish until thousands of years later (see Sigerist, 1951). The recorded testimonies of the great Egyptian civilization are its papyri, deciphered by Jean-François Champollion (1790-1832).[3] I came across a note titled "Egyptians, not Greeks were true fathers of medicine" on the University of Manchester website;[4] the note says, "The research team from KNH Centre for Biomedical Egyptology at the University of Manchester discovered the evidence in medical papyri written in 1,500 BC-1,000 years before Hippocrates was born." I fully concur with the conclusion of the Manchester scientists.

Hippocrates is almost universally acclaimed to be the father of medicine; this, I think, is an injustice to history in general and to history of medicine in particular. Indeed, no one is the father of medicine. In reality, modern medicine is the achievement of the collective effort of thousands of peoples across continents; and yet this obvious truth is effectively ignored by so many historians. I am somewhat amazed at the culture of identifying a father for every branch of science. Is Thales of Miletus (620-540 BC) really the father of physics, and is Jabir (Geber) Ibn Hayyan (AD c.721-815) the father of chemistry? Or does this merely reflect our propensity for a father? Why father? Why not mother or parents? Is it because only men can pioneer science? As mentioned in Chapter 4, medicine started with women and not men.

Notwithstanding the undue importance given to Hippocrates and Galen or even Harvey in any narrative of the history of medicine, most serious texts on the subject do refer in a laudatory tone to the Egyptian contributions to medicine. Of the ones I have come across, the book *History of Medicine V.1: Primitive and Archaic Medicine* by Henry E. Sigerist (1951) is, by far, the most comprehensive and beautifully written. In the 156-page-long text with 591 notes in all, Sigerist details and analyzes the impact of the Great Nile, the state intervention in water management, weather, geography, different dynasties, economics, external and internal threats, wars of aggression and maritime commerce, on the evolution of Egyptian medicine. Obviously, Sigerist had studied all the papyri,[5] especially those by Edwin Smith (1822-1906) and George Moritz Ebers (1837-1898), the works of Jean François Champollion, the travelogue of Herodotus of Halicarnassus (484-418 BC), and many other texts on Egyptology. Robinson (1931b) devotes the second chapter of his book *A Story of Medicine* to a narrative of medicine in Egypt, from which the above quote is taken. Volume one of *Introduction to the History of Science* by George Sarton (1927) starts from Homer (700-800 BC) and naturally goes straight to Greek science although he does say:

> The golden age of Egyptian science seems to have occurred about the twentieth to fifteenth century B.C., and though we know that the Greeks were influenced by the Egyptians in many ways, it is impossible to tell with any completeness or precision how Egyptian lore was transmitted to Greece.

What follows in this chapter is mainly based on the writings of Sigerist (1951) and Robinson (1931). Although the book *Ancient Egyptian Medicine* by John F. Nunn (2002), has re-evaluated papyri and provides some additional material, I found the books by Sigerist and Robinson sufficient on all accounts. Some other historians of medicine too have a high esteem for Egyptian medicine. For example, Sir William Osler (1921), in his book *The Evolution of Modern Medicine*, recognizes that "Egypt became the centre from which civilization spread to the other peoples of the Mediterranean." *The History of Medicine* by David Allyn Gorton [1832-1916] (1910), and *History of Medicine* by Fielding H. Garrison [1870-1935]) (1929), mention Egyptian medicine admiringly. On the other hand, Max Neuburger (1868-1955), in his book, *History of Medicine* dismisses not only Egyptian but also all ancient medicine in the following words: "Western medicine in the early Middle Ages, is strictly speaking, hardly a subject for the historian of science who would present a coherent picture of progressive events . . ." (Neuburger, 1910). Daniel Le Clerc seems too preoccupied with gods to be objective (Le Clerc, 1910). Albert H. Buck uses Neuburger's (1910) scheme to divide the evolution of medicine into nine epochs and treats Egyptian medicine as part of Oriental medicine in the second epoch, along with Babylonian medicine; the only additional point he makes, which is not clear in the narratives of Sigerist and Robinson, is that Egyptian gods might as well be real people of stature (Buck, 1917). Roy Porter (1946-2002) is quite off the mark when he writes, "As with Mesopotamia, Egypt's imposing political regime made for an organized medical practice. It is, however, with Greek civilization that evidence of recognizable medical discourse first appears" (Porter, 1997). In any case, none of the books cited above add much more either in substance or in analysis to what Sigerist (1951) and Robinson (1931) had done.

Egyptian civilization is at least as ancient as Mesopotamian, if not older, and certainly older than Indian civilization. But there is a qualitative difference between these civilizations, and this difference, to my mind, affects the evolution of medicine. Jawaharlal Nehru,[6] in a letter to his daughter Indira Gandhi (1917-1984) dated January 9, 1931, reflects on the rise and fall of ancient civilizations in the following words (Nehru, 1982):

> Egypt, Knossos, Iraq, and Greece – they have all gone. Their old civilizations, even as Babylon and Nineveh, have ceased to exist. What, then, of the two other ancients in this company of old civilizations? What of China and India? As in other countries, they too have had empire after empire. There have been invasions and destructions and looting on a vast scale. Dynasties of kings have ruled for hundreds of years and then were replaced by others. All this has happened in India and China, as it did elsewhere. But nowhere else, apart from India and China, has there been a real continuity of civilization.

While Nehru's remarks are generally held valid, the decline in medical sciences in Egypt occurred while Egyptian civilization was still intact. There are two distinct phases in Egyptian medicine and paradoxically the regressive aspect, namely the spiritual aspect as summarized by Robinson above, follows rather than precedes the materialistic aspect as highlighted by Sigerist. How can that happen? Are there other parallels of this kind?

I think materialism and spiritualism are dialectical opposites. They have always coexisted as they do now. The question, rather, is which of the two is dominant at a given stage in society. Just take note of the popular and scientific culture of the twentieth and very early twenty-first centuries. Medicine has made gigantic progress and might be on the verge of not only discovering a cure for cancer but, *frighteningly, also on the verge of creating life from elements.*[7] Yet, other schools of medicine, from chiropractic to acupuncture, have a sway (Singh and Ernst, 2008).

That is not all. The comments on the efficacy of intercessory prayer (unknown to the patient) on the well-being of patients undergoing coronary artery intervention (Krucoff et al., 2005) was not only published by the prestigious medical journal *Lancet*, but *Lancet* also deemed it necessary to make the following comments editorially (Editorial, 2005): "The contribution that hope and belief make to personal understanding of illness cannot be dismissed so lightly. They are proper subjects for science, even while transcending its known bounds." In reality, this comment by *Lancet* might be the inner voice of the editor. More than a hundred years earlier, a person of no less a stature than Sir Francis Galton argued that the efficacy of intercessory prayer on healing should be scientifically studied although he did not find much validity in this theory; Galton found that the life span of kings, for whom the population at large prays, is shorter rather than longer than those in other occupations (Galton, 1872). In India, almost until the mid-twentieth century, there were professional mourners. When someone of status died, they were hired to accompany the coffin shedding tears and beating their chests. Who can vouch that an institution of prayer renderers would not emerge in the scientific West to pray for the well-being of the patient as a part of their godly duty? And who can say that generous grants would not be awarded to undertake clinical trials to assess the healing efficacy of intercessory prayers? Sloan and Ramakrishnan (2006) have questioned the conclusions of the *Lancet* study cited above, but it is unlikely to end the pursuit of the role of divination in healing. So if this is happening in the twenty-first century, it is easy to understand why Egyptians, starting from a materialistic medicine, embraced demons and divinity for cures and healing.

Notwithstanding what I have just written, the factors that reintroduced divinity and incantations, mystery and magic, demons and deities alongside the evolution of sciences are complex and reflect the totality of societal culture. What these factors were in the case of Egypt is presented below as a tentative outline based on details narrated by Sigerist (1951).

The Great Nile and Egyptian Dynasties

The lifeline of the Egyptian civilization was the river Nile, just as the Tigris and Euphrates were central to the Mesopotamian civilization. Without these natural gifts, the two ancient centres of civilization would have remained just deserts, fit only for camels. It is no wonder that the historian and traveller Herodotus considered Egypt as "a gift of the river;" he also noted that Egyptians "are the healthiest of all men, next to the Libyans" and attributed this state of affairs to the fact "that the climate in all seasons is the same."[8]

Menes, the founder of the city of Memphis, most probably established the first dynasty in Egypt around 3,000 BC. However, villages and cemeteries characteristic of the chalcolithic period (4500-3500 BC) had existed long before the founding of the first dynasty. Menes' dynasty lasted until about 2600 BC. Sigerist (1951b) writes, "It was a period of great cultural advances of which the most significant undoubtedly was the development of the Egyptian alphabet from pictorial signs and also the invention of suitable writing material."

Writing is a powerful tool for transmitting knowledge from one generation to another and far more superior than oral history. For this reason, one can assume that medical information of one generation was further enriched by the next generation. Moreover, the establishment of organs of governance by the founding dynasty required leaders in the different areas, very similar to the current institutions of government cabinets and the body of ministers. Such institutions may have been unique to Egypt and perhaps existed elsewhere with the emergence of nation states, but Egypt might well be the first nation state.

What seems unique in Egypt was that its cabinet included a physician, who was not simply a physician for the royalty but, rather, in charge of the health of the population at large, which was not the case in other civilizations and which constitutes a very advanced concept in public health-care system, currently practiced only in Cuba.

During the succeeding four Memphite dynasties (III to VI) from about 2600 to 2200 BC, wonders of the world were created in Egypt in the form of pyramids, sphinxes, and tombs that continue to attract huge numbers of archeologists, science historians, and tourists. It is during this period that the legendry Imhotep, physician and architect of the twenty-seventh century BC, did many things including the construction of the pyramid complex at Saqqara. Imhotep, by no means a member of the royalty, came to occupy a central position in the conduct of government affairs. In the combined role of physician and architect, Imhotep could have supervised effective water management for safeguarding the interests of the population during the inundation and shrinking of the Nile. Even if Imhotep did not foresee the effects of his water management, his actions would most certainly have spared Egyptians from malaria and other waterborne parasitic infestations like hookworm (*Ancylstoma duodenale*,[9] the cause of anaemia) or bilharziasis (in Egypt, mainly caused by the parasite *Schistosoma hematobium*). It is worth noting that this would certainly have had important health benefits given the fact that effective drug therapy of hookworm and Bilharzia infestations was not discovered until the1980s.

The age of the pyramids was followed by many dynasties during which Egypt faced the breakdown of central authority and the emergence of local rulers, which disrupted the proper management of the waters of the Nile, with grave consequences for every aspect of Egyptian life, including health. It was not until Ahmose ascended the throne around 1550 BC that Egypt again had a golden age. It became stronger and wealthier. The magnificent tomb of Tutankhamen was created during this period, about which Sigerist (1951c) remarks, "It is highly developed, refined art that reveals the full mastery of techniques, but it cannot be denied that it shows the early signs of decadence." What could be these signs of decadence? During the eighteenth dynasty, Amenhotep IV attempted to establish a monotheistic religion. He abolished cults and established a state religion, which gave rise to the institution of official priesthood with immense power and wealth. Thereafter, Egyptian civilization steadily declined until the country was conquered in 323 BC by Alexander the Great (356-323 BC).

Certain conditions in Egypt were very different from those in other contemporary civilizations. Perhaps because of the centrality of the river Nile to the economic and social foundations of Egypt, the country remained relatively static even after the dawn of the Christian era. According to Harry Reginald Holland Hall (1873-1930),[10] "the life of the fellah of the XIIth or even the IVth Dynasty is the same as it is to-day. The change of religion to Christianity and then to Islam has altered nothing but the form of prayer; the changes of political allegiance have mattered nothing at all. The agricultural and urban classes were differentiated just as they are to-day."

Social Institutions

In Egypt, marriages occurred at the age of twelve or thirteen in the case of girls, and slightly older in case of boys. This, however, is not specific to Egypt. In India, for example, infants were married off and the system hardly changed despite legal restrictions on child marriages by the British rulers, and even later in independent India. What is very special in the case of Egypt was the system of marriages between brothers and sisters. Even by the second century AD, Sigerist (1951d) writes that "two-thirds of the inhabitants of the city of Arsinoe were married to brother or sister." Although this custom most likely started with the royalty to retain blood lineage, I am not aware of the impact of this practice on population growth and health in Egypt; non mixing of the genetic pool has to have consequences. Indeed, the current Zoroastrian population, one of the most prosperous communities, is approximately only one hundred thousand, which is considered to be the result of inbreeding.

Monogamy was the rule in Egypt and sex was freer than under any other religious system. Nudity defied modesty preached by other religions. Prostitution was an accepted institution to serve the needs of travellers and soldiers.

As in any agricultural society with high infant mortality, having many children was considered desirable. Circumcision was not universal as is the case among Jews and Muslims, which implies that it was not based on religion; Herodotus attributed this practice to a sense of cleanliness. Egyptians were obsessed with cleanliness; they drank from cleaned bronze pots, wore washed linen, and even used emetics and enema to clean the intestinal tract. They were equally obsessed with black hair and had devised all kinds of liniments from blood and body part of animals against hair greying and loss, which were probably as ineffective as our present day hair tonics, but certainly they were not magical formulae. Robinson writes (1931b), "Moreover the Egyptians, by their extensive use of animal remedies, became the forerunners of organotherapy: much more testicular, ovarian, hepatic, adrenal and thyroid extract are consumed in the world today than when the Pharaohs were in power."

The Egyptians had worked out some system of diagnosing early pregnancy by the change of gait of the woman and even the sex of the unborn child by the effect of the woman's urine on the sprouting of wheat and barley seedlings. It might be faulty, but was certainly not without basis; it required a knowledge of some chemical change in the urine of a pregnant woman, which could affect the sprouting of gentle seeds like that of wheat and barley. It was the expression of a materialist approach and not of spiritualism, and is in stark contrast to the practice in certain countries, including modern India, of appeasing certain deities in order for the unborn baby to become male. The Egyptians also used knots, usually assumed to be characteristic of indigenous American people (Day, 1967). They developed veterinary medicine as well. The *Veterinary Papyrus of Kahun* was most likely composed during the Twelfth dynasty, that is, around 1900 BC (Sigerist, 1951e).

Medical Papyri

There can be no doubt that Egyptian medical papyri are an eye-opener in any survey of the history of medicine. The Edwin Smith, Ebers, Kahun (Fayoum), and Hearst papyri were scribed sometime between 2000 and1500 BC, which makes them the oldest written medical texts, more than one thousand years before the Hindu Ayurveda, or anything that Hippocrates wrote. Obviously, Hippocrates did not have access to these papyri, most of which were discovered in the nineteenth century. These papyri describe pathology and the method of diagnosis of numerous diseases and their treatment, as well as the ethics of the relationship between the physician and the patient in no uncertain terms. In the art of diagnosis, Egyptian doctors did very much what is done today and what was done by Charak of Ayurveda or by Hippocrates of Greece. Physicians asked relevant questions of the patient or the relative, looked at the patient's face, examined his pulse, which shows they were aware of the relationship between the pulse and the heart, and the appearances of urine, faeces, and any blood that might have been expelled. There already existed specialists for different kinds of ailments; there were surgeons and there were dentists. What Hippocrates wrote might reflect his independent thoughts, but the similarity between Hippocrates' text and those of the Ebers papyrus are striking. It is noteworthy that the method for correcting a dislocated jaw as described by the Egyptians is identical to the one by Hippocrates in his treatise *On Articulations* and the one practiced now.

Most historical texts about Egyptian medicine, including that by Sigerist (1951), describe Egyptian medicine to be an amalgam of materialist medicine and magic. There is no doubt that magic occupied an important place in ancient Egypt. Indeed the papyrus in the British Museum in London (No. 10059) is primarily magical in its orientation. The Berlin papyrus also contains evidence of a magician acting as a physician. Sigerist (1951f) writes, "Horus, the child of Isis and Osiris, appeared frequently in the incantations ...Stung by a deadly scorpion he was saved by the powerful spells of the gods and thus acquired special faculties to cure people bitten by venomous animals." It is very likely that the scorpions considered deadly were indeed not deadly. It is also possible that Horus recovered from the scorpion bite by squeezing out or sucking the poison and then repeated the same on other victims of scorpion bites. It is also most likely that the magical part of the proceedings was a social ritual concerning the conduct of the physician and his interaction with the patient, but not the actual treatment, which comprised certain medicines to be consumed by the patient and certain rules regarding the diet and other activities to be followed by the patient. Given this understanding, I come to the conclusion that Egyptian medicine was primarily a materialistic and not a spiritualistic medicine. Whether or not any of the medicines used by the Egyptian physicians had therapeutic merit is difficult to ascertain, but then, no medicine, with the exception of a few, were of any therapeutic value until the end of the nineteenth century in any part of the world.

Mystical stories have a way of finding a place in history, often without substance. It is said that the Indian mathematician Srinivasa Ramanujan (1887-1920) found solutions to complex mathematical problems in his dreams from the goddess of Namagiri (Kanigel, 1992). The chemistry genius August Kekule (1829-1896) is said to have discovered the ring structure of chemicals, requiring carbon-to-carbon bonds, because he dreamt of a snake swallowing its own tail and thus forming a ring structure. Most likely, these great personalities were so engrossed in the subject matter of their investigation that they even dreamt of it in some modified form. In short, magical stories and true science can coexist, but that does not imply any direct link between the two. It is thus very likely that an abundance of gods and a richness of medicine existed as independent disciplines in the Egypt of early years – at least from 3000 BC to 1500 BC. On the other hand, empirical medicine free from gods and magic also existed in Egypt and did so long before anywhere else in the world.

Thus it may be concluded that despite all the fancy of the early Egyptians for gods and magic, they were the founders of empirical medicine, which existed along with spiritual medicine. As a service to their own history and a gift to the world, Egyptians scribed much of their medical knowledge, and this knowledge was transmitted to us, thanks to celebrated historians like Edwin Smith and George Moritz Ebers, who recognised the exceptional merit of the papyri and purchased them from unlikely sources in Egypt, and James Henry Breasted (1865-1935), who translated important medical papyri. Breasted (1922) was the first to report on the marvels of Egyptian surgery contained in the Edwin Smith Papyrus; the impact of this publication led historian Sigerist (1951g) to write:

> If this book[11] had been written before 1922, I should never have thought of discussing Egypt's magico-religious and empirico-rational medicine in separate chapters. We knew at that time, of course, that there was more to Egyptian medicine than incantations and amulets, and that in addition to the magician there was a physician who treated his patients primarily with drugs. We also had some evidence of surgical interventions, literary as well as paleopathological. We knew, moreover, that Egyptians had made a first attempt to explain the phenomena of health and disease philosophically rather than mythologically. Yet this entire rational sector was limited . . .But then in 1922 James H. Breasted published two preliminary accounts of the papyrus Edwin Smith, which created a sensation among students of ancient medicine.

Obviously, no civilization can be limited to an accomplishment in a single field. The Egyptians were a marvel in almost all the areas characteristic of the age of civilization. Egyptians made bricks, baked bread, brewed beer, made glass and tanned leather, domesticated plants and animals, made bronze out of copper and tin, and above all, determined that the solar year consists of 365 days (Robinson, 1931c). In short, the Egyptians moved civilization from the Stone Age to the Bronze Age.[12] The accomplishments of no civilization can be completely documented in written texts. Obviously there is more to Egyptian civilization than is revealed in retrieved papyri. The great river Nile, which built and destroyed much of Egypt also washed away much of the evidence about Egyptian history.

Given these dimensions of Egyptian civilization, it could be expected that they would break away from spiritualism to materialism in medicine. But they did not. Indeed, they gave rise to a mixture of the two; their physicians were invariably priests, and the gods were always present. Even the most learned Egyptians, mathematicians, and astronomers worshipped the sacred bull. However, despite all this fascination with divinity, Egyptians searched for physical remedies for their illnesses. One can only conclude that for Egyptians, a mixture of gods and earthly remedies accomplished more than either alone. One papyrus reads, "Welcome, remedy, welcome, which destroyed the trouble in this my heart and in these my limbs. The magic of Horus is victorious in the remedy, . . ." (Robinson, 1931d). Fascination with the curative value of animal and human parts including excreta is not limited to Egyptians, but they certainly excelled in this, especially because wild animals from lions to hippopotami, snakes to crocodiles were abundant in Egypt. British and French pharmacopoeias of the seventeenth and eighteenth centuries also describe the therapeutic value of animal parts and excrements.

The embalming technique used by Egyptians reveals that they were aware of what to let remain and what to remove in order to preserve the body for eternity. This is also true of the Chinese. The mummies reveal the diseases that prevailed in ancient Egypt. Arterial lesions, including blockages by blood clots, suggest that hypertension existed. "The humpbacked priest of Ammon, with characteristic spinal protrusion and psoas abscess, shows that tuberculosis existed among Egyptians" (Robinson, 1931e). Although beautiful slaves were exploited for sexual purposes and orgies were common occurrences, there is no evidence of the existence of gonorrhoea and syphilis.

Veterinary and gynaecological papyri from Kahun date back to 2160-1788 BC. They reveal that Egyptians had devised methods of contraception as well as being aware of the fertility of women based on the texture of the breasts. The papyrus of the Mother and Child, according to Robinson (1931f) "is predominantly magical" and "the source from which Moses borrowed his fairy-tales."

"The Surgical Papyrus written about 1600 B.C. is over fifteen feet in length when unrolled, and originally was considerably longer. The writing in black ink is beautiful, and the important words and subsections are in red – the first rubrics;" the papyrus describes 48 cases "beginning with injuries of the head and concluding with the feet" (Robinson 1931f). Each case records symptoms, diagnosis, treatment, and prognosis. Interestingly, this papyrus is a copy of an older text written a thousand years earlier, which makes Egyptian written medicine at least 4,500 years old, long before any record of medicine in India. Although the text is very realistic and free from demonology, the back of the papyrus contains a magic formula, and two columns are devoted to the "incantation of transforming an old man into a youth of twenty" (Robinson, 1931f).

The Therapeutic Papyrus of Thebes was written in 1552 BC and was at least sixty feet long; it discusses the treatment of tumours, obstructive diseases, diseases of the eye and ear, pain, diseases of children and women, baldness, burns, sores, and gangrene and includes numerous cosmetic prescriptions. It includes seven hundred remedies including opium, castor oil, copper salts, squill, acacia, calamus, coriander, saffron, hyoscyamus, colchicum, gentian, pomegranate, olive oil, and salts of various metals. Almost all these were used in modern medicine even as late as the early twentieth century, and some are still in use (Robinson, 1931f).

Pulsation is compared with inundations of the Nile. While pulse is central to the diagnostic approach of the Indian and Unani-Tibb medicine,[13] it has received significant attention in Egyptian medicine as well. The Therapeutic Papyrus writes: "There is in the heart a vessel leading to every member of the body. If the physician places his finger on the head, neck, arms, hands, feet or body, everywhere he will find the heart, for the heart leads to every member, and speaks in the vessels of every member" (Robinson 1931f).

"Egypt was the medical centre of the ancient world" (Robinson (1931g). However, it could not advance; it in fact became backward in the later centuries. "The earlier papyri contain more medicine and less magic, while in the later scrolls the incantations are predominant" (Robinson, 1931h). This reversal in the advance of medicine in Egypt coincides with a general decline of the Egyptian civilization as a result of several factors, two of which are noteworthy.

In some respects, the history of Egypt is similar to that of India. In both countries, a central authority could not be maintained, and both countries suffered. Unlike the case of India, however, the lifeline of Egypt was solely the Nile. Like India, Egypt encountered many invasions. Egypt was conquered by the Assyrians in 669 BC, the Persians in 525 BC, by Alexander the Great in 332 BC, and by the Romans in 31 BC. This was not all. The Arabs conquered Egypt in AD 642; it became a part of the Ottoman Empire in the early sixteenth century; Napoleon

Bonaparte attacked it in 1798, and by the late nineteenth century, Egypt came under the control of the British. Not until Gamal Abdul Nasser (1918-1970) overthrew the rule in 1952 did Egypt gain its independent status. Unlike India, almost all the invaders ruled Egypt as foreigners, while for India, this was the case only with the British.

Aside from these instances of political turmoil, Egyptian geography limited its pharmaceutical resource domain, which was bountiful in places like Peru, China, and India. This could be the reason why Egyptian medicines were mainly of animal parts and chemicals, and not herbs.

Principal Weakness of Egyptian Medicine

Robinson (1931h) writes:

> Mother Egypt tended the cradle of civilization: her wonderful children possessed considerable empirical knowledge, but viewing nature through an inscrutable veil of mystery they could not investigate the laws of science or understand the principles of medicine. Egypt transmitted no scientific legacy to posterity; ...From the pyramid fields, the silent Sphinx of Giza gazes eastward over the Nile valley, and has no message for the younger generation.

Egyptian medicine differed fundamentally from Indian, Chinese, and Greek medicine. However faulty the Chinese, Indian, and Greek postulates for the causes of diseases may have been, they constituted a theoretical framework that could be refined to greater and greater precision, given an overall social, economic, and political development. *The main weakness of Egyptian medicine is that it did not formulate a general theory of health and disease.* Had it done so, and had Egyptians had sufficient basis to do so, even the most enthusiastic admirers of Greece would have had difficulty in calling Hippocrates the father of medicine. Nonetheless, in my opinion, Egypt – and not India, not China, and certainly not Greece – is the birthplace of medicine.

Notes

1. Sigerist, H. E. *A History of Medicine V.1: Primitive and Archaic Medicine* (Oxford: Oxford University Press, 1951a), 359.

2. Robinson, V. *The Story of Medicine* (New York: Tudor Publishing, 1931a), 12-13.

3. Jean-François Champollion (1790-1832) deciphered Egyptian hieroglyphics in 1822.

4. *ScienceDaily*, May 19, 2007; University of Manchester KNH Centre for Egyptology website.

5. Edwin Smith, Ebers, Kahun, the Ramesseum IV and V, Berlin, the London Medical, the Hearst, Chester Beatty, The Carlsberg, and the Brooklyn Papyri.

6. Nehru was the first Prime Minister of independent India from 1947-1964; he wrote two monumental books from the prisons of British India, *Glimpses of World History* (Allahabad: Kitabistan, 1934-1935) and *The Discovery of India* (Calcutta: Signet Press, 1946). Had he done nothing else, Nehru might well have be treated as a historian of standing.

7. This text on creating life in the laboratory was originally written in the summer of 2009, months before the scientists led by Craig Venter announced in May 2010 that they had actually created life in the lab (Gibson, D. G., Glass, J. I., Lartigue, C. et al. "Creation of a Bacterial Cell Controlled by a Chemically Synthesized Genome," *Nature Methods 11(2010): 887-889.* Science doi:10.1126/science.1190719;2010).

8. Quoted by Sigerist: *A History of Medicine V.1: Primitive and Archaic Medicine* (Oxford: Oxford University Press, 1951), 222.

9. Larvae of hookworm enter through the toenail and find their way into the intestine; as mature worms, they suck enough blood to cause iron-deficiency anaemia. Wearing shoes, not drugs, proved the most effective preventive measure.

10. *Cambridge Ancient History. Vol. 1,* p. 317, quoted by Sigerist (1951, 238).

11. Sigerist. *A History of Medicine, Volume 1* (Oxford: Oxford University Press, 1951).

12. Dr. Julius Ernst Lips (1895-1950) in his book *The Origin of Things*, abridged (New York: Fawcett Publications, 1956, 55-68), argues against chronological characterization of different Ages because gathering and hunting as a means of procuring food did not cease to exist with the domestication of animals and agriculture. However, a chronological description of Ages may be valid because a new Age is defined by the emergence of a new social order and not by the disappearance of the old or the remnants of the old social order. He is undoubtedly correct.

13. Unani-Tibb medicine is an offshoot of Galenic medicine; this is described in some detail in Chapter 10 titled Islamic Medicine.

References

Buck, A. H. *The Growth of Medicine from the Earliest Times to About 1800* (New Haven: Yale University Press, 1917), 18-19.

Breasted, J. H. "The Edwin Smith Papyrus." *Quarterly Bulletin. New York Historical Society* 6 (1922): 1-31.

Day, C. L. *Quipus and Witches' Knots* (Lawrence: The University of Kansas Press, 1967).

Editorial. "Mantra II: Measuring the Unmeasurable?" *Lancet* 366 (2005): 178.

Galton, F. "Statistical Inquiries into the Efficacy of Prayer." *Fortnightly Review* 12 (1872): 125-135.

Garrison, F. H. *An Introduction to the History of Medicine* (Philadelphia: W. B. Saunders, 1929).

Gorton, D. A. *The History of Medicine, Philosophical and Critical: From its Origin to the Twentieth Century* (New York: G. P. Putnam's Sons, 1910).

Kanigel, R. *The Man Who Knew Infinity: A Life of the Genius Ramanujan* (New York: Washington Square Press, 1992).

Krucoff, M. et al. "Music, Imagery, Touch, and Prayer as Adjuncts to Interventional Cardiac Care: the Monitoring and Actualisation of Noetic Training (MANTRA)II Randomised Study," *Lancet* 366 (2005): 211-217.

Le Clerc, D. *Histoire de la médecine.* Nouvelle ed. (Amsterdam: Aux depens de la Compagnie, 1723).

Nehru, J. L. *Glimpses of World History* (New Delhi: Indraprastha Press [1934], 1982), 12.

Neuburger, M. *History of Medicine*, Trans. Ernst Playfair (Oxford: Oxford University Press, 1910).

Nunn, J. F. *Ancient Egyptian Medicine* (Norman: University of Oklahoma Press, 1996).

Osler, W. *The Evolution of Modern Medicine* (New Haven: Yale University Press, 1921), 10-11.

Porter, R. T*he Greatest Benefit to Mankind: A Medical History of Humanity* (London: W. W. Norton, 1997), 50.

Robinson, V. *The Story of Medicine* (New York: Tudor Publishing, 1931a).

Ibid., 1931b. 15.

Ibid., 1931c. 11.

Ibid., 1931d. 13.

Ibid., 1931e. 17.

Ibid., 1931f. 19-23.

Ibid., 1931g. 25.

Ibid., 1931h. 26.

Sarton, G. *Introduction to the History of Science V.I: From Homer to Omar Khayyam* (Huntington, New York: Robert E. Krieger Publishing, 1927), 52.

Sigerist, H. E. *A History of Medicine V.1: Primitive and Archaic Medicine* (Oxford: Oxford University Press, 1951a).

Ibid., 1951b. 227.

Ibid., 1951c. 232.

Ibid., 1951d. 239.

Ibid., 1951e. 300.

Ibid., 1951f. 288.

Ibid., 1951g. 297.

Singh, S. and Ernst, E. *Trick or Treatment?: Alternative medicine on trial* (London: Transworld Publishers, 2008).

Sloan, R. P. and Ramakrishnan, R. "Science, Medicine and Intercessory Prayer." *Perspectives in Biology and Medicine* 49 (2006): 504-514.

CHAPTER 6

The Transition to Materialist Medicine: Ayurveda

Bharadvaja, the mighty ascetic, in search of (the science of) longevity approached Indra, having deemed him, the lord of immortals, worthy of suit. Daksha Prajapati (the progenitor) first obtained the Science of Life in its entirety as promulgated by Brahma (the Great One, the Creator) and from him in turn the Ashwin Twins obtained it. From the Ashwin Twins the god Shakra (Indra) acquired it. Therefore Bharadvaja bidden by the sages approached Shakra. When diseases arose like so many impediments to austerity, fasting, study, continence and the vows of the embodied souls, then the great sages, the doers of good, keeping compassion for creatures foremost, met together on the sacred slopes of the Himalayas.

Charaka Samhita[1]

The Buddhist king, Asoka, was the first builder of hospitals for man and beast; these animal-hospitals throw light on the Hindu injunction that the physician should refuse medical advice to criminals and to hunters who trap animals and ensnare birds. Buddhism is the gentlest and wisest, the most sceptical and scientific of religions – and the only one that does not worship the sword – and had it continued to prevail, Asiatic history would be different. But with the reestablishment of Brahmanism, Buddhist hospitals and tolerance were destroyed.

Victor Robinson[2]

Introduction

There are many similarities between Egypt and India[3] and, of course, many differences as well. The Pre-Aryan Indus valley civilization (3000-1500 BC) is a contemporary of the Egyptian and Mesopotamian civilizations. Egypt has its Nile, Mesopotamia its Tigris and Euphrates, and India its Sindhu and Ganges.[4] All these rivers shaped the histories of the lands that they spanned, but the Ganges did not determine the fate of India as much as did the rivers of Egypt and Mesopotamia. And yet the Ganges occupies an important spiritual place, especially among India's majority Hindu population. All invaders, with the exception of the British, were drawn toward India by the fertile plains of its rivers. But unlike in Egypt, all those who came, with the exception of the British,[5] made India their permanent home.

The Indus Valley civilization (c. 3000-1500 BC), of which Mohenjo-daro in Sind and Harappa in Punjab (both now in Pakistan) are impressive examples of advanced civilization, predates the Aryan-Hindu civilization; its discovery in the 1920s puzzled the world. The people of the Indus Valley were Dravidians, distinct from the Aryans. The Aryans pushed the Dravidians southward, and the Indus Valley settlements were turned into ruins (Eraly, 2000; Nehru, 1946; Sigerist, 1961; Thapar, 1966; Kosambi, 2002).

The Indus Valley people must have had some form of medical discipline; their sophisticated water drainage system and communal baths indicate their awareness of hygiene. Many Indus valley seals (Sigerist, 1961a) were very similar to those in Egypt and the representation of the mother figure on these seals was far more frequent than that of the father figure. However, we do not know much about the medical system of the Indus valley civilization. On the other hand, we do know of the medical system known as Ayurveda, which originated some 1500 years later, after the arrival of the Aryans and the advent of the Vedic Age (1500-500 BC).[6] Also, the arrival of the Aryans gave rise to the Indo-European language in this region, which was distinct from the original inhabitants of the Indus valley.

The Dawn of Materialistic Medicine

Buddhism reached its pinnacle in India during the reign of Emperor Asoka (304-232 BC) from 270-232 BC (Thapar, 2009). As a tribute to this period, Asoka's insignia of four lions atop a wheel (Chakra) was adopted as the national symbol of independent India. According to Robinson (1931) :

> The chief period of Indian medicine is coincident with the rise of Buddhism and corresponds with the classic age of Greece, and the parallelism between Hellenism and Hinduism is one of history's disputed problems.

Ayurveda postulated that disease is the result of Tridoshas (imbalance between three bodily systems); the significance of this postulate does not lie in its correctness or otherwise, but rather in its materialist approach. Similar developments also took place in China (*Yang-Yin* theory) and Greece (Hippocrates' theory of four humours) at about the same time.

In short, the most revolutionary shift in the history of medicine in the form of laying the foundations of a materialist approach to medicine occurred approximately at the same time in India, China, and Greece.

Situating Ayurveda in Indian History

Ayurveda was born in India between the seventh and sixth century BC (Majumdar, 2004); its popularity reached a peak during the Buddhist Maurya dynasty (321 BC-184 BC). Following the end of the Maurya dynasty and the decline of Buddhism, the popularity of Ayurveda or, more accurately, the state concern for the well-being of its people began to decline.

Thus the stagnation of Ayurveda coincides with the decline of Buddhism and the reassertion of Vedic Hinduism; it did not occur during the Moghul and British (1526-1857) periods as Majumdar (2004a) claims. The British did introduce modern medicine but the factors leading to the decline of Ayurvedic medicine are many, of which British rule, in my opinion, might only be one of the indirect factors (see Berger, 2007; Hardiman, 2009; Kumar, 1995, 2001a; Leslie, 1992; Panikkar, 1992; Sivaramakrishnan, 2006). The British did not administratively suppress Ayurveda, though contrary views also exist (Arnold, 2000); rather, Ayurveda became and remains less attractive than modern medicine (Ramanna, 2002). There is a vigorous attempt to revive Ayurveda in independent India, which might be a consequence of the rise of Hindu nationalism (Sivaramakrishnan, 2006), elaborated by Jaffrelot (1993).

Indeed the impact of British rule on healthcare is very important, but it has nothing to do with the colonial attitude towards the indigenous medical system comprised of Ayurveda and Unani-tibb. Rather it has a lot to do with the impact of British colonialism and the state of nutrition. Most likely there was an abundance of food until almost the end of the Mughal period (Habib, 1999). Food availability to the population declined during the British rule for a variety of reasons, such as the role played by the market, emphasis on cotton production, and neglect of irrigation systems as explained by Marx (1853) and in general the impact of British colonialism on Indian economy. Voltaire (François-Marie Arouet, 1694-1778) condemned the British rule in the following words: "As soon as India became a little known to the barbarians of the West and the North, she became the object of their cupidity. This was all the more so when these barbarians, becoming civilized and industrious, created new needs for themselves" (Bedi, 1937). India, like China, faced annual famines till the end of the British rule, the worst being the 1943 Bengal famine in which two to three million people died in Bengal (current Bangladesh plus the West Bengal part of India) (Mukerjee, 2010).

Differing Visions of Ayurveda

In what follows, I will attempt to describe the theoretical framework of Ayurvedic medicine as well as the factors that currently promote this system, and how its materialist approach had got embroiled in spiritualism.

There are many books on Ayurveda, briefly summarized in the footnote.[7] Some of them are written like promotional material (Chopra, 1991, 1995; Sharma, 1993; Sharma et al. 2002) and attribute benefits to Ayurveda not attainable by any other system of medicine; its primitiveness is made its biggest virtue. Some books, like the one by Atreya (1999), are stories of specific individuals who benefited from Ayurveda almost, like the popular "before and after" advertisements. The book *Boundless Energy* by Chopra (1995) relates bodily functions with quantum physics, almost as if he has proof for this, and then goes on to describe various Yogic exercises for the acquisition of limitless energy. In contrast, the book *Ayurveda Revisited* (Dahanukar and Thatte, 1989) tries to explain fundamental Ayurvedic concepts in accordance with the principles of modern medicine without being as assertive as the book by Majumdar (2004).

The following description of Ayurveda is mainly but not exclusively based on Dr. Ashok Majumdar's book (2004) *Ayurveda: The Ancient Science of Healing*. This is because his book is as good a description of the theory and practice of Ayurveda as any. Besides, like Dr. Deepak Chopra, Dr. Majumdar also has a modern medical degree (MBBS; Bachelor of Medicine and Bachelor of Surgery, equivalent to the American MD) in addition to a degree in Ayurveda. In the preface to the book, he uses his two degrees and his ancestry of Ayurvedic doctors to add credence to his authority on Ayurveda (Majumdar, 2004b); just as Dr. Chopra, hooked up with Maharishi Mahesh Yogi (1914-2008) of *Transcendental Meditation*, uses his MBBS (MD) degree to boost his credentials. Although the book of Dr. Majumdar is more substantive than the *Perfect Health* by Dr. Chopra, the first lines of both books are strikingly similar.

Dr. Majumdar (2004a) begins his book with the sentences:

> Ayurveda, one of the ancient medical sciences in the world, adopts a holistic approach. It treats a human being as a complex whole and strives for harmony between a human being and the entire environment that surrounds him.

Dr. Chopra (1991a) starts as follows:

> There exists in every person a place that is free from disease, that never feels pain, that cannot age or die. When you go to this place, limitations which all of us accept cease to exist. They are not even entertained as a possibility.
>
> This is the place called perfect health.

Most books on Ayurveda are written by Indians of Hindu faith, who often also take the opportunity to assert their devotion to Hinduism. Dominik Wujastyk (1998) is an exception, and his book *The Roots of Ayurveda* is free from religiosity and provides a virtually literal description of drugs and diseases as mentioned in the original Sanskrit texts; his description does not match the hyperbolic pronouncements of Chopra (1995) such as: "Ayurveda, which in Sanskrit means 'science of life,' is the most comprehensive system of mind/body medicine ever devised." Sharma et al. (2002) assure a cancer-free life if only the diet and life style advised by them were followed; Sharma (1993) discovered the term Maharishi Ayur-Ved and implies that the use of anti-oxidants is a gift of Ayurveda, although he does mention Pauling who introduced this field in medicine (Pauling, 1970).

Aside from the link of Ayurveda with Vedic Hinduism, there are additional factors that make a historical narrative of Ayurveda complex. One aspect of this complexity is the chronology. All claims that Ayurveda is the oldest medical science are utterly false, just as are the claims that the Vedas are the earliest written text. Egyptian medicine and Egyptian papyri are older than Ayurveda and Vedas.

The Philosophic Foundations of Ayurveda

Most historians agree that the Ayurveda is entrenched in the Hindu holy texts of theVedas (knowledge) and Upanishads (teaching of), which is the cause of its complexity (Majumdar, 2004b) as well as its acclaimed validity for "thousands of years" (Majumdar, 2004c). There is some dispute over the time line of Vedas as well as the specific Veda from which the Ayurveda was born. Some say Vedas are five thousand years old (Atreya, 1999; Chopra, 1991; Frawley, 1998; Tripathi et al., 2000), others date it to about 500 BC (Berger 2007; Hardiman, 2009; Majumdar, 2004; Sigerist, 1961; Wujastyk, 1998).

My research on this matter leads me to agree with Kenneth G. Zysk (1986) according to whom "Vedic religious tradition ...covers a period from about 1500 B.C. to 200 B.C." within which Vedas, Upanishads, and ritual texts (Sûtras) were composed...."there is the period from 200 B.C. to A.D. 300, in which we see the first, classical medical texts: the *Caraka Samhitã* and the *Susruta Samhitã*."

Susruta was a surgeon and belonged to 700-600 BC and not earlier (Johnson-Saint, 1929; Baskaradoss and Jose, 2006). Surgery is a technique and it cannot usher the discipline of medicine. Trepanation involves surgery and was common in many cultures but is not credited with the origin of medical discipline. On the other hand, if one believes that Ayurveda started with god Brahmä (the creator) as stated by Majumdar (2004d), obviously then Ayurveda started in untraceable antiquity.

There are four Vedas. Rigveda is the oldest (c. 2000-1500 BC) and wholly devoted to sacrifices to gods, all of which are not from the same period; some seem borrowed from the Indus valley civilization and some are the same as in old Iran and Mitanni (Western Asia). These were followed by Yajurveda and Samaveda, which are full of hymns and rituals and none of them have a direct link with Ayurveda (Chand, 2007, 2009, 2010; Griffith, [1896] 1995; Sigerist, 1961b). The last Veda is Atharvaveda, composed in about 1000 BC; although this too does not directly refer to the term *Ayurveda,* it has an outspoken magic character and does not glorify gods; it contains verses "to protect the people against enemies, witchcraft, lightning, worms and all kinds of disease, or to provide for them welfare and long life, freedom from fear, recovery of virility, the love of a girl, a husband, fecundity, successful pregnancy, a male child, relief from insanity and other diseases, or even take care of such trivial matters as to fasten and increase the hair" (Chand, 2007; Sigerist, 1961c). In other words, linking Ayurveda with Atharvaveda has some basis; Sigerist (1961b) contends that Atharvaveda "reminds us very strongly of certain Egyptian and Mesopotamian texts."

In summary, according to Majumdar, the creator Brahma passed on knowledge of Ayurveda to Punarväsu Atreya, who passed it on to his six disciples including Agnivesha, and each of these six wrote a treatise. The treatise by Agnivesh is known as *Agnivesh Samhita,* which was revised by Charaka in the first century AD and deals with internal medicine. Because early Aryans ate meat of oxen, sheep, goats, and horses (Sigerist 1961c) and dissected horses and humans, Susruta's description of human and horse anatomy is quite accurate (Zysk, 1986). If *Susruta Samhita* is treated as an Ayurvedic text, Ayurveda began in the seventh century BC, which would be the same period as that of *Agnivesh Samhita,* which was revised by Charaka. In short, Ayurveda is a contemporary of Chinese and Greek medicine rather than significantly more ancient.

The Ayurvedic concept of Tridoshas (imbalance between three bodily systems) has a much-clearer physical representation than the Chinese yin and yang and Hippocrates' theory of four humours.

Nonetheless, the significance of these three schools in the history of medicine lies neither in their being the oldest because Egyptian medicine predates them by almost two thousands years, nor in being scientifically valid, which they are not; but rather in the fact that they signify, for the first time after thousands of years, a departure from spiritualism to materialism, and opened up avenues for modern medicine.

In its early period, Ayurveda was as scientific as possible. Because it formulated a physical basis of disease, it developed a system of diagnosis in which the pulse rhythm played a critical role and sought physical remedies in herbs and diet rather than only in incantations and magic. Indeed, Susruta recommended the use of all the five senses for the diagnosis. He deserves no less credit than does Hippocrates. By taste, the Indian physicians knew that the urine of a diabetic patient is sweetish long before its recognition by European physicians. Susruta preached the use of the sense of hearing to determine whether the contents of an abscess are frothy or gaseous, which can provide some clue to the nature of an infecting micro-organism. The sense of touch could identify if the skin is hot or cold, rough or smooth, thick or thin – all of which can give an insight to what the problem is. The sense of sight can determine corpulence or emaciation and energy. The sense of smell can recognize the characteristic perspiration of many diseases.[8]

Ancient Indian surgery was quite advanced. Surgical tools included steel knives, reed-like catheters, fluid-removing trocars, bone-dividing nippers, polypus forceps, cupping glasses, and almost one hundred blunt instruments. There is a reference to plastic surgery; Susruta's description of repairing a severed nose is fundamentally the same as what is being done now; he insisted that some pipe be inserted into the nostrils during healing. Ayurveda also developed a pharmacopeia of herbs and minerals.

In short, Ayurveda was a complete medical system; it dealt with the cause, diagnosis, treatment, and prognosis of diseases.

Current Relevance of Ayurveda

The divorce of Ayurveda from spiritual medicine must be seen in the context of the tenets of Hinduism. Hinduism is not a monotheistic religion but a mix of spiritualism and materialism; it has a provision, indeed a necessity, to worship mountains, rivers, animals, and so on, all of which deliver some benefit to humans. Take just one phrase from the Oath of Initiation in *Charaka Samhita*; it says, "If thou desirest success, wealth and fame as a physician and heaven after death, thou shalt pray for the welfare of all creatures beginning with the cows and Brahmanas."[9]

I think that Ayurveda began as a science but matured as metaphysics. The question therefore is *how* and *why*. What, then, led to its stagnation and return to an amalgam of materialism and spiritualism?

Basically, Ayurvedic history can be divided into four phases – its beginning as spiritual-materialistic medicine, its transformation to primarily materialist medicine during the Buddhist period, its reversal to its spiritual-materialistic roots with the defeat of Buddhism and the reassertion of Vedic Hinduism, and finally its revival in independent India in its spiritual-materialistic form.

A recent article (Valiathan, 2009) attempts to analyze the evolution, achievements, and the decline of Ayurveda and the current attempts to resurrect it. Little do the proponents of Ayurveda realise that the functions of the body do not depend upon our knowledge. There can be only one correct understanding of health and disease; there can be multiple speculations. Ayurveda, like all other primitive medical sciences, attempted to answer this puzzle out of which grew an entirely new discipline bypassing everything, including Ayurveda.

The Principal Weaknesses of Ayurveda

Majumdar (2004e) tells us that Ayurveda possesses "1,000 single drugs and 8,000 compound formulations" which belong to two groups, one of plant origin and the other consisting of metals and minerals. This is most likely true. Certainly, Ayurveda possesses many more drugs than used by modern medicine or perhaps any other school of medicine. *The Cambridge World History of Human Disease* (Kiple, 1993) lists 158 diseases; there might be a few more. Why did Ayurveda need so many drugs? Is it because therapy was based on the assumption that if many drugs are given, some might work? Rational medicine strives to identify the drug of choice not an array of drugs for any ailment.

Moreover, why does Ayurveda need 8,000 compound drugs? Almost all plant preparations in their native state contain more than a single active chemical. So 8,000 compound drugs might add to many times more molecules. For example, *Rauwolfia serpentine* (source of reserpine and a discovery of India), ergot compounds (derived from fungus *Claviceps purpurea*), and St John's wort (*Hypericum perforatum*), each contain many active ingredients and different constituents produce different effects. Take the case of ergot; it contains so many different chemicals that it has been termed a "veritable treasure house of pharmacological constituents". Ergot`s constituent ergonovine (ergometrine) can cause abortion and ergotamine can relieve migraine. This means that if a pregnant woman with migraine consumes crude ergot preparation for the relief of migraine, she risks abortion.

Majumdar (2004f) and many others claim that Ayurvedic drugs do not produce side effects; this is a preposterous statement because there cannot be a drug without side effects. Even penicillin, the least toxic of all known drugs, can produce toxicity and, in the event of allergy, even death. Even oxygen, salt, and water can produce toxicity; it is a matter of dosage. It must be noted that some of the useful pharmaceuticals of India like Neem (*Azadirachta indica*), turmeric (*Curcuma longa*), and garlic (*Allium sativum*) are a part of Indian folk medicine and not specific contributions of Ayurveda. Moreover, some of the important drugs of plant origin such as quinine, opium, aspirin's ancestor salicin, atropine, quinidine, digitalis, ephedrine, or the anti-malarial Chinese drug artemisinin, are not the gifts of Ayurveda.

The second category of Ayurvedic drugs mentioned by Majumdar (2004f) includes metals such as mercury, gold, silver, copper, iron, tin, lead, and zinc; it is interesting that arsenic, an effective ancient drug against syphilis, is not mentioned. It might be that syphilis did not exist in India until the arrival of Portuguese in sixteenth century.

Metals (e.g. iron, zinc, copper) and non-metals (e.g. iodine) in trace amounts do play an important role in plants, animals, and humans. Ferrous iron is used as a drug for the treatment of iron-deficiency anaemia, quite common in India and other developing countries. However, the most important metal in Ayurvedic therapeutics is mercury. Mercury and arsenic were used in medicine in the past in Egypt and Europe as well. Their toxicity was well known, but alternatives did not exist. The discovery of penicillin eliminated the need for arsenic in the treatment of syphilis and gonorrhoea, and newer diuretics (thiazides, furosemide) made mercurial diuretic a thing of the past. Even mercury vapour can cause toxicity so that mercury batteries in electronic gadgets are no more legal. However, Majumdar (2004f) writes:

> Mercury is an excellent catalytic agent. After its purification and detoxification it is mixed with other purified metals and plant products to make various types of compound medicines based on prescribed formula in the texts. These products retain their medicinal property for a good period and gives [give] very good therapeutic benefits without any side effect. Side effects of metals and minerals are observed, when they are not properly purified or prepared by incompetent and unscrupulous people not having proper Ayurvedic medical background.

Majumdar (2004f) contends that the purer the mercury, the less toxic it is; he does not mention the exact therapeutic effect of mercury but does say that it is "an excellent catalytic agent." I trust that he knows the meaning of the word *catalytic* because he also has a modern medical degree. In chemistry and biological science, the term *catalytic* is used to describe acceleration of a reaction, mostly the interaction between an enzyme and its substrate. There is no known enzymatic activity that is catalyzed by mercury. If anything, mercury inhibits the activity of sulfhydryl (SH)-containing enzyme systems; that is why it works as a diuretic. Majumdar's conjecture that properly purified mercury is non-toxic defies overwhelming scientific evidence to the contrary. Indeed, a compound, dimercaprol (British antilewisite), was specifically developed to treat toxic effects of mercury and other heavy metals during World War II and is still used to treat mercury toxicity.

Much is made of the distinctive feature of Ayurveda as a holistic system, attending to both body and mind, which has lately received extra attention from Dr. Deepak Chopra. However, it is fraudulently attributed as an exclusive Ayurvedic concept claim; every system of medicine from witchcraft to modern medicine follows a holistic approach. Each system of medicine pays attention to diet, life style, and environment, and each system reinforces the will of the patient to fight the disease, including in cases of cancer.

Majumdar (2004g) writes:

> The fundamental principle of Ayurveda is based on the theory that a living body is composed of five basic elements or "Building Blocks" of existence, ...which are Kshiti (earth), Ap (water), Teja (fire), Marut (air) and Vyom (space) ...the functions of human body are governed by three bioregulating principles, namely Vayu, Pitta and Kapha. When these three principles are in normal state (or in perfect balance) in the body, they are called Tridhatu. However, they are never found in perfect equilibrium in the body; hence they are called Doshas because their disequilibrium is the root cause of disease. The three bioregulatory principles are, therefore, commonly called Tridosha, which may be translated as the three main sources that cause disease.

First of all, the living body, even of Indians (!), is not made up of the five elements – earth, water, fire, air, and space. Neither is there any evidence that the human body could be compared with the waveform of quantum physics as done by Chopra (1995). All body constituents can be identified as protein, lipid, carbohydrate, water, and minerals; and except for the last, each of them is a complex of elements of the periodic table. Benton (2008) says: "Life is essentially water (H_2O) with carbon."

I referred to the definition of life by Bernal (1967) and Spencer (1875) in Chapter 1, which is as close to reality as we know so far. It was perfectly scientific to speculate on what the living organism was made of, but the concept needed modification as knowledge advanced. However, Majumdar (2004g) writes that "when *vayu, pitta*, and *kapha* (could mean respiratory, digestive, and circulatory systems) are studied with the new scientific or equivalent terminology as 'bioregulatory principles,' the study of Ayurveda becomes very meaningful ...What Ayurveda stated thousand of years ago is still valid and does not differ from the modern medical findings."

The most revolutionary aspect of the Ayurvedic system is its theory of disease. According to Ayurveda's Tridosha theory, disease is the result of an imbalance between the three systems – *vayu, pitta*, and *kapha*. I still assert that this materialistic approach to disease was a breakthrough in medical science, but I also think it is faulty just like the theory of the four humours of Hippocrates. The concept of Tridoshas (*vayu, pitta*, and *kapha*) of Ayurveda is not verifiable. The argument that *vayu, pitta*, and *kapha* represent a bioregulatory system is an assertion because the notion of the latter does not have a precise definition and can mean nothing or everything.

Assuming that *vayu, pitta,* and *kapha* are some equivalent of a bioregulatory system, their imbalance cannot cause disease; rather, it is the disease that causes imbalance of the bioregulatory system. For instance, streptococcal lung infection can cause pneumonia, which, in turn, produces fever, deficiency in oxygen-carbon dioxide exchange, malaise, and, unless cured by itself or by drugs, death. No possible imbalance between *vayu, pitta,* and *kapha* can cause pneumonia or add bacteria to lungs.

By and large, Ayurveda exists as a method used by its practitioners with no possibility of renovation (Obeyesekere, 1992). Ayurvedic texts assume that the Ayurvedic system of medicine is both complete and eternally valid; to add credence to this assertion, they vouch by the authority of sages. In so doing, they negate the fundamental materialist concept of Ayurveda; they invoke faith and not science. There is more merit to Susruta's surgery than to Charaka's internal medicine because it is difficult to mystify surgery.

Reason for the Popularity of Ayurveda

The current popularity of Ayurveda is based on three cardinal arguments. First, there is invariably a spiritual appeal without necessarily invoking any specific god or prophet. Second, the therapeutic regimen is all natural – herbs, specific exercise, most commonly yoga and diet. Third, its efficacy is guaranteed, no ifs, or buts; "proof" is provided by the narration of personal experiences. There is an additional feature of Ayurveda, which is specific to India.

In India, it has also become an aspect of nationalism both by zealot Hindus who see Ayurveda as a god-bestowed gift of the Vedas, as well as by a substantial section of the educated well-off elite, for whom the worship for Ayurveda is an act of anti-imperialism and an assertion of the traditional wisdom of India. A good example of this national pride is a review article "Ayurvedic Medicine and Epilepsy" (Tripathi et al., 2000); the four authors are based at the neuroscience centre of the prestigious All India Institute of Medical Sciences, New Delhi, and they ought to be aware of diphenylhydantoin (dilantin), which opened a new era in the control of tonic-clonic (grand mal) epilepsy without causing sedation (Putnam and Merritt, 1937).

Ayurvedic description of epilepsy (Manyam, 1992) is undoubtedly quite realistic and a bit more detailed than that by Hippocrates in his essay "On the Sacred Disease." It was perfected to minute detail by John Hughlings Jackson (1835-1911); in the 100 years since Jackson, "little has been added to his concepts except for the electrical proof of their correctness" (Goodman and Gilman, 1958). However, Tripathi et al. (2000) and Manyam (1992) contend that Charaka Samhita "written in Sanskrit about 5000 years ago" describes everything about epilepsy before Hippocrates. This is obviously false on two accounts; first, because Charaka Samhita was scripted in the first century AD, more than five hundred years after Hippocrates. Second, even today everything about epilepsy is not known.

About the therapy of epilepsy, Tripathi et al. (2000) describe an amalgam of multiple herbs devised by Charak.[10] It is very likely that some of the herbs in this amalgam are anticonvulsant, but the contention that they are as good as the currently available anticonvulsant drugs defies rational thinking. There are different types of epilepsies. No single molecule is the drug of choice against all kinds of epilepsies; briefly, phenytoin (dilantin) against tonic-clonic and valproate against absence seizures and other forms of epilepsy are the most commonly used. Given the method in which Charak's concoction is prepared and the ingredients it uses, it is unlikely that two batches of the same concoction are ever identical. One can only hope that Tripathi and his colleagues do not teach students at his medical school the Charak way of treating epilepsy!

There are other methods by which credence is given to the Ayurvedic approach. One example is a 231-page book *Practical Ayurveda: Secrets for Physical, Sexual & Spiritual Health*. The name of the author is Atreya (1999). The term *sexual* in the subtitle might not be innocuous. The author's name Atreya is also probably adopted for its effect because the name appears in the lineage of the evolution of Ayurveda. The foreword is by Dr. David Frawley, a doctor of Oriental medicine (OMD), who also has another name – Pandit Vamadeva Shastri. Frawley runs the American Institute of Vedic Studies in California and wears a beard like the 'holy men' of India.

The author of the book, Atreya (1999), says that he developed an ulcer as a result of aspirin (albeit a natural herb) and almost bled to death; but that was in the past. In so far as the present is concerned, he writes (Atreya, 1999a):

> Should you be interested in a medical system that dates back at least 5000 years? Is there really any practical use in using ancient method of health care? Can the Ayurvedic system help you in your busy everyday life?
>
> The answer is definitely, yes, to all the above questions. I found out through personal experience that the Ayurvedic medical system is very applicable today. Had I understood my Ayurvedic constitution I could have avoided all the problems I mentioned. I have now been able to cure myself of duodenal ulcer, reverse deterioration of the kidneys, correct chronic intestinal problems, and alleviate continuous back pain through Ayurvedic methods. The natural therapies I use have left me healthier, happier, and with a greater knowledge of myself and the universe; and most importantly, my relationship to that universe.

Atreya has a chapter on "Sexual Rejuvenation Methods" in which he decides that a woman should write about female sexuality, because being a man, he cannot do justice to the subject. The woman writer narrates that the book *The Function of Orgasm* by Wilhelm Reich (1897-1957) changed her life. She became determined "to find some way to be able to live and enjoy that energy released by orgasm" (Atreya, 1999b). The narration of this woman contributor to Atreya's book is not convincing because Reich (1983) deals with orgasm but provides no recipe for general use.[11]

Fossilization of Ayurveda

Ayurvedic physicians persist in believing that their system of medicine emanates from the Vedas, the Hindu equivalent of the Bible and Qur'an. This puts insurmountable constraints on the discipline of Ayurveda and is a big hindrance to scientific investigation and any renewal of concepts. It allows the search for more herbs but does not allow conceptual advances. Moreover, the various social-religious and political factors that hindered the evolution of India into modernity, also put a constraint on Ayurveda.

The population of greater India at the time of the founding of Ayurveda was approximately 25 million sparsely scattered people. Even by the end of the sixteenth century AD, greater India's population was 100 million and approximately 150 million by the time it was formally annexed as part of the British Empire in 1857 (Sigerist, 1961e). Life expectancy was short, perhaps less than thirty years since it was still less than forty years at the time of independence in 1947. Ayurveda developed in the context of illnesses prevalent in India thousands of years ago. Many diseases have made their way with the increase in population. There is an allergic component to asthma, and many allergens have been introduced with the industrialization of society; it is very likely that the currently prevalent childhood asthma did not exist at the time of the birth of Ayurveda.

A great deal has changed since then, especially since the industrial revolution, and even more with the advent of wireless communication and computers. But Ayurveda has not changed much, and its practitioners see no need to change. Experimentations or trials that led to the discovery of remedies thousands of years ago had limitations. Indeed Ayurveda's principal objective was to maintain good health and not to treat diseases as was the case with Hebrew medicine. Treatment was a secondary aspect of Ayurveda. While the protocol for maintaining good health changes little, the method of treatment needs continual innovation to make it better and better.

Ayurveda ceased to be a living science a long time ago, and several factors contributed to this state of affairs.

First, the advance of Ayurveda was hindered by the Brahmanical culture, which exerted adverse effects not only on medicine but also on other scientific pursuits. One characteristic of Brahmanical culture was that knowledge must only be transferred to deserving select pupils and not to the general public and never to the people belonging to the low caste (Trawick, 1992). Buddhism tried to break it and introduced more accessible learning institutions, but it was then routed from India, partly by force and partly because it was not mystical enough. The guru-shishya (teacher-pupil) culture is ingrained in every science and art form in India. It even influenced Muslim practitioners of Unani-Tibb medicine and also classical musicians. This is the single most binding constraint placed on Ayurveda, which prevented its evolution. In some way, this practice existed in Greece and Europe as well, but there it soon gave way to teaching in institutions. Ayurvedic institutions did not exist until the beginning of the 20th century.

If one traces the profile of Ayurveda practitioners, almost all of them, until recently, were caste Hindus, which excludes a large section of the population from higher learning. Abha Sur (2010) has elegantly described the perilous impact of the caste system on Indian science and society.

The second deterrent to the advance of Ayurveda was the culture of secrecy in knowledge transfer. An Ayurvedic practitioner almost never wishes to divulge the full secrets of his prescription. If feeling the pulse – the diagnostic approach in Ayurveda – can tell more than listening to the heart rate and rhythm, this special knowledge is, by and large, non-transferable. Any knowledge that is not transferable is doomed; it cannot evolve into a living science. Some of these constraints have been eliminated with the introduction of formal Ayurvedic schools.

The third factor that led to the ossification of Ayurveda, which is also true for other intellectual and scientific pursuits in India, is the stagnation of Indian society due to the long persistence of a feudal mindset. In Chapter 16, I deal with why feudalism survived for so long in India and why, with all their culture and development, India and China were not the first to accomplish the Industrial Revolution. Feudalism is a shackle against science. All branches of science grew with the turmoil and success of the Industrial Revolution in the West.

Finally, Ayurvedic practitioners tend to specialize in treating diseases that are vague or nonexistent, such as purifying blood, increasing libido, freshening mind (*Mastishk*), increasing strength (*shakti*), et cetera, some of which have been elaborated by Zimmermann (1992). If one reads *Boundless Energy* by Deepak Chopra (1995), one can get an idea of how convincing the treatment is of a disease that is not real.

Indeed, in modern India, all emergencies and serious cases that reach the Ayurvedic Hospital are at once referred to modern medical hospitals. Even the Yoga Guru Baba Ramdev who claims to treat AIDS and cancer with his Yoga and Ayurvedic medicine had to be rushed to a modern hospital when he collapsed after a short period of a hunger strike in June 2011.

An unintended offshoot of the nationalism that led to India's independence was revivalism, which had many expressions; rejuvenating Indian therapeutics and Ayurveda was one of them. The Indian state encouraged research in indigenous drugs of plant origin partly to meet nationalist sentiment and partly in the hope of providing cheap drugs to meet national needs. The government also established training centres in Ayurvedic medicine and nearly three hundred of them exist today. They attend to minor diseases that will probably respond to any non-toxic drug but do not meet the need of the population suffering from serious ailments. The culture of revivalism has created a climate conducive to an increase in the popularity of Ayurveda and the support of Ayurveda by the Indian government.

There is not much one can do to stop irrational therapeutics or the love for godless spiritualists as a symbol of national rejuvenation. A scientific approach to the evolution of medical science must assess the merits and demerits of each medical discipline.

Conclusion

While Ayurveda was an early attempt to take medical science from mysticism to materialism, it was, as could be expected, not a thorough break. In years to come, the materialist aspect of Ayurveda was to be drowned in the mystic aspect primarily because of the prevailing Brahmanical culture. Its backbone now is national chauvinism within India and the current culture, which grossly exaggerates the evils of industrialization and equally grossly worships what is natural and ancient.

Notes

1. From *The Charaka Samhita*, Vol. 2, Trans. and published by Shree Gulabkunverba Ayurveda Society in six volumes, Jamnagar (India), 1949.

2. From Robinson, V. *The Story of Medicine* (New York: Tudor Publishing Co, 1931), 141.

3. India was partitioned into India and Pakistan in 1947; unless specifically required, all references to science, technology, philosophy, and religion in India refer to undivided India.

4. The Ganges, Sindhu, and Brahmaputra, originating from the Himalayas, are legendary rivers of the subcontinent.

5. There were many other invasions, mainly for plundering and assertion of military might, such as by Alexander the Great in 327 BC, by the Persian Mahmud Ghazni between AD 997-1030, and by others. British rule in India can be divided into three phases. It began with the arrival of the East India Company in 1612, which had considerable influence especially in Eastern India. The East India Company became the de facto ruler of parts of India in 1757 following the defeat of Bengal's Siraj-ud-Daulah by Robert Clive in 1757. East India Company rule lasted till 1857. In 1857, Indian soldiers and princes launched an armed rebellion under the leadership of the last Mughal Emperor, Bahadur Shah Zafar, which is described as the 'First War of Independence' by many Indian historians and Mutiny by many British historians. The rebellion was crushed and India was brought under the direct British rule in 1857. India achieved its independence on August 15, 1947. Briefly the three phases of British Raj are 1612-1757; 1757-1857; 1857-1947.

6. The timeline of the Vedic Age and also the origin of Ayurveda, especially of the surgeon Sushruta, remain disputed by thousands of years (Atreya, 1999; Baskkaradoss and Jose, 2006). All the Vedas were originally written in Sanskrit; English translations are available in most major libraries.

7. (1) *Anti-Aging Herbal Drugs of Ayurveda* by Dr. Gyanendra Pandey (Indian Books Centre, Delhi, India, 2002), which, aside from a list of anti-aging drugs, also talks about the pathophysiology of aging and the care of the elderly; (2) *Realms of Ayurveda by 19 Scholars*, edited by Pundit Shiv Sharma (Arnold Heinemann, 1979), which illustrates the principle of Ayurveda, Ayurvedic pharmacopeia, and how it differs from modern medicine; (3) *Ayurveda, the Oriental Healing Science* by Dr. S. B. Ranade and Dr. M. H. Paranjape, edited by Dr. David Frawley (Shripad Offset, Navi Peth, 1991), which goes into the history, philosophical basis, and fundamental principles of Ayurveda; (4) *Synopsis of Ayurveda* by G. D. Singhal and T. J. S. Patterson (Oxford University Press, Bombay, Calcutta. Madras, 1993), which contains subjects as does any modern book of internal medicine, surgery, ophthalmology, obstetrics and gynaecology, paediatrics and toxicology – all in one; (5) *Principles of Ayurvedic Therapeutics* by Atmakuri Vinaya Kumar (Indian Books Centre, Delhi, India, 1995), which deals with the fundamentals of the Ayurvedic view on causes and classification of diseases and the role of Yoga; (6) *Scientific Basis for Ayurvedic Therapies*, edited by Lakshmi Chandra Mishra (CRC Press, 2004), which deals with many specific disease states such as thyroid dysfunction, obesity, arthritis, allergies, asthma, liver diseases, Alzheimer, epilepsy, Parkinson's, ischemic heart disease, and indigestion; (7) *Ayurveda; The Ancient Science of Healing* by Dr. Ashok Majumdar (Macmillan India, Delhi, 2004); this book

is dealt with in some detail in this Chapter; (8) Deepak Chopra's *Perfect Health* (New York: Harmony books, 1991) and too many others; (9) *Ayurveda, State and Society in Colonial North India*, 1895-1940 by Rachel Berger (Cambridge: Cambridge University, PhD Thesis, 2007) is an excellent critical examination of political determinants of Ayurvedic practice in the context of evolving Indian nationalism; (10) *Glossary of Indian Medicinal Plants* by R. N. Chopra, S. L. Nayar, and I. C. Chopra catalogues the majority of Indian herbs with indications; it was produced by the Council of Scientific and Industrial Research, 1956, and is used by most pharmacology departments in India to assist them in their research on indigenous drugs; (11) and (12) *The Ayurvedic System of Medicine*, or an *Exposition, in English, of Hindu Medicine*, by Kviraj Nagendra Nath Sen Gupta (two Volumes); it provides introduction to the system, and catalogues many herbs (New Delhi: Logos Press, 1906, 1919); (13) *Aryan Medical Science: A Short History* by H. H. Bhagvat Sinh Jee; this is an excellent text of 280 pages with an extensive index, a history of India and of Ayurveda, as well as a description of Indian Materia Medica and surgery (Delhi: Low Price Publications, 1895).

8. It is related that in a village in the province of Uttar Pradesh in North India, there lived a very famous Vaidya, who could diagnose cases of tuberculosis and prescribe medicaments. He could not travel all over to see patients, and patients with tuberculosis were too weak to make long journeys. This Vaidya demanded that some of the patient's clothes be brought to him and he would diagnose the disease by the smell of the clothing and prescribe the drugs accordingly. I did not hear of anyone getting cured.

9. Cows and Brahmins were singled out because cow is considered sacred by Hindus, so much so that a movement exists to ban cow slaughter; Brahmanas enjoy the highest status in the Hindu caste system, and on auspicious occasions, they are feasted in India even now. The food has to be cooked by Brahmans because they do not eat cooked food touched by any other caste.

10. Charaka described the commonly advocated formulation called *mahapanegvya ghrta*. Both *pancamudas triphala*, both types of *haridra kutaja* bark, *saptaparna, apamarga, nilini, katurohini, aragvadha, phalgu (root), puskaramula* and *duralabha* were used. Eighty grams of each should be boiled with 10.24 litres of water until it reduces to one-fourth. Ten grams each of *bhagri, patha, triaktu, trivert, nicula, gajapippali, adhaki, murva, Rohini, danti, kiratatikta, citraka,* two types of *sariva, Rohini, bhutika and madayantika* should be powdered and added as paste. To this (decoction and paste) 640 g of ghee is added and the mixture is cooked with equal quantities of cow dung juice, sour curd, milk, and urine. This is known as *mahapanegvya ghrta* and is like ambrosia. It is efficacious in epilepsy and should be taken daily.

11. Wilhelm Reich (1897-1957) was a scientist of the view that suppression of sexuality acted as a major instrument of suppression of democracy and promoted Fascism. In the book, *The Function of the Orgasm*, he philosophises about orgasm and his intellectual interaction with Sigmund Freud. Reich despised Hitler and left Germany for the USA, where he distributed his books that were confiscated, and he was put in jail during the McCarthy era. In perhaps the largest censorship in history, the Food and Drug Administration burned tons of his books. Reich died in a US prison.

References

Atreya. *Ayurveda: Secrets for Physical, Sexual & Spiritual Health* (Delhi: Jaico Publishing House 1999).

Ibid., 1999a. xiv-xv.

Ibid., 1999b. 170.

Baskaradoss, V. K. and Jose, R. M. "Life and Times of Susruta: Fact and Fiction," *Indian Journal of Plastic Surgery* 39 (2006): 109-110.

Bernal, J.D. *The Origin of Life* (London: Weidenfeld and Nicholson, 1967), xv.

Benton, M. J. *The History of Life: A Very Short Introduction* (Oxford: Oxford University Press, 2008).

Berger, R. *Ayurveda, State and Society in Colonial North India 1895-1940*, PhD Thesis, Cambridge University, Cambridge, 2007.

Chand, D. *The Atharvaveda: Sanskrit Text with English Translation* (New Delhi: Munshiram Manoharlal Publishers, 2007).

——. *The Samveda: Sanskrit Text with English Translation* (New Delhi: Munshiram Manoharlal Publishers, 2010).

——. *The Yajurveda: Sanskrit Text with English Translation* (New Delhi: Munshiram Manoharlal Publishers, 2009).

Chopra, D. *Perfect Health: The Complete Mind/Body Guide* (New York: Harmony Books, 1991a), 3.

——. *Boundless Energy: The Complete Mind-Body Programme for Overcoming Chronic Fatigue* (New York: Three Rivers Press, 1995), 14.

Dahanukar, S. and Thatte, U. *Ayurveda Revisited* (Bombay: Popular Prakashan, 1989).

Eraly, A. *Gem in the Lotus: The Seeding of Indian Civilization* (London: Phoenix, 2004).

Frawley, D. *Ayurveda and the Mind: The Healing of Consciousness* (Delhi: Motilal Banarsidass, 1998), 4.

Griffith, R.T.H. *The Hymns of The Rigveda: Translated with a Popular Commentary*.V.I and II [1896] (Delhi: Low Price Publications, 1995).

Hardiman, D. "Indian Medical Indigeneity: From Nationalist Assertion to the Global Market," *Social History* 34 (2009) 263-283.

Jaffrelot, C. *The Hindu Nationalist Movement in India* (New York: Columbia University Press, 1993).

Johnson-Saint, P. "An Outline of the History of Medicine in India," *Indian Medical Records* 49 (1929): 289.

Kiple. K. F. Ed. *The Cambridge World History of Human Disease* (Cambridge: Cambridge University Press, 1993).

Kosambi, D. D. *Combined Methods in Indology and Other Writings*. Ed. B. Chattopadhyaya (Oxford: Oxford University Press, 2002).

Kumar, D. *Science and the Raj: A Study of British India* (Oxford: Oxford University Press, 1995), 19.

———. "Science and Society in Colonial India: Exploring an Agenda," *Science Technology Society* 6 (2001a): 375-395.

———. (Ed.) *Disease & Medicine in India: A Historical Overview* (New Delhi: Indian History Congress, Tulika Books, 2001b).

Leslie, C. "Interpretation of Illness: Syncretism in Modern Āyurveda". In *Paths to Asian Medical Knowledge*. Ed. C. Leslie and A. Young (Berkley: University of California Press, 1992), 177-208.

Majumdar, A. *Ayurveda: The Ancient Science of Healing* (Delhi: Macmillan India, 2004).

Ibid., 2004a. 1.

Ibid., 2004b. Preface, 1st edition.

Ibid., 2004c. Preface, 2nd edition.

Ibid., 2004d. 7.

Ibid., 2004e. 220-221.

Ibid., 2004f. 230.

Ibid., 2004g. 2.

Manyam, B. V. "Epilepsy in Ancient India," *Epilepsia* 33 (1992): 473-475.

Nehru, J. *The Discovery of India* (Calcutta: Signet Press, 1946), 69-72.

Obeyesekere, G. "Science, Experimentation, and Clinical Practice in Āyurveda." In *Paths to Asian Medical Knowledge*. Ed. C. Leslie and A. Young (Berkley: University of California Press, 1992), 160-176.

Panikkar, K. N. "Indigenous Medicine and Cultural Hegemony: A Study of the Revitalization Movement in Kerala." *Studies in History* 8 (1992): 283-308.

Pauling, L. *Vitamin C and the Common Cold* (London: Pan/Ballantine, 1970).

Putnam, T. J. and Merritt, H. H. "Experimental Determination of the Anticonvulsant

Properties of Some Phenyl Derivatives. *Science* 85 (1937): 525-526.

Reich, W. *The Function of the Orgasm* (1942) (London: Souvenir Press, 1983).

Robinson, V. *The Story of Medicine* (New York: Tudor Publishing Co., 1931),139-141.

Sharma, H. *Freedom from Disease* (Toronto: Veda Publishing, 1993).

Sharma, H., Mishra, R. K. and Meade, J. G. *The Answer to Cancer is Never Giving a Chance to Start* (New York: Select Books, 2002).

Sigerist, H. E. *A History of Medicine, VII: Early Greek, Hindu, and Persian Medicine* (Oxford: Oxford University Press, 1961).

Ibid., 1961a. 140.

Ibid., 1961b. 138.

Ibid., 1961c. 150-151.

Ibid., 1961d. 151-152.

Ibid., 1961e. 127-128.

Sivaramakrishnan, K. *Old Potions, New Bottles: Recasting Indigenous Medicine in Colonial Punjab 1850-1945* (New Delhi: Orient Longman, 2006).

Spencer, H. *The Principles of Biology, V. 1* (New York: D. Appleton and Company. 1875), 69.

Sur, A. *Dispersed Radiance: Caste, Gender, and the History of Physics 1900-1960* (New Delhi: Navayana Publications, 2010).

Thapar, R. *A History of India, V.1.* (London: Penguin Books, 1966).

——. "Asoka: A Retrospective", *Economic and Political Weekly*, Mumbai, November 7, 2009.

Trawick, M. "Ayurveda, Cosmopolitan Medicine, and Other Traditions in South Asia." In *Paths to Asian Medical Knowledge*. Ed. C. Leslie and A. Young (Berkley: University of California Press, 1992), 98-128.

Tripathi, M., Maheshwari, M. C., Jain, S. and Padma, M. V. "Ayurvedic Medicine and Epilepsy," *Neurological Journal of Southeast Asia*. 5 (2000): 1-4.

Valiathan, M. S. "An Ayurvedic View of Life." *Current Science* 96 (2009): 1186-1192.

Wujastyk, D. *The Roots of Ayurveda* (London: Penguin, 1998).

Zimmermann, F. "Gentle Purge: The Flower Power of Ayurveda." In *Paths to Asian Medical Knowledge*. Ed. C. Leslie and A. Young (Berkley: University of California Press, 1992), 209-223.

Zysk, K. G. "The Evolution of Anatomical Knowledge in Ancient India, with Special Reference to Cross-Cultural Influences," *Journal of the American Oriental Society.* 106 (1986): 687-705.

CHAPTER 7

The Transition to Materialist Medicine: Chinese Medicine

The attachment of Chinese medicine to its own culture is so strong that it has not yet entirely come out of it. All the sciences of ancient times and the Middle Ages had their distinct characteristics, whether European, Arabic, Indian or Chinese. Only modern science has subsumed these ethnic entities into a universal mathematised culture. But while all the physical and some of the simpler biological sciences in China and Europe have long ago fused into one, this has not happened with medical systems of the two civilisations.

Joseph Needham[1]

And if simple mechanical change of place contains a contradiction, this is even more true for the higher forms of motion of matter, and especially of organic life and its development ... life consists precisely and primarily in this – that is a being is at each moment itself and yet something else. Life is therefore also a contradiction which is present in things and processes themselves, and which constantly originates and resolves itself; and as soon as contradiction ceases, life, too, comes to an end, and death steps in.

Frederick Engels[2]

Introduction

The history of China is unique; its development is fiercely independent, far less influenced by the outside world, than the civilizations of India, Egypt and Greece. At the same time, as in the case of Indian civilization, there is continuity from ancient times. This is not to say that Chinese scholars were not in contact with Indian and Arab scholars and philosophers; they very much were. However, by and large, and especially in medicine, the developments in China are largely of Chinese origin.

There were only two major external interventions[3] in the progression of China from antiquity to the twenty-first century. The first was the entry of Buddhism brought by Indian monks at the beginning of the first century during the Han Dynasty (AD 25-220), followed by visits of Chinese pilgrims to India. According to Needham (1954), four visits to India by the Chinese are particularly significant: the first by Fa-Hsien (AD 399-414), the second by Hui-Seng and Sung Yun (AD 518-522), the third by Hsuan-Chuang (or Xuanzang) (AD 600-645), and the fourth by I-Ching (AD 671-712). It is the journey of Xuanzang in search of Buddhist enlightenment, which is the subject of Sun Shuyun's beautifully written book *Ten Thousand Miles without a Cloud* (Shuyun, 2003).

The dialogue between the Indian Buddhist monks of Nalanda and the visiting Chinese monk Hsuan-Chuang in the seventh century, as described by Hui-Li, are illustrations of Indian chauvinism and Chinese humility as well as a sense of pride. Hui-Li writes,

> *The monks of Nalanda, when they heard of it* [the decision of Hsuan-Chuang to return to China], *begged him to remain, saying: "India is the land of Buddha's birth,*[4] *and though he has left the world, there are still many traces of him ...Moreover, China is a country of mlecchas* [menials, untouchables], *of unimportant barbarians, who despise the religious and faith. That is why Buddha was not born there. The mind of the people is narrow, and their coarseness profound, hence neither saints nor sages go there. The climate is cold and the country rugged – you must think again."*
>
> *The Master of the Law replied, "Buddha established his doctrine so that it might be diffused to all lands. Who would wish to enjoy it alone, and to forget those who are not yet enlightened? ...Moreover, how deep and mysterious is their knowledge; their wisdom equals that of spirits. They have taken the Heavens as their model, and they know how to calculate the movements of the Seven Luminaries; they have invented all kinds of instruments, fixed the seasons of the year, and discovered the hidden properties of the six tones and of music. This is why they have been able to tame or drive away all wild animals, to subdue the demons and spirits at their will, and to calm the contrary influences of the Yin and the Yang, thus procuring peace and happiness for all beings ...How then can you say that Buddha did not go to my country because of its insignificance?* (Needham, 1954).

The second major foreign influence found its way into China some 1,500 years later in the twentieth century, when Marxist ideology, born in Europe and nurtured in Vladmir Ilyich Lenin's (1870-1924) Soviet Union, made inroads into China. Thus, the land of Confucius became the land of Gautama Buddha (563-483 BC) and then of Karl Marx. Perhaps there is something common between these three great men – neither of them relied on God, and they all held the well-being of humanity as one of their principal objectives. One might not be entirely wrong in saying that even Mao Zedong (1893-1976), the most prominent Chinese Communist leader, was more of a Chinese than a Marxist.[5] The starkly different course of the developments in the now extinct Soviet Union and the emergence of China as an economic giant by the late twentieth century show that the Russian Lenin and the Chinese Mao understood their acclaimed mentor Karl Marx differently.

There is yet another important way that China is different from any other civilization. The three religions of China prior to the intrusion of Christian missionaries in the eighteenth century are Confucianism, Taoism, and Buddhism. And yet, religion has not been a powerful force at any time in Chinese history. Philosophy is in China what religion is in most countries and the scope of philosophy in China is wider than just Confucius (563-483 BC) and Lao-Tzu (570-490 BC) (see Yu-Lan, 1948; Bodde, 1948; Musunaga and Ohashi, 1977). The impact of Christianity on the cultural milieu of China is minimal. Even the Falun Gong, which made its presence in the 1990s, does not have the classical features of a religion, such as some form of obligatory worship.

This single factor, that is the relative insignificance of religion, has had a far-reaching influence on all other developments in China, including that of medicine; my guess is that this single factor might propel China to become the most powerful country overtaking the USA in very near future.

Commentaries on the Chinese Concept of Health and Disease

Consistent with its prevailing philosophic outlook, China founded the yang-yin system of medicine, which bears some resemblance to the Ayurvedic thesis of Tridosha (see, Chapter 6) and the Hippocratic postulate of the four humours (see, Chapter 8). The obvious similarity between these three systems, as well as the fact that they were formulated within a few hundred years of one another, might not be a mere coincidence. Rather, comparable levels of social, economic, and philosophical progress in these three countries generated similar or identical material development, which has been postulated as a general theory of civilization by Freeman (1896). In a far-fetched analogy, it can be said that sociological developments are in harmony with the Darwinian thesis that identical environmental conditions determine the evolution of species in an almost identical manner.

While the developments in medical science in India, Greece, and China are similar in content, they differ in form. This too is important. However, literature on the philosophical and historical context of Chinese medicine is relatively scarce; what is there is not as easy to comprehend, which is not the case with Egyptian, Indian, and Greek medicine. George Sarton refers to Chinese science and civilization but barely mentions Chinese medicine in his three volumes of *Introduction to the History of Science* (Sarton, 1927, 1931, 1948). Victor Robinson deals in excruciating detail with Indian, Persian, Greek, Roman, Egyptian, and European medicine in his book *The Story of Medicine* (Robinson, 1931) but says nothing about Chinese medicine. The medical historian Henry E. Sigerist promised to "discuss Chinese medicine in Volume III of his series *A Story of Medicine* especially since the uncertainties of the early chronology of China require detailed examination."[6] Unfortunately, Sigerist died in 1957, and even the second volume was published posthumously in 1961. If I were to imagine what Sigerist would have wanted to do but did not do, I feel confident that he would have done a better job of describing Chinese medicine than anyone else I can think of. This is because Sigerist knew both medicine and history, and he had a clear dialectical-materialist viewpoint without a Western bias in historiography.

The perceptions of historians about Chinese medicine differ widely. For example, Roy Porter (1997) devotes a chapter in his book to Chinese medicine and gives a brief summary; he, however, thinks that Chinese medicine "is not wholly indigenous." Professor William Bynum of the University College of London did not even use the word China or Chinese in his book on the history of medicine; for him, there was Hippocrates and no one else (Bynum, 2008). Some historians are scornful of Chinese medicine. Fielding H. Garrison (1929) writes, "Chinese medicine has been what our own medicine might be had we been guided by medieval ideas down to the present time, that is, absolutely stationary. Its literature consists of a large number of works, few of which are of the slightest scientific importance." Likewise, Duffin (1999) has only this much to add about Chinese medicine: "Concepts similar to this imbalance, such as disharmony or conflict in the natural components of the body, can be found in the medical systems of ancient India and China" (he is referring to Hippocrates' four humours). The book by Charles Greene Cumston (1868-1928) has chapters on Egyptian, Hindu, Persian, Greek, Islamic, and even Chaldean medicine but says nothing about Chinese medicine (Cumston, 1926). Albert H. Buck is not as dismissive and disrespectful of Chinese medicine, but he is not respectful either; he writes (Buck, 1917):

> The isolation of China with respect to those countries which were within comparatively easy reach and in which there was a civilization that, already several thousand years before the Christian era, had attained a remarkable degree of development (India, Babylonia, and Egypt, for example); her [China's] blind belief in authority; her unwillingness to tolerate any influence that seemed to emanate from foreigners; and her complete satisfaction with her own methods of doing things, with her own beliefs, and with her own natural and manufactured products – these, it is generally believed, were the most important factors in keeping this remarkable nation in a state of immobility as regards at least some departments of human knowledge and accomplishment. This is particularly true in respect of the science and art of medicine.

In their book, *Tricks or Treatment? Alternative Medicine on Trial*, Singh and Ernst (2008) adhere to the theme embodied in the title. Acupuncture is the first target of their criticism, and even the cover page has delicate fingers sticking needles on letters *C* and *K* of the title word *Trick*. They take pains in 61 of the 410 pages of the book to provide evidence that acupuncture is devoid of medicinal benefits. However, given its physical nature (sticking a needle in certain parts of the body), acupuncture cannot be subjected to strict double-blind evaluation. In any case, the issue is not whether acupuncture is effective against everything as claimed by its practitioners, but rather, whether it is effective against any ailments at all. If that is the case, the acupuncture practitioner is merely boasting about the benefits of the procedure, which is a characteristic of all professions including those practicing modern medicine.

A detailed investigation into the merits or demerits of acupuncture would reveal scientific bases for its efficacy in certain ailments. Just take the example of bloodletting as a therapeutic measure; it has some place in therapeutics. Finally, Singh and Ernst (2008), like many others from lay persons to experts, wrongly think that placebo effects are spurious effects. There is immense literature on the pharmacology of placebos, and I refer to two early articles here by experts in clinical pharmacology (Lasagna et al., 1954; Wolf, 1959).

Theory of Chinese Medicine

What I am writing in this chapter is mainly, though not exclusively, based on *The Web That Has No Weaver* by Ted J. Kaptchuk (2000), the monumental undertaking *Science and Civilisation in China* by Sinologist Joseph Needham and *Knowing Practice* by Farquhar (1994). The book *The Theoretical Foundation of Chinese Medicine* by Manfred Porkert (1978) religiously abides by the title of his book. He carefully explains the philosophic context of each aspect of Chinese medicine. However, it is not an easy book to follow, which perhaps is a testimony to the complexity of the general theory of the Chinese yin and yang and not the fault of the author. As another China expert Nathan Sivin writes (1971) in the foreword to the book: "Dr. Porkert combines knowledge of modern medicine with an extremely sound grasp of philosophy, the lamentably dying art of digging out what words really mean ...Dr. Porkert's working knowledge of the literature of theoretical medicine is in orders of magnitude greater than that of any previous writer." I personally do not have a sound grasp of Chinese philosophy nor do I expect the readers of this book to have it. Consequently, I have tried to extract only such aspects of Porkert's narrative as, I think, would be easily understood by the readers of this book. The book *How to Harmonize Yin and Yang for Better Health* by Musunaga and Ohashi (1977) tends to simplify Chinese medicine into a practical tool for health.

It would be appropriate to make some additional comments on Needham's contribution toward popularizing Chinese science. Professor Needham's series on *Science and Civilization in China* is in seven volumes, each with many parts totalling twenty-seven in all; volume 6 is entitled *Biology and Biological Technology* and part VI of this series, 224 pages-long, deals with medicine. In the concluding volume 7, Needham briefly reflects on Chinese medicine again. It is clear from Needham's books that Chinese science, if anything, was ahead of sciences of not only the north-west of Egypt and Persia but of India as well, at least up to the seventeenth century. Indeed, the scientific achievements of China compelled Needham to pose what became known as the "Needham Question." The essence of Needham's question is, why did China, with so much to offer in the past, fail to keep pace with the West after the seventeenth century? I have attempted to address this Needham dilemma in Chapter 16.

There is a room for bias without being grossly untruthful in historiography, especially that of ancient civilizations. Historians of Chinese science and medicine tend either to exaggerate or to undermine its merits. Take, for example, Harvard professor Kaptchuk (2000a). He writes that traditional Chinese medicine did not "recognize *Streptococcus pneumoniae* as a pathological cause of pneumonia, yet before the discovery of antibiotics, its treatment seems to offer a reasonable and relatively effective response." Kaptchuk quotes a paper by Liu and Douglas (1998) to support his statement; however, the authors of this quoted paper, Liu and Douglas (1998), concluded that "it is difficult to recommend the use of CHMs (Chinese herbal medicines) in ARIs (acute respiratory infections)."

Pneumonia is a very old disease (Duffin, 1993); however, until Louis Pasteur and Robert Koch provided evidence for the germ theory of diseases in the 1860s, no system of medicine, including that practiced by Hippocrates, considered pneumonia to be caused by a micro-organism, and yet all of them, not only Chinese medicine, had some treatment for pneumonia. I doubt if any of these treatments were effective. However, even in the absence of any treatment, all cases of pneumonia do not degenerate into lobar consolidation and death. Many recover from pneumonia without any treatment.

This is not to say that herbs cannot treat pneumonia or even AIDS and cancer. The therapeutic efficacy of drugs is historically determined and cannot be considered in absolute terms. Thus, many drugs were the drugs of choice at one time but have been completely discarded following the arrival of new ones. Countless examples can be cited; arsenic is no longer used to treat syphilis, chloroform is no longer used to induce general anaesthesia, and so on.

The number of ancient Chinese herbs that are still of value is limited; the Chinese artemisinin, effective against chloroquine-resistant malaria, may be the sole undisputed drug in this category – not ephedrine, not ginseng, and not caffeine. There is nothing special about Chinese herbs, and there is no scientific ground for condemning herbs as a source of medicine either. Unschuld (1992) reports how a child unable to even lift chopsticks because of muscular atrophy was able to walk up stairs following the use of certain Chinese herbal preparations. Anti-malarial quinine from Peru and artemisinin from China were the only agents that could cure (not just cause relief) until sulphonamides were discovered in the 1930s. What is, perhaps, special about the Chinese medical system is its failure to recognize micro-organisms as one of the causes of pneumonia even in the twenty-first century.

Unlike Porkert's *The Theoretical Foundations of Chinese Medicine*, Dr. Kaptchuk's *The Web That Has No Weaver* is very lucid; he introduces the history of medicine in China as follows (Kaptchuk, 2000b):

> The Huang di Nei-jing or Inner Classic of the Yellow Emperor (hereafter referred as the Nei Jing) is the source of all Chinese medical theory, the Chinese equivalent of the Hippocratic corpus. Compiled by unknown authors between 300 and 100 B.C.E., it is the oldest of the Chinese medical texts. The knowledge and theoretical formulations it contains are the basic medical ideas developed and elaborated by later thinkers.
>
> The Nei Jing has been called the bible of Chinese medicine, and the rest of Chinese medicine can be compared to rabbinical exegesis of interpretation of doctrine by church fathers. Just as, in the Jewish tradition, later authorities needed to explain theoretical issues raised by the Torah, so Chinese commentators added glosses on the Nei Jing that elucidated or even amended its seminal ideas.

The central feature of Chinese medicine is based on the yang-yin theory. The construct yang-yin as two complementary opposites is philosophically similar to the world outlook of dialectical materialism, advanced by Frederick Engels (1820-1895) in his 1878 classic *Anti-Dühring* (1947) and the *Dialectics of Nature* (1940), both published posthumously; the latter book was assembled through a painstaking effort by the eminent geneticist and statistician Professor John Burdon Sanderson Haldane (1892-1964), born as British national, who died as an Indian in India. Engels makes references to Francis Bacon, Immanuel Kant, Leibniz, and John Locke, but not to the yang-yin theory. This may be because Chinese experience and literature were not available to European thinkers. However, even Mao Zedong, who frequently refers to Chinese history and Chinese episodes to illustrate political points and who is a follower of Karl Marx and Frederick Engels, does not mention yang-yin in his book *On Contradiction* (Zedong, 1937). It would thus seem that Mao Zedong either did not want to show disrespect to his mentors Marx and Engels or did not understand the philosophical dimensions of his native yang-yin.

None of the historians make an issue of witchcraft in describing Chinese medicine. However, in antiquity, Chinese medicine must also have had equivalents of witchcraft as in other civilizations, notably by Incas, Mayans, and North American Indians. Needham (1956) writes, "Superstitious practices flourished in China just as in all other countries. Divination of the future, astrology, geomancy, physiognomy, the choice of lucky and unlucky days, and the lore of spirits and demons, were part of the common background of all Chinese thinkers, both ancient and medieval." Unlike mathematics, astronomy and engineering, which belonged to elite orthodoxy, Needham writes (2000a):

> Medicine and the studies which supported it, such as pharmacy and the anatomy of the acupuncturists, constituted a fully borderline case ... Therapists could be found at every level from the imperial court to the most isolated mountain temple, and the varieties of healing were correspondingly manifold. Our concern is learned medicine and its written traditions, but it is advisable to keep in mind that this was only the tip of the iceberg of ancient health care.

I have not come across any reference to witch hunts in China similar to what was practiced in the Americas, Africa, Europe, and much of Asia. If I am right, this would be a testimony to Chinese civility in contrast to the barbaric witch burning practices of Europe and elsewhere.

In any case, the switch from spiritualist to materialist medicine represented by yang-yin must also reflect the advances in Chinese civilization, as was the case for India and Greece. However, unlike the Indian *Tridoshas* and Hippocrates' four humours, which relate to medicine and biology, the Chinese yang-yin is a universal philosophical approach and not limited to medical science. Yang and yin are not physical entities. According to Kaptchuk (2000c), "Yin and Yang, necessarily, contain within themselves the possibility of opposition and change." Yin represents the shady side of a slope while Yang represents the bright side.

The five principles of yang-yin are the following: (1) All things must have a yang and yin, such as the front and the back of the body; (2) Each yin can be further divided into yin and yang and so can the yang; a logical extension of this would be that there is no fundamental particle like the electron and proton because they should be further divisible, as they probably are; (3) Yang and yin can be distinguished but cannot be separated; (4) Yang and yin control each other; (5) Yang and yin transform into each other.

It was the idea of yang-yin being two fundamental forces that led the royal physician Ho (540 BC) to divide diseases into six classes caused by an excess of yang or yin. Needham's (2000b) views on this subject can be summed up as follows: "Excess of yin ...causes ...(cold illness), excess of yang ...(hot illness), excess of wind ...(affliction of the extremities), excess of rain ...(affliction of the belly), excess of twilight ...(illness involving confusion) and excess of the brightness of the day ...(illness of the heart and mind)." Needham interprets that the "first four of these are subsumed in the later classification under ...diseases involving fever; the fifth implies psychological disease, and the sixth cardiac disease." This is different from the view of naturalists who classified "all natural phenomena into five groups associated with Five Elements or Five Phases" (Needham 2000b).

The yang and yin concept is represented by the Taoist symbol, which is a circle of which one half is black and the other half white, and within the white circle there is a black spot just as within the black circle there is a white spot. Based on original Chinese literature, Porkert (1978a) summarizes the complementary relationship between yin and yang in these words:

> In yin there is again a yin, in yang there is again a yang. Thus the hours from sunrise to noon correspond to the yang of heaven (i.e., of day) and at the same time to yang in yang because the hours of daylight are yang and those of darkness yin; the hours from noon to sunset correspond to the yang of heaven and to yin in yang because the hours of the setting sun are yin; the hours from nightfall to the first cry of the cock (i.e., midnight) correspond to yin of heaven and yin in yin; and the hours from the first cry of the cock until sunrise correspond to yin of heaven and to yang in yin.

The Chinese philosophy and yang and yin do not require postulating a cause of disease, for it is internal to the being itself. Consequently, Chinese medicine does not emphasize the diagnosis of a disease but rather tries to map out the entire state of the body as a consequence of any ailment. Kaptchuk (2000d) illustrates this by quoting studies published in the *Journal of Traditional Chinese Medicine* in which six patients with complaints of stomach pain were diagnosed as suffering from peptic ulcer by the use of modern diagnostic techniques while the same six patients were placed in six separate categories by physicians of Chinese medicine. In a way, it resembles homeopathy. Different diseases can have identical treatment. Conversely, the same disease can have different treatments because in the Chinese holistic approach, the same disease can affect different people differently.

The Chinese State and Chinese Medicine

There is another feature of ancient medicine that seems specific to China – the role of the state. This can be inferred from the writings of Shun-yü I of the second century BC as stated by Needham (2000c). Chinese feudalism was essentially nonhereditary. Governors and magistrates of China were equivalent to earls and barons of Europe and England. Thus, the "Chinese invented the 'career open to talent' a millennium before it appeared in France" (Needham, 2000d). Consequently, the state took over the health-care system by opening hospitals and centres for training physicians; this was the earliest formalization of the profession of medicine.

Finally, no other country seems to have combined continuity and change as well as China; this is true in practically all aspects of Chinese life (Leslie ad Yong, 1992), including medicine (Farquhar, 1992).

Chinese Therapeutics

While it is possible to comprehend the essence of the yang-yin theory of health and disease, it is not as obvious how this constitutes the philosophic basis of Chinese therapeutics. Chinese therapeutics uses two different approaches – one by herbs and the other by acupuncture.

Needham talks about Chinese visiting India in search of herbs, and it is very possible that chaulmoogra oil, the only effective remedy against leprosy until very recent times, was brought from India (Needham, 1954) although there is some evidence that it was brought to India from Burma (current Myanmar). However, in any discussion of Chinese medicinal herbs, it is relevant to consider that the environmental factors in China, unlike in Egypt, are conducive to rich herbal flora.

Landmarks in Chinese Herbal Medicine

Here I describe a few of the landmarks in herbal medicine in China, which perhaps point to many others that have yet to be noted by modern medicine. However, before I do this, I must point out that neither the number of herbs, nor their nature, constitute the foundation of medical discipline, for they are not unique to any specific country or medical discipline.

There are many books on Chinese herbal medicine (Beinfield and Korngold, 1991; Bensky and Barolet, 1990; Liu et al., 2004; Michell, 2003; Tierra, 1997), which not only list a large number of herbs to treat practically all diseases but also attempt to create the impression of their high efficacy and relative safety. Some are like recipe books (Beinfield and Korngold, 1991; Tierra, 1997); they seem to be written to produce physicians of Chinese medicine and describe herbs for all possible symptoms, but none for a specific disease. However, the most significant aspect of the mammoth compendium is more a testimony to the immense pharmacological curiosity of Chinese physicians rather than a proof of the therapeutic value of many of these herbs. Rarely does a therapeutically useful drug of plant origin remain completely neglected by modern medicine; however, only a few of the Chinese herbs have gained prominence because of their proven therapeutic efficacy. I describe them below.

Ephedrine was isolated from *Ephedra Vulgaris Helvetica* (Chinese Ma Huang) by Professor K. K. Chen (1898-1988) before he moved from China to the United States (Chen, 1927). Ephedrine shares many of the properties of adrenaline, but unlike adrenaline, it is effective orally. Two important effects of ephedrine are bronchial dilatation and stimulation of the central nervous system. Because of its ability to dilate bronchi, ephedrine remained an important drug in the treatment of bronchial asthma; indeed it's the structure and pharmacological profile of ephedrine that ultimately led to the synthesis of drugs like albuterol (Ventolin), which are currently the mainstay of asthma therapy. The second major activity of ephedrine is stimulation of the central nervous system, which served some therapeutic purpose but which is now the basis of an array of illicit ecstatic drugs or weight-reducing regimens; it is still a constituent of many cold remedies.

The second drug of major importance is artemisinin, used in the treatment of malaria; it is derived from the plant *Artemisia annua* (qinghaosu), which has been grown in China for over two thousand years and was used to treat cold and fever. Writings from 1596 show the first use of qinghaosu (source of artemisinin) for the treatment of malaria (Klayman, 1985). It was rediscovered by Chinese scientists four hundred years later to deal with the debilitating effect of malaria on the Vietnamese liberation army during the Vietnam War in 1960s. In the 1980s, the US military sponsored research on *Artemisia annua*, which was grown in the Washington area; however, climatic conditions have some effect on the therapeutic efficacy of the plant so that the Washington variety was not as good as the Chinese one. Currently, the main sources of *Artemisia annua* are still China and Vietnam. Artemisinin and its derivatives are unique because they are effective against malaria caused by all the four species of *Plasmodium*. The major significance of artemisinin is that it is effective against chloroquine-resistant malaria as well (WHO, 1998). However, there is a growing risk that malaria parasites will develop resistance against artemisinin because a good number of its manufacturers are ignoring WHO guidelines that the drug not be used singly.

Coffee originated in Arabia and tea in China. Tea, the leaves of *Thea sinensis*, contains caffeine and theophylline. Caffeine (also present in coffee) is a stimulant of the central nervous system. The other component, theophylline, has been used as a diuretic, anti-angina, and antiasthma drug; it still has a place in certain situations in asthma but has lost its therapeutic standing, at least in modern medicine. The legend about the discovery of tea reveals Chinese awareness of its stimulant activity; it is narrated as follows by Goodman and Gilman (1941):

> Bodhidharma, the son of a king of India and an apostle of Buddhism, travelled to China to spread his belief. There he lived under the open sky, mortified his flesh, tamed his passion, and subsisted on leaves. He sought sanctity by attempting to stay awake for nine years while contemplating the virtues of Buddha. After three years of this practice, he fell asleep. Upon awakening, overcome with chagrin, he cut off his eyelids so that his sin might not be repeated. A plant sprang up where his eyelids had fallen. He ate its leaves and found that he could return to his worship with renewed vigor. This plant was the tea plant.

The other Chinese herb popular in China, Korea, Japan, and, increasingly, in the West is ginseng since it is supposed to give energy; it is difficult, if not impossible, to ever be definite about its effectiveness and, consequently, it will remain in use for a long time. Ginseng-equivalent herbs are known in many countries. Ayurvedic and Unani medicine promote energy-giving herbs in a big way.

Rhubarb, perhaps the first to be imported from China by other countries, is undoubtedly an effective laxative.

Two comments are, perhaps, in order. First, as in the past, so also in the present and the future, herbs can be an additional source of safe and effective remedies. There are no theoretical reasons for assuming that drugs tailored by giant pharmaceuticals would invariably be superior to those provided by nature itself. The second, and even more important point, is that there is absolutely no reason to assume that herbs or other natural products are non-toxic. A recent warning by Corns (2003) of the potential toxicity of herbal medicine, including Chinese herbs, is worthy of all the attention; aside from the toxicity of contaminants such as lead, chromium, and so on introduced during the formulation of herbal medicine both in India and China, the herb itself can be toxic. End-stage renal failure, a fatal condition has been reported from the use of Chinese *Aristolochia* to treat minor skin conditions (Lord et al., 1999).

While it is true that "nowhere else, apart from India and China, has there been a real continuity of civilisation,"[7] it is also true that the two medical systems founded by these civilizations have maintained their continuity as well. The most important feature of Ayurveda that kept it alive until today is Yoga. The equivalent of Yoga in the popularity of Chinese medicine is acupuncture although Tai Chi is also in competition with Yoga. However, unlike Yoga, which is a set of exercises, which can be done by the subject in isolation, acupuncture is administered by someone else while the recipient marvels about the painlessness of the tiny prick; both can have healing effects.

Acupuncture is specific to China and has been in use for about 2,500 years. It caught the attention of the world because of the novelty of the approach and its repute as a drug-free method of inducing analgesia-anaesthesia. There is no confirmed evidence that acupuncture can produce general anaesthesia or even local anaesthesia of sufficient magnitude to allow major surgery although many people vouch having witnessed such interventions. Acupuncture consists of penetrating points or loci in defined parts of the body with needles of varying lengths and thicknesses. Closely related procedures are *acupressure* and *laser* acupuncture. The number of these points has varied over the years between 450 and 650, but the most commonly employed points number about 100. There are varied explanations for the selection of specific points, all of them difficult to comprehend in modern anatomical terms. It is even more difficult to comprehend that they were based on any knowledge of the anatomy of the human body, given the fact that they originated in China 2,500 years ago. There is no conceivable method of identifying as many as 650 points or even 100 points, the piercing of which by trial and error can cure or ameliorate a disease; it follows that these points must have been identified by trial and error.

I am more inclined to think that an intuitive application of pressure at points in some proximity with the site of pain, such as at the eyebrows in the case of migraine-like headache, may have given rise to the idea that blossomed into the whole discipline of acupuncture. There is no equivalent concept in modern medicine with which acupuncture points or the flow of message from a specific point of acupuncture to the affected part can be verified. The closest to acupuncture in modern medicine is the external application of counterirritants. However, in therapeutics, the final test is the efficacy of a drug or a procedure and not our understanding of how it works. Modern medicine uses many drugs of which the mechanisms of action are not fully known. Given this premise, the issue of whether acupuncture produces the desired effects can only be ascertained by an objective evaluation of clinical efficacy, requiring a very large and tedious protocol. There is no reason to dispute the role of the brain in almost any event occurring in the body. Likewise, there is no reason to reject the possibility that, in certain cases of acupuncture, pain can be relieved. Indeed, a study by Goldman et al. (2010), published in the prestigious journal *Nature Neuroscience*, provides a role of the chemical adenosine long recognized as a neurotransmitter in mediating pain (Burnstock, 2007) in mice subjected to acupuncture; the report was significant enough to appear as a news item in *Nature* (Cressey, 2010).

In general, however, patients seek acupuncture therapy for relatively vague and non-life-threatening ailments that are more subject to placebo effects than are diseases like infection, cancer, diabetes, and so on. Consequently, it is difficult to establish unequivocally whether acupuncture is an effective therapeutic intervention. Dismissal of any therapeutic role of acupuncture by Singh and Ernst (2008) is unsound because their premise that their book is based on the Hippocratic principle and evidence-based medicine is unsound.

Acupuncture has been accepted as a complementary medicine by the World Health Organization and has received sufficient attention by modern medicine as signified by international scientific conferences on the subject (NIH Consensus Conference, 1998). If judged on the basis of the extent of its use, Chinese medicine would perhaps be on top. This is for two reasons. First, acupuncture is quite popular all over the world. Second, the Chinese, who account for almost one-fifth of the world population, are much more prone than any other people to adhere to their traditional practices in everything from food and exercise to medicine. Almost every Chinese student coming to the West for higher education brings an array of Chinese medicaments, especially balm for the relief of headache. The balm is like acupuncture without a needle, and when applied to the forehead, it evaporates, which probably acts as a counter-irritant and therefore relieves pain. Generations of Chinese who settled in India, often no more than one to two families in small towns, practicing dentistry or mending shoes, continue to use the Chinese language at home, both written and spoken. The Chinese, more than anyone else, believe in Tai Chi, acupuncture, and Chinese herbs, which are flourishing in Chinatowns in every major city in the West. Fortunately, Chinese nationalism focuses more on personal cultural attributes than on proclaiming superiority over other ancient traditions and nations.

As I mentioned earlier, the yang-yin concept is more compatible with health and disease than with therapeutics. Hypothetically, suppose the yang-yin construct is true and suppose they are opposite of each other, it follows that in every therapeutically effective herb, there must also exist a harmful or, at the very least, an ineffective constituent. How is it then possible that the native herb can exert only one kind of effect?

It is unfair to attribute motives other than scientific curiosity and interest to the scholarly writings of different authors. At the same time, it is quite natural that if someone specializes in Chinese or Indian medicine, critical appraisal gets intertwined with professional interests by varying degrees. When it comes to Chinese medicine and science, the readers of this book are urged to read the work of the late Joseph Needham, Chicago anthropologist Judith Farquhar, Professor Manfred Porkert, and others to understand China. In my view, there is little to differentiate between Chinese and Ayurvedic medicine on scientific grounds; these disciplines stand today where modern medicine was during the European renaissance.

Notes

1. Needham, J. *Science and Civilization in China, Vol.6* (Cambridge: Cambridge University Press, 2000), 38. Needham's series on science and civilization is a classic. He was persuaded to undertake this task by visiting scientists from China to his laboratory at Cambridge, England.

2. Engels, F. *Anti-Dühring,* 1878 (Moscow, Progress Publishers, 1947), 138. Engels did most to develop dialectical materialism. Levins and Lewontin dedicated their book *The Dialectical Biologist* to Engels with the following words: "To Frederick Engels, who got it wrong a lot of the time but who got it right where it counted."

3. Japan's brutal war from 1937 to 1941, then World War II until 1945, had little cultural impact. Likewise, the Mongol invasion was no more than a transient episode.

4. Actually, Buddha was born in Lumbini, in present day Nepal, and not in India; but Nalanda monks and many Indians even today think of Nepal as just an extension of India.

5. In his book, *Prisoner of the State, The Secret Journal of Zhao Ziyang* (New York: Simon & Schuster, 2009), Zhao Ziyang, who was general secretary of the Communist Party of China (CPC) at the time of Tiananmen crisis and was deposed for his sympathies with the democracy movement, says that Mao favoured socialism with a Chinese face as opposed to a socialism of the Soviet Union type.

6. Sigerist, H. E. *A History of Medicine, V. II* (Oxford: Oxford University Press, 1961), Note 1.7.

7. Nehru, J. L. *Glimpses of World History* (New Delhi: Indraprastha Press (1934), 1982), 12.

References

Beinfield, H., and Korngold, E. *Between Heaven and Earth: A Guide to Chinese Medicine* (New York: Random House, 1991).

Bensky, D. and Barolet, R. *Chinese Herbal Medicine: Formulas and Strategies* (Seattle: Eastland Press, 1990).

Bodde, D. *Fung Yu-Lan: A Short History of Chinese Philosophy: A Systematic Account of Chinese Thought From its Origin to the Present Time* (New York: The Free Press, 1948).

Buck, A. H. *The Growth of Medicine from the Earliest Times to About 1800* (New Haven: Yale University Press, 1917), 38-39.

Burnstock, G. "Physiology and Pathophysiology of Purinergic Neurotransmission," *Physiological Reviews* 87 (2007): 659-797.

Bynum, W. *The History of Medicine: A Very Short Introduction* (Oxford: Oxford University Press, 2008).

Chen K. K. "A Study of Ephedrine," *British Medical Journal* 2 (1927): 593.

Corns, C. M. "Herbal Remedies and Clinical Biochemistry," *Annals of Clinical Biochemistry*, 40 (2003): 489-507.

Cressey, D. "Acupuncture for Mice," *Nature* 465 (2010): 538.

Cumston, C. E. *An Introduction to the History of Medicine: From the Time of the Pharaohs to the End of the XVIIIth Century (1926)* (New York: Dorset Press, 1987).

Duffin, J. "Pneumonia," In *The Cambridge World History of Human Disease*. Ed. K. F. Kiple (Cambridge: Cambridge University Press, 1993), 938-942.

——. *History of Medicine: A Scandalously Short Introduction* (Toronto: University of Toronto Press, 1999), 71.

Engels, F. *Anti-Dühring. (1878-1894)* Trans. Emile Burns (Moscow: Progress Publishers, 1947).

——. *Dialectics of Nature* (New York: International Publishers, 1940).

Farquhar, J. *Knowing Practice: The Clinical Encounter of Chinese Medicine* (Oxford: Westview Press, 1994).

——. "Time and Text: Approaching Chinese Medical Practice through Analysis of a Published Case." In Leslie, C. and Yung, A. *Paths to Asian Medical Knowledge.* (Berkeley: University of California Press, 1992),62-73.

Freeman, E. A. *Comparative Politics, 1896* (Danvers, MA: General Books, 2009).

Garrison, F. H. *An Introduction to the History of Medicine* (Philadelphia: W. B. Saunders, 1929), 73.

Goldman, N., Chen, M., Fujita, T. et al. "Adenosine A1 Receptors Mediate Local Anti-Nociceptive Effects of Acupuncture," *Nature Neuroscience*. doi.10.1038/nn.2562.

Goodman, L. and Gilman, A. *The Pharmacological Basis of Therapeutics* (New York: Macmillan Company, 1941), 274.

NIH (National Institutes of Health) Consensus Conference. "Acupuncture," *Journal of American Medical Association* 280 (1998): 1518-1524.

Kaptchuk, T. J. *The Web That Has No Weaver; Understanding Chinese Medicine* (New York: McGraw-Hill, 2000a), 2.

Ibid., 2000b. 25.

Ibid., 2000c. 8.

Ibid., 2000d. 4-5.

Klayman, D. L. "Qinghaosu (Artemisinin): an Antimalarial Drug from China," *Science, New Series.* 228 (1985): 1049-1055.

Lasagna, L., Mosteller, F., von Felsinger, J. M. and Beecher, H. K. "A Study of the Placebo Response," *American Journal of Medicine* 16 (1954): 770-779.

Leslie, C. and Yung, A. *Paths to Asian Medical Knowledge* (Berkley: University of California Press, 1992).

Lieu C., Tseng, A., and Yang, S. *Chinese Herbal Medicine* (New York: CRC Press, 2004).

Liu, C. and Douglas, R. M. "Chinese Herbal Medicine in the Treatment of Acute Respiratory Infections: a Review of Randomised and Controlled Clinical Trials," *The Medical Journal of Australia* 169 (1998): 579-582.

Lord, G. M., Tagore, R., Cook, T., Gower, P., and Pusey, C. D. "Nephropathy Caused by Chinese Herbs in the UK," *Lancet* 354 (1999): 48-482.

Masunaga, S. and Ohashi, W. *Zen Shiatsu: How to Harmonize Yin and Yang for Better Health.* (Tokyo: Japan Publications, 1977), 10.

Michell, C., Trans. Shu-De, J. *Ten Lectures on the Use of Medicinals from the Personal Experience of Jia Shu-De* (Brookline, MA: Paradigm Publications, 2003).

Needham, J. *Science and Civilization in China, Vol. I* (Cambridge: Cambridge University Press, 1954), 207-210.

——. *Science and Civilization in China, Vol. 2* (Cambridge: Cambridge University Press, 1956), 346.

——. *Science and Civilization in China, Vol. 6. Biology and Biological Technology: Part VI: Medicine.* Ed. Nathan Sivin (Cambridge: Cambridge University Press, 2000).

Ibid., 2000a. 40.

Ibid., 2000b. 43.

Ibid., 2000c. 51.

Ibid., 2000d. 52-53.

Porkert, M. *The Theoretical Foundations of Chinese Medicine; Systems of Correspondence* (Cambridge: The MIT Press, 1978).

Ibid., 1978a.32.

Porter, R. *The Greatest Benefit to Mankind: A Medical History of Humanity* (London: W. W. Norton & Co. 1997), 147-162.

Robinson, V. *The Story of Medicine* (New York: Tudor Publishing, 1931).

Sarton, G. *Introduction to the History of Science.* (V.1, 1927; V.2, 1931; V. 3, 1948) (New York: Robert E. Krieger Publishing Co., 1975).

Shuyun, S. *Ten Thousand Miles Without a Cloud* (London: Harper Perennial, 2003).

Singh, S. and Ernst, E. *Trick or Treatment? Alternative Medicine on Trial* (London: Transworld Publishers, 2008.54-113).

Sivin, N. Foreword (1971). In Porkert, M. *The Theoretical Foundations of Chinese Medicine; Systems of Correspondence* (Cambridge: The MIT Press, 1978), XI-XVI.

Tierra, L. *Healing with Chinese Herbs* (Freedom, CA: Crossing Press, 1997).

Unschuld, P. U. "Epistemological Issues and Changing Legitimation: Traditional Chinese Medicine in the Twentieth Century". In Leslie, C. and Yung, A. *Paths to Asian Medical Knowledge* (Berkley: University of California Press, 1992).

Yu-Lan, F. *A Short History of Chinese Philosophy.* Edited by Derk Bodde (New York: Free Press, 1948).

WHO (World Health Organization). *The Use of Artemisinin and its Derivatives as Anti-Malarial Drugs: Report of a Joint CTD/DMP/TDR Informal Consultation.* Geneva, 1998, June 10-12.

Wolf, S. "The Pharmacology of Placebos," *Pharmacological Reviews* 11 (1959): 689-704.

Zedong, M. (Mao Zedong) "On Contradiction" (1937). In *Selected Works of Mao Tse-Tung.* Vol. 1 (Peking: Foreign Language Press, 1975), 311-347.

CHAPTER 8

The Age of Materialism: Greek Medicine

The libertarians, on the other hand, with the exception of the extreme anarchists, have tended to be scientific, utilitarian, rationalistic, hostile to violent passion, and enemies of all the more profound forms of religion. This conflict existed in Greece before the rise of what we recognize as philosophy, and is already quite explicit in the earliest Greek thought. In changing forms, it has persisted down to the present day, and no doubt will persist for many ages to come.

Bertrand Russell[1]

What is important is that the Hippocratic attitude toward medicine threw off the religious aspect of suffering and made a beginning toward the scientific study of disease.

Francis Adams[2]

Introduction

If one were to compile adulations of Hippocrates by historians of medicine and occasional commentators on Google and *Wikipedia*, one could easily write a book more voluminous than Francis Adams's translation of the corpus of Hippocrates (Adams, 1939). Robert B. Downs, in his *Books That Changed the World* (Downs, 1956), declared: "Greek medicine culminated, about 420 B.C., in the school of Hippocrates, who had an approach to the art far in advance of anything preceding it and similar in spirit to modern medical theory and practice." The chapter on Greek medicine in the book *The Evolution of Modern Medicine* by Sir William Osler (1921) states: "Let us come out of the murky night of the East, heavy with phantoms, into the bright daylight of the west, into the company of men whose thoughts made our thoughts, and whose ways made our ways – the men who first dared to look nature with the clear eyes of the mind." Such contempt for the East was quite acceptable in 1920s – indeed applauded.

I must therefore say at the start that in this chapter, I am dealing with something extraordinary in the history of medicine. I am dealing with Greece and the icon of medicine, Hippocrates.

Hippocrates belonged to the school of Cos. There were two other notable schools of medicine in that period, the school of Cnidos in Ionia and the school of Sicily (Sarton, 1927). Hippocrates' school is obviously the most well known. Although almost all historians write that Hippocrates' corpus was authored by more than one person, over a period of time, the only person credited for this is Hippocrates. Almost any book on the history of medicine deals extensively with Greek medicine, and authors show no restraint in praising Hippocrates. Even books on the history of philosophy and other sciences almost unanimously proclaim the pioneering and exclusive contribution of the Greeks. Socrates (c. 469-470 BC), Hippocrates, Plato and Aristotle along with a few others, elevated Greece almost to the level of mythology. I suppose this view compelled Conner (2005) to write, "According to the Greek Miracle doctrine, the Greeks of classical antiquity were the creators of philosophy, of science, of mathematics, of medicine, of politics, of theology – indeed, of everything of intellectual value." Pingree (1992) coined the phrase "Hellenophilia versus the History of Science," which ridiculed the concept by saying "that the only sciences are those that accredited Greeks recognized as such."

There is not much more that I can add to praise the Greek contribution than what has already been written by eminent medical historiographers (Gorton, 1910; Garrison, 1913; Buck, 1917; Osler, 1921; Cumston, 1926(1987); Robinson, 1931; Sigerist, 1961; Porter, 1997; Duffin, 1999; Bynum, 2008) and many others; indeed, much is not needed. Likewise, I can hardly add much to the critique of this nearly unanimous adulation of Greece, which would add to or improve upon what was done by Conner (2005) and Pingree (1992). Therefore, I would write about Greek medicine only what is needed to place the rest of what I have to say in some context. Moreover, I would place the achievements of Greece in an historic context rather than as a sudden outburst of genius in a solitary island named Greece.

My main objectives are to answer four questions: (1) Why did the separation between scientific and religious medicine most explicitly happen in Greece rather than in India and China? (2) Why did a small island country like Greece make a greater contribution to science and philosophy in a span of about one thousand years (700 BC to AD 200) than any other contemporary civilization? (3) Is modern medicine really an extension of Hippocratic medicine or does this reflect a western bias in historiography? (4) If Greece was the birthplace of science and philosophy, why are there no birthmarks – less than in India and China?

The Separation of Scientific and Religious Medicine

It is clear from the writings of Hippocrates that it is much more materialistic than Hindu medicine, but only in detail and not in essence. Even so, why and how did Greek medicine evolve as materialistic medicine divorced from the religious overtones inherent in Indian Ayurveda and the abstract ideas integral to Chinese medicine? Inevitably, there are almost always different explanations for any sociological phenomenon, and often it is difficult to establish, which, if any, is correct. My explanation is closer to, but not identical with, that of the historian Sigerist (1961); however, my reservations regarding the uniqueness of Greece as the all-time epitome of excellence in philosophy and science are closer to those of Conner (2005). Nonetheless, the Greek puzzle is important not because it concerns medicine but because it concerns philosophy and science in general.

Without in the least intending to deride physicians of both modern and other schools of medicine, it must be admitted, as discussed in Chapters 2 and 3, that medicine is the least rigorous of all the sciences. Indeed, medical science is even less rigorous than other biological sciences because the social aspects are more important in the former than in the latter. The science historian Sarton (1935) wrote that "however scientific it (medicine) be or may become, it is also and will always remain an art." However, this view has been challenged, in particular, by Warner (1995).

In order for medicine to detach itself from religiosity, all other branches of science ought to become materialistic. Since the forerunner of any branch of science is philosophy, the breakthrough must first occur in philosophy. Like medicine, philosophy too is a very old discipline although not generally realized. Therefore, the main question is: When and why did philosophy emerge as a materialistic discipline, relatively free from divination and the occult, both of which reigned supreme all over the world, including Greece, from antiquity to the time of Buddha?

Religion is also a very old construct and has existed in various forms. Religion is an institution; it is fundamentally opposed to science although the introduction of the culture of secularism has allowed advances in science. Spiritual medicine or witchcraft grew during the era of no religion or folk religion characterized by belief in the supernatural, powerful spirits, and magic, leading to the worship of rivers, trees, and mountains, which serve some purpose; it offered no true solution, but did not prevent anyone from venturing beyond the horizon. The most restrictive are the monotheistic religions. Most of what Greece accomplished really took place before the beginning of the Christian era and centuries before the birth of Islam. True, Judaism was around, although not in Greece, until the founding of Alexandria;[3] but Judaism, though a monotheistic religion, is introvert and not expansionist and hence not a shackle in scientific advances. Jews, by and large, were looking after the welfare of a tribe rather than of a state, and as other citizens of Alexandria were eager to learn rather than be a hindrance to scientific pursuits – that was a unique culture. Hebrew medicine is limited to what is contained in the Old Testament and, as Max Neuburger (1910) writes, primarily concerns "prophylaxis and suppression of epidemics, suppression of venereal disease and prostitution, care of the skin, which undoubtedly was known to the Greeks, baths, food, housing and clothing, regulation of labour, sexual life, discipline of the people, etc." Egyptian religiosity was of the primitive type and hence, as I said before, not a shackle. Thus, Greece was already blessed with one prerequisite for the evolution of materialistic philosophy, namely the absence of strong religious bondage. India of that time was not. Although the teachings of Buddha had no mystic aspect, Buddhism could not completely detach itself from the mysticism of Vedantic Hinduism; consequently, Ayurveda, though primarily a materialistic medicine, carried remnants of mysticism.

Although religion influenced every aspect of human activity, it is practically incorporated in medicine. Consequently, the founding of the scientific discipline of medicine and separating it from religion, must be treated as a major and very significant development, no matter which country and who did it. The next major breakthrough in this direction came with the publication of the *Principles of Biology,* by Herbert Spencer (1875) and *On the Origin of Species,* by Charles Darwin (1859).

Magic and the occult were becoming powerless in offering universal explanations for natural events by the beginning of the last millennium of the pre-Christian era. So the stage was set – indeed ripe – for the birth of materialistic philosophy and science. This is no surprise.

Why Did Greece Become the Birthplace of Nonreligious Medicine?

Why did a tiny country like Greece accomplish so much in less than one thousand years from Thales of Miletus to Hippocrates to Galen, superseding much larger countries with much older civilizations like India and China? Certainly, science and health sciences did not start in Greece, but it was undoubtedly in Greece that they matured from a set of sporadic discoveries or even rational explanations into a materialistic discipline. The question still remains – why not in India and China, with civilizations older than that of Greece?

The culture of India was religion and not science for the greater part of its history, and to a great extent, it is so even now. True, like Greece, India too is a country of immigrants. However, the earliest immigrants, that is, the Aryans, came to India from a highly religious background via Persia, and their first task was to formalize a religion. The climate favoured a mixture of materialism and divinity.

China, on the other hand, was never very religious. However, for both geographic and historic reasons, it was self-contained and self-satisfied; it rested on the glory that they already had an answer to every puzzle, from natural phenomena to matters of biology, in the philosophy of Confucius, Lao-Tzu, and Taoism (see Bodde, 1948) and the yang-yin theory. Culturally, therefore, China was, and one might add, remained somewhat static until the entry of Marxism in the early twentieth century.

What did Greece achieve during the same period while India and China were not yet fully awake? Chronologically, Thales of Miletus, Pythagoras of Samos, Democedes of Croton (550-460 BC), Herodotus of Halicarnassus, Socrates (469-399 BC), Democritus (460-370 BC), Plato (427-347 BC), Hippocrates of Cos, Thucydides (460-400 BC), Aristotle (384-322 BC), Galen, and many others represent a continuum of increasing political, scientific, and philosophical advances not known in any other country within such a short time frame.

Russell (1945) writes, "Philosophy begins with Thales ...Philosophy and science – which were not originally separate – were therefore born together at the beginning of the sixth century." Robinson (1931a) says that Thales "created geometry ...laid the basis of physics ...founded astronomy ...opened the story of electricity." Thales's friend Anaximander (610-546 BC) was the first evolutionist, 2,500 years before Darwin; he speculated that man developed from aquatic animals. Thus, for Thales and Anaximander, the world and world events were physical without any room for gods. If medicine arose from them, which in a way it did, it arose out of worldly matters, unlike the Indian Ayurveda that descended from the creator Brahma, whom no one can see or touch. The legacy of Thales went to Democedes of Croton (550-460 BC), not a scientist but a very skilled physician.[4] The materialistic phase of philosophy, mathematics, and medicine began from this time on in the island of Greece. The most prominent initiator of materialist medicine in Greece was Hippocrates.

Geographically and demographically, Greece is quite unique, which might have something to do with the quality and speed of its progression from Thales to Galen. Continental Greece, in antiquity, was not much more than 65,000 sq. km and is still only about 130,000 sq. km, with about 110,000 sq. km being the mainland and 20,000 sq. km being a set of islands (Sigerist, 1961). If civilization could be numerically quantified and expressed as a function of per unit land mass, it would baffle the wildest dreamer when it comes to Greece. For a time, Greece was a capsule of wisdom – in philosophy, mathematics, medicine, and literature – even in the world of sports.

According to Toynbee (1946a), the closest country comparable to Greece, albeit in a different way, is England – with a land mass of only, approximately, twice as large. England ushered in the Industrial Revolution, established parliamentary form of governance, made gigantic overseas expansions, changed the course of history of many nations, popularized the English language, and much more. I will not dwell on this subject other than to say that the geographic constraints placed upon both Greece and England might have something to do with their accomplishments, whatever their quality. While making this statement, I am neither implying that the rest of the world got civilized because of Greece, nor denying independent developments of a very high order in ancient Egypt, Persia, India, China, Peru, and Mexico.

I think that the historian Arnold Toynbee is on the mark when he writes that the modern state of world civilizations is not a consequence of diffusion, a theory propagated by Dr. Grafton Elliot Smith (1871-1937) (Smith, 1911). A closer examination of different civilizations would prove the correctness of the postulate of Freeman (2009 [1896]) that civilizations evolved independently. This does not mean that one civilization does not lend to or borrow from another but, rather, that the central aspect is invariably indigenous.

In a way, Greece is a land of immigrants as India was and as the new world was to become after the seventeenth century. If judged purely on the basis of scientific and technological progress and not on the basis of the social deprivation of indigenous people, the factors that led to mass emigration also were the stimulus for innovation and scientific progress. In Greece, Achaeans came from the north Danube region sometime around 2000 BC. The Dorian acquisition of the Greek mainland and Crete occurred toward 1200 BC. The Aegean Islands were colonized by the end of 1000 BC; these three groups spoke different dialects (Sigerist, 1961).

Geographically, the three continents – Asia, Africa and Europe – embrace one another at the Mediterranean to lend to and borrow from the islands of Greece and Crete. As only 23 percent of their land is arable, the

Greeks either depended on trade or on the sea, for sustenance. Sigerist (1961b) says:

> Access to sea always opens wide horizons, stirs the people's imagination, and makes them dream of foreign lands. Greece, however, not only has access to the sea, it is dipped into the sea …Thanks to the sea, Greece did not remain a small peninsula but became a world …Crete did not share in the wars of Asiatic and African mainland. Unlike their oriental neighbors, the Cretans were neither afraid of the dead nor haunted by the fear of ghosts … the Cretan's attitude toward nature and life was outspokenly rational. To the Greek, sailing was not only a necessity, but a passion …Navigation is always a stimulus to science.

Expansionist, unethical and victorious wars by Alexander the Great – notably the victory over Persia and Egypt and the founding of Alexandria – added to the vibrancy of Greece and possibly to its subsequent decline. It is also possible that despite initial reverence for Homer and the *Iliad*, Alexander himself might have developed respect, if not understanding, of philosophy, science, and medicine while he was a student of Aristotle. Alexander the Great died very young. Usually, youthful zeal is very intense though not very rational; it so happens that Alexander unified and expanded Greece, did not dampen its science, and might have even given it a boost.

Nevertheless, Greek medicine did not start as materialist medicine; it became so only with the immigrations mentioned above. Indeed, until the time of Thales and Hippocrates, it was as much, if not more, loaded with spirituality of the wilder type as anywhere else. Quite often, there is a reference to Homeric medicine; Sigerist (1961) even has a whole chapter with that name in his book. References to disease or wound, which were plentiful in the epics *Iliad* and *Odyssey*, have been interpreted as a commentary on disease and healing. Galen and many others even treat Homer as a physician. All this, I do think, reflects bias and not rational historiography.

The epics *Iliad* and *Odyssey* are poems depicting the fury of Achilles, the Trojan War, and the exploits of *Odyssey*; they are not medical texts. If there is a war, there would be injuries and something would be done to heal wounds, depending upon the hierarchy of the injured. To convert such descriptions into aspects of medicine is far-fetched. Texts more or less comparable to the *Iliad* and the *Odyssey* can be found in other civilizations such as the Indian epics *Ramayana* and *Mahabharata*.[5]

According to Robinson (1931a), Greece was not different from Egypt. It was in Crete, the Greek island of great intellectual activity, where Zeus was born and his offspring Minoans had built a civilization as early as 4000 BC. However, by the time of Homer, about 1000 BC, the Minoan civilization had already been vanquished. It is said Aesculapius, linked to Apollo, could cause havoc with his medicine when he was displeased and treated other gods; he listened to the advice of his talking raven. Temples were famed with tales of miraculous cures; abandoned crutches prove the spontaneous setting of broken bones – a miracle that can still be witnessed at many shrines. When a girl suffered from dropsy (accumulation of fluid in the body most often due to heart or kidney failure) and asked for help, "Aesculapius cut off her head, turned her upside down until the fluid ran out and then replaced her head." Even this episode has an Indian parallel.

Anyone who has visited India or Indian establishments in the West must have noted a statue, a figurine, or a calendar with a potbellied youthful human with an elephant's head; that is Lord Ganesha, and the tale of how he got the elephant's head is similar to the decapitation of the girl by Aesculapius.[6] So what the Greek Aesculapius did had been done elsewhere long before him. In any case, Greek medicine had a very long way to travel from Homer's fancy and Aesculapius's occult to modern medicine. But it did.

In short, geographical and demographic factors as well as close contact with the achievements of Egypt, Persia, and India, and the relative absence of religious constraints were major factors in the achievements of Greece at that period.

The Legacy of Hippocrates

One of the many legacies of the ascendancy of the West in defining world politics was to name medicine as Hippocratic medicine. The late Professor Robinson (1933) prepared a *Syllabus of Medical History*, which consisted of specific questions and answers. Question no. 5 is: "Who is the Father of Medicine? Why does he deserve this title?" Robinson's answer, which students were expected to know was: "We properly call him [Hippocrates] the Father of Medicine because he 'emancipated medicine from the gods,' 'founded clinical medicine,' argued that 'nature heals; the physician is only nature's assistant,' discarded 'polypharmacy,' 'inaugurated pharmacology,' and gave 'medicine its ethical basis' through the Oath." Osler (1921) is equally emphatic. Hippocrates burnt the library of Cnidos, the rival school of medicine, to conceal his plagiarism; he set Athens on fire to stop the plague (Robinson, 1931); but these episodes are ignored in bestowing to him the highest honour in medicine. Robinson (1931b) does describe the genius of the Persian physician Rhazes (c. 850-932) as a physician and medical ethicist but does not find him equal to Hippocrates.

Only a few have challenged the notion of Hippocrates as the father of medicine (Conner, 2005; Pingree, 1992).

Hippocrates' contributions to medicine can be placed in two categories: (1) A general theory of health and disease formulated as the theory of the four humours; (2) The medical treatises known as *Corpus Hippocraticum*, which most likely resulted from the contributions of several authors.

Hippocrates' Theory of the Four Humours

The most significant contribution of Hippocrates was his doctrine of the four humours (yellow bile, black bile, phlegm, blood), corresponding to the four seasons (autumn with black bile, spring with blood, winter with phlegm, and summer with yellow bile); according to this theory, health is a state of balance between them and disease reflects imbalance. There is no doubt that this is a materialist concept and most likely influenced "by the philosophy of nature and the scientific outlook of the pre-Socratics, and particularly by the Pythagoreans and Sicilians" (Sigerist 1961b). Nonetheless, Sigerist (1961b) asserts that Hippocrates' postulates were not only "a perfect scientific view" in the past but also "a correct view and one that we still hold today."

However, the theory of the four humours is, in essence, similar to the Hindu Ayurvedic theory of the three imbalances (*Tridoshas*) and the yang-yin theory of China. But is the four humours theory also a rational description of what really causes disease? One can stretch the meaning of yellow bile, black bile, phlegm, and blood, as Sigerist (1961) does, and conclude in the affirmative; but this, to my mind, requires reverence of the Greek contribution, and even rational people like Sigerist have got carried away. Sigerist writes, "Give a drug that acts on phlegm and the individual will vomit phlegm"; he does not give the example of any such drug that existed at the time of Hippocrates, or even in the present; in any case, if there is such a drug, it is the property of a drug and not the basis of any disease.

I do not wish to use as many words to refute the scientific rationale attributed to the four humour theory by Sigerist (1961b), Osler (1921), Porter (2005), and many others but I do think that Hippocrates' theory of disease is less rational than the Ayurveda's theory of *Tridoshas* and the Chinese theory of yang-yin. Hippocrates' much applauded speculation about the relationship of seasons to disease, as the origin of medical geography cannot stand scrutiny. Lung cancer, pneumonia, bronchial asthma, emphysema, pleurisies, pulmonary hypertension, pulmonary tuberculosis, and anaphylactic reactions – all involve lungs; but what kind of air or anything else can account for all of them? Seasons vary less in some places than in others.

If the Hippocratic theory were valid, disease would have to be and would have to remain integral to human life. Perhaps for these reasons, almost two thousand years later, one of the greatest physiologists of all times, Claude Bernard (1813-1878)[7] said that seeking the essence of disease was "pursuing a phantom. The words: life, death, health, disease, have no objective reality." Therefore, attributing virtues to Hippocrates' four humours' theory of disease is like resurrecting a phantom. More on Hippocrates' theory is presented below in connection with a discussion of his treatises.

Corpus Hippocraticum

Hippocrates' writings have been translated into English by Francis Adams (1796-1861) under the title *The Genuine Works of Hippocrates*, which contains seventeen chapters (Adams, 1939). Hippocratic physicians wrote much more, of course; maybe as many as sixty treatises.

However, the ones mentioned here provide the basic elements of Hippocratic medicine.

There is no element of god in any of these books, and there are profound projections to the future of medicine. Unlike the texts of Ayurveda, Hippocrates does not claim to have written the last word, and no one who expresses allegiance to him claims so either. At the same time, there does not exist sufficient evidence to their accuracy and relevance. I will briefly dwell on all these seventeen essays of Hippocrates (Adams, 1939).

I will first discuss the chapter "On Airs, Waters, and Places" in some detail for two reasons. (1) It is theoretical. Just as the theory of four humours speculates on the cause of disease, the book *On Airs, Waters, and Places* defines why people are what they are. (2) In my opinion, almost nothing written in this chapter conforms to the actual characteristics of people in the real world. I would rather use the inference of historian Arnold J. Toynbee (1946b) than my own to illustrate the fallacies of Hippocrates. Toynbee knew Greek and wrote his own translation of Hippocrates. Toynbee (1946b) writes:

> The Egyptian and Scythian might be far apart from each other and from their Greek observer (Herodotus, for example) in the manner of life, but they were not physically different from him in the sensational way in which the Negro of West Africa and the Red Man of America differed from the European. It was natural, therefore, that the Greeks should find some factor other than biological inheritance of physical characteristics, i.e. race, to account for the differences of culture they observed around them. They found their explanation in differences of geographical habitat, soil and climate.
>
> There is a treatise entitled Influences of Atmosphere, Water and Situation, dating from the fifth century B.C. and preserved among the collected works of the Hippocratean School of Medicine, which illustrates Greek views on this subject. Here we read, for example, that Human physiognomies may be classified into the well-wooded and well-watered mountain type, the thin-soiled waterless type, the meadowy marshy type, the well-cleared and well-drained lowland type ...Inhabitants of mountainous, rocky, well-watered country at a high altitude, where the margin of seasonal climatic variation is wide, will tend to have large-built bodies constitutionally adapted for courage and endurance ...Inhabitants of sultry hollows covered with water-meadows, who are more commonly exposed to warm winds than to cold, and who drink trepid water, will, in contrast, not be large built or slim, but thickset, fleshy and dark-haired, with swarthy rather than fair

> complexion, and with less phlegm than bile in their constitutions. Courage and endurance will not be innate in their characters to the same degree, but will be capable of being produced in them by the co-efficient of institutions ...Inhabitants of rolling, wind-swept, well-watered country at a high altitude will be large built and un-individualized, with a vein of cowardice and tameness in their characters ...In the majority of cases, you will find that the human body and character vary in accordance with the nature of the country.

Toynbee (1946b) goes on to add: "Both the race theory and the environment theory try to account for the observed diversity in the psychical (intellectual and spiritual) behaviour and performance of different fractions of mankind by supposing that this psychical diversity is fixedly and permanently correlated, in the relation of effect to cause, with certain elements of the observed diversity in the non-psychical domain of nature."

Surprisingly, almost all the historians who proclaim Hippocrates as the father of medicine, either say nothing about the book *On Airs, Waters, and Places* or say as little as possible. Buck (1917), Osler (1921), and Sigerist (1961) do not comment on this treatise. Garrison (1913a) writes, "The excursus *On Airs, Waters and Places*, is at once the first book ever written on medical geography, climatology, and anthropology." Robinson (1931c) says that *On Airs, Waters, and Places* "is the first treatise on public health, medical geography, climatology, physiotherapy and balneology. It contains the earliest observation on urinary calculi, and the first account – a masterly one – of sexual impotence." Cumston (1926) writes that this treatise is "immortal" because "it relates the quality of water to health and disease including infections and advises the use of boiled water." Porter (1997a) does link the treatise *On Airs, Waters, and Places* with Hippocrates' theory of the four humours and goes on to add, "*Airs, Waters, Places* also attributed national characteristics to bile and phlegm: the pasty, phlegmatic peoples of the North were contrasted with the swarthy, hot, dry, bilious Africans. Both were judged inferior to the harmonious Greeks in their ideally equable climate." Porter is truthful to what Hippocrates says, but what Hippocrates says is hardly meritorious.

Hippocrates did not travel much. It seems he had only seen Greeks, Egyptians, Libyans, and Sicilians or read Herodotus, who found both Egyptians and Libyans very healthy. If one stretches Hippocrates' thesis, one must encounter giant-size Nepalese around the Himalayas and weaklings in West Africa, who are not fit to be trapped as slaves years later.

Here is another absurd conjecture of Hippocrates in *On Airs, Waters, and Places*:

> I will pass over the smaller differences among the nations, but will now treat of such as are great either from nature, or custom; and, first, concerning the Macrocephali. There is no other race of men which have heads in the least resembling theirs. At first, usage was the principal cause of the length of their head, but now nature cooperates with usage. They think those the most noble who have the longest heads. It is thus with regard to the usage: immediately after the child is born, and while its head is still tender, they fashion it with their hands, and constrain it to assume a lengthened shape by applying bandages and other suitable contrivances whereby the spherical form of the head is destroyed, and it is made to increase in length. Thus, at first, usage operated, so this constitution was the result of force: but, in the course of time, it was formed naturally; so that usage had nothing to do with it; for the semen comes from all parts of the body, sound from the sound parts, and unhealthy from the unhealthy parts. If, then, children with bald heads are born to parents with bald heads; and children with blue eyes to parents who have blue eyes; and if the children of parents having distorted eyes squint also for the most part; and if the same may be said of other forms of the body, what is to prevent it from happening that a child with a long head should be produced by a parent having a long head? (Adams, 1939a)

By claiming that such important changes introduced in the body can be genetically transferred, Hippocrates puts Russian Trofim Lysenko (1898-1976) to shame. It is redeeming that no one has called Hippocrates the father of genetics, displacing Gregor Johann Mendel.

Other books of Hippocrates are concerned with specific diseases, therapies, or the conduct of physicians. The treatise *On Ancient Medicine* is interesting for two reasons. First, it argues that "whoever …laid down some hypothesis …such as hot, or cold, or moist, or dry, or whatever else they choose (thus reducing their subject within a narrow compass, and supposing only one or two original causes of disease or of death among mankind), are clearly mistaken in much that they say." I do not know how to reconcile it with the fact that Hippocrates is actually admired, most of all, for his four humour theory of diseases. The rest of the treatise elaborates how the quality of food is critical to health and disease. *The Book on Prognostics* is basically a set of general instruction to physicians on bedside manners, on diagnostics and therapy. The book *On Regimen in Acute Diseases* reinforces what is said in *On Ancient Medicine* and *The Book on Prognostics* has additional instruction on certain parasitic diseases. *Of the Epidemics* relates diseases to the season with a number of case histories, which has a good measure of truth. In the book *On Injuries of the Head*, Hippocrates describes the external anatomy of the head, the nature of possible injuries and treatment, including surgery and trepanning, with a warning against the application of any liquid except when the injury is on the forehead. The books, *On the Surgery, On Fractures, On the Articulations*, and *Mochlicus*, (bone structure) provide detailed and rational instruction for the management of injuries, fractures and dislocation of joints with then-existing tools. The book, *Aphorisms,* starts with the sentence: "Life is short, and the Art long; the occasion fleeting; experience fallacious, and judgment difficult." This is followed by the therapeutic relevance for purging, vomiting, food, sleep, cleanliness, role of seasons, and so on. In *The Law*, Hippocrates warns against training scoundrels as doctors. The books, *On Ulcers, On Fistulae,* and *On Haemorrhoids*, deal with their possible causes and also describe therapy with potions. Undoubtedly, by and large, these descriptions are rational, and the surgical interventions are similar to those described by Susruta of India.

The book, *On the Sacred Disease,* attacks priestly attitudes toward disease; this book is most emphatic against religion in medicine. It essentially describes tonic-clonic (previously known as grand mal) epilepsy and forcefully argues that it is as physical as any other disease. Since epilepsy by the very nature of its symptoms had been much more closely related to spiritualism than were other ailments, Hippocrates makes a very strong argument against mixing magic with medicine. However, his explanation for the cause of epilepsy is as far from truth as can be, and to some extent, it was due to his incorrect understanding, expressed as follows: "When a person draws in air by the mouth and nostrils, the breath (*pneuma*) goes first to the brain, then the greater part of it to the internal cavity, and part to the lungs, and part to the veins, and from them it is distributed to the other parts of the body along the veins; and whatever passes to the stomach cools, and does nothing more; and so also with regard to the lungs." It is worth mentioning that a much more sophisticated description of epilepsy, including aura-accompanying tonic-clonic seizures, can be found in Indian Ayurvedic texts along with some form of treatment, predating Hippocrates (Manyam, 1992; Tripathi et al., 2000).

Overall, the writings of Hippocrates are based on experience, observation, and deduction, beyond doubt. Robinson (1931d) is correct in saying that by "demonstrating that disease was not dependent upon supernatural causes, Hippocrates emancipated medicine from the gods." But I do not think this should lead to the inference that modern medicine is Hippocratic medicine.

Hippocrates and Modern Medicine

This brings me to the critical question I posed in the beginning: is modern medicine an extension of Hippocratic medicine? It is easier to envision the link between Galileo's physics and Einstein's physics. It neither requires reverence of Galileo nor of Einstein although both deserve it. As to the link between Hippocrates and modern medicine, the link is no more obvious than is the link between modern medicine and witchcraft. In my opinion, modern medicine is founded on the cumulative and evolving efforts of thousands upon thousands dealing with the often encountered disease, and it would be more accurate to look at medicine as a continuum, with some accomplishments playing a bigger role than others.

Indian and Chinese physicians made significant contributions, and there is nothing extraordinary about Hippocrates. Separating medicine from magic is important. But almost everything that Hippocrates said or did was said and done by Indians and Chinese within the same time frame. Although Hindu medicine is not completely divorced from spiritualism, Chinese is. As far as written texts are concerned, *Agnivesh Samhita*, written a few hundred before and *Charaka Samhita* compiled a few hundred years before are comparable to *Corpus Hippocraticum*, if not superior.

Galen

Hippocratean tradition was taken many steps forward by Galen; there were Diocles of Carystus (c. 375-300 BC), Herophilus of Alexandria (335-280 BC), Erasistratus of Chios (304-250 BC), pharmacologist Pedanius Dioscorides (AD 40-90) and others in between. They were materialist and experimentalist.

Galen belonged to Asia Minor and studied philosophy and mathematics before starting his medical training. Just as Aristotle was forced to waste seven years of his life by Alexander the Great, though the latter learnt nothing from the former, Galen too was retained for an extended period by the emperors of Rome. Nevertheless, Galen travelled extensively, including to Alexandria, once a city of knowledge. While the contributions of Hippocrates were primarily based on his observations and analysis, Galen introduced experimental approach to medical science (see Robinson, 1931e; Porter, 1997a); in this sense, Galen's contribution to the evolution of modern medicine is far more significant than the speculations of Hippocrates. Galen also put due emphasis on the role of philosophy and ethics.

The study of natural philosophy allowed the physician insight into both human nature and the nature of the universe. The Galenic body was fluid because it was composed of humours – blood, black bile, yellow bile, and phlegm – which were formed by the same elements that constituted the cosmos (fire, water, air, and earth).

Indeed, Galen's elaboration of the four humours is much more specific than that by Hippocrates and also more specific than the *Tridoshas* of Ayurveda. It is not just imbalance – for minor imbalances must be occurring all the time – but it is the predominance of one over the other that causes a disease. That is why modern medicine emphasises a normalcy range rather than a single figure.

Galen emphasized the importance of logic as a tool in diagnostics; to some extent it is common practice to elicit history and identify the distinct aspect of a disease from numerous symptoms narrated by the patient. Hence both reason and sense experiences were essential for the discovery and confirmation of the true nature of things. Logic also led to the search for causes within a teleological cosmology that demanded the inference of the invisible from the visible; the hidden causes from the manifest signs (Nutton, 1993).

Ethics was the domain of human action and conduct. In Galenism, the patient, the physician, and their mutual relation were subjected to an elaborate *askesis* aimed at cultivating certain dispositions and habits (*hexis*) to restore the balance of body and soul (Edelstein, 1967). Galenic therapeutics throughout the Middle Ages placed a strong emphasis on *dieta*, the art and craft of morals and somatic virtues. Health required the good ordering of the *naturals* (elements, humours, parts of the body, and faculties) and the regulation of the *non-naturals* (rest, motion, food and drink, evacuation, passions, and errors of the soul). The virtuous character of the physician hastened the healing powers of nature by forging a relationship of trust and friendship (Entralgo, 1967). In short, Galen took the vistas of medicine opened by Hippocrates to new heights. Galen combined philosophy with the science of medicine and thereby became the leader of a battle on two fronts – against servility to religion and against demonology in medicine.

Galen's main area of research was anatomy. Dissection of the human body was not allowed during Galen's times. However, merely on the basis of dissection of animals, Galen described human bones and muscle. He was the first to describe the physiology of muscle contraction, heart valves, and the structural differences between arteries and veins. He demonstrated that severing the spinal cord would cause paralysis, that the laryngeal nerve controlled the function of the larynx, and that urine passed from the kidneys to the bladder. Galen pioneered the diagnostic use of pulse rate and described cardiac arrhythmias. Galen also collected therapeutic plants in his extensive travels and explained their uses.

Galen correctly recognized that blood passes from the right to the left side of the heart through blood vessels but was not able to recognize the role of pulmonary circulation, which remained unknown for the next 1,400 years until William Harvey unravelled the physiology of circulation. Only a very few medical scientists have achieved so much in a single lifetime and that too, 1,800 years ago. Galen wrote extensively although only about 120 of his writings have survived.

However, Galen could not achieve final victory against obscurantism. But this is no discredit to him – it has not been achieved even as we enter the twenty-first century. Compared with the last 700 years before the birth of Christ – which witnessed such greats as Thales, Buddha, Confucius, Pythagoras, Plato, Hippocrates, Charaka, and many more – the 1,400 years that passed between Galen and William Harvey are a period of relative quiescence as far as medical science is concerned. Several factors must have contributed to this interlude but two deserve attention. Hippocratic medicine ended with Galen. What was revived after the dawn of the Renaissance was a new kind of approach, not only characterized by the absence of gods and magic but also supplemented by logic and experimental verification of conjectures. Since the current concept of the causes of diseases has nothing to do with Hippocrates' four humours theory, modern medicine is hardly a continuum of Hippocratic medicine; either way, it is an innocuous postulate.

Whatever Happened to Greek Medicine, Science, and Philosophy?

Toynbee (1946) has done a deep study of civilizations – how they emerged and how a few of them became extinct. Of course, Hellenic civilization remains one of the nineteen live civilizations like Western, Chinese, Indian, Egyptian, etc. Yet within any civilization there are periods of ups and downs, the causes of some can be identified and of others are evasive. I think it is generally agreed that the period of about 1,000 years from Thales to Galen, on both sides of the Christian era, was the high point of the Greek civilization. Why did it not continue? If modern medicine is indeed the continuity of Greek medicine, why did it have to find a home in England, Germany, and France? Why the great civilizations failed to carry their own accomplishments to yet higher a stage, and why they did not retain their superiority for all time, is a complex question.

Science, or even philosophy and romance, cannot grow unless overall productive forces develop. Economics seems to condition politics, politics in turn philosophy and science. Indeed, economics and politics are conjoint twins. Therefore, a more appropriate answer to my question is that productive forces did not grow in Greece but rather in England, Germany, and France, which were to overtake Greece in everything by a big margin.

Besides philosophy and medicine, among the well-known achievements of Greece were its wars of conquest under the leadership of Alexander the Great. These wars united Greece and expanded it, and gave rise to the intellectual centre of Alexandria in Egypt. However, the empire built by Alexander was destined to break down since it was more like the conquests of Genghis Khan (1162-1227) and Kublai Khan (1215-1294), without an internal base, and not like the later conquests by England and other colonial powers. Greece was reduced to city-states.

Just as certain socio-political factors are prerequisite for the birth of new ideas, they are also needed for the maturity and progress of these ideas. Materialist medicine does not solve the problems of health and disease. Quackery is also materialist medicine. Materialist medicine is a precondition for scientific advances. Medicine is not, and cannot be, a determining force in the social transformation of a society. What transforms a society is the development of its productive forces. In order for medicine to progress, it needed the breakdown of the feudal order. The breakdown of feudalism required many other developments, which were not evident in the Greece of Socrates, Plato, and Hippocrates. Nor did they become evident any time soon after. Greek sustenance was the sea, and Greek commerce was limited to neighbouring countries. Consequently, it was not in Greece but elsewhere in Europe that feudalism was coming under attack. The Industrial Revolution, an essential prerequisite for the evolution of the sciences, occurred elsewhere. Just as Greece woke up from approximately 700 BC to AD 200, it soon went to sleep basking in its past glory, neither prepared nor suited for further progress.

Notes

1. Russell, B. *The History of Western Philosophy* (New York: Simon & Schuster, 1945), xxii-xxiii.

2. Francis. A. *The Genuine Works of Hippocrates* (Baltimore: Williams & Wilkins, 1939). Introduction vi. Adams is the first translator into English of Hippocrates' Greek texts.

3. It has been said that there were more Jews in Alexandria (in Egypt but really as a Greek colony) than in Jerusalem.

4. Democedes was captured by Darius (550-486 BC), the Zoroastrian King of Persia. When Egyptian physicians of Darius failed to fix his twisted foot, Democedes was summoned. The Greek Democedes fixed Darius's twisted foot and in return his life was spared, but Democedes had to agree to become Darius's physician. Fortunately, Darius's wife got sick, and Democedes agreed to cure her if she could arrange his freedom, which is what happened.

5. *Ramayana* (written c. 300 BC and again in the sixteenth century) is a story of lord Rama (c. 2000 BC). The most popular version is in verse and is one of the holiest texts of Hindus. One episode in *Ramayana* is as follows: One of the three wives of Rama's father, Dashrath, wanted her son Bharat to inherit the kingdom and not the eldest son Rama as was the custom. Rama was sent into exile; his wife, Sita, and the younger brother, Lakshman, accompanied him. While in exile, Sita, was abducted by Ravana, the king of Lanka (the present Sri Lanka). Rama, assisted by his brother Lakshman and an army of monkeys led by the monkey god Hanuman, attacked Lanka to rescue Sita. In the ensuing war, Lakshman got seriously injured. The official healer pronounced that the life of Lakshman could be saved if, and only if, a certain herb (*Sanjivani*) be brought from a Himalayan mountain peak (*Dronagiri*), approximately three thousand kilometres north of Lanka. The Rama devotee, Hanuman, quickly reached the relevant mountain but could not recognize the herb in the midst of the thriving greenery, so he brought the entire mountain. The physician identified the relevant herb and Lakshman recovered.

The epic *Mahabharata* is the world's longest poem, with about 100,000 verses and its core was composed between the 5th and 6th centuries BC (Mulay, 2010). The great battle of Mahabharata, the subject of Peter Brook's play and films, was fought with chariots and bows and arrows as is the case in Homer's epics. There is a story of how Dronacharya, the greatest archer of all times, was killed deceptively. *Mahabharata* also contains the Hindu philosophical text *Bhagavad Gita*, which is essentially a sermon by Lord Krishna on the battlefield telling his favourite Arjuna that it is perfectly okay to fight against his cousins, the *Kauravas*.

It is said that Dronacharya, who was fighting on the side of the *Kauravas* could not be killed while armed. Lord Krishna devised a plan to disarm him. There was an elephant named Ashwathama, also the name of Dronacharya's son. Krishna got the elephant killed and the news was to be conveyed to Dronacharya. One of the five Pandava brothers who was on Lord Krishna's side was Yodhistir, who was known to never lie. He was therefore sent to Dronacharya to announce Ahwathama's death. In front of Dronacharya, Yodhistir pronounced that Ashwathama had been killed – but was it the elephant or …As soon as he finished the word killed, as per Krishna's instruction, there was a loud sound of a conch and trumpets, so Dronacharya could only infer that it was his son who had been killed. He surrendered his arms and was killed. The story goes that Dronacharya did not grow in a womb but outside it, in a jar, from the semen of a sage. Should one give a medical meaning to such episodes in the epics *Ramayana* and *Mahabharata*, as has been done to Homer's *Iliad* and *Odyssey*, and affirm, as some indeed do, that India had a herb that could revive the almost dead?

Should one conclude that the authors of these two Indian epics were physicians like Homer? Should one conclude that something faster than a jet existed in the India of antiquity to provide a return journey to the monkey god Hanuman with the heavy load of a mountain over a distance of about three thousand kilometres? Should one conclude that India had knowledge of *in vitro* fertilization thousands of years ago because Dronacharya grew up in a jar and not in the womb? In my opinion, the *Iliad* and the *Odyssey* have nothing to do with medicine; these are tales told in poems and, when translated into English, become more popular, more understandable, and more fascinating to Western audiences than would happen to similar tales from other lands.

6. Ganesh is the son of Shankar (Shiva, the destroyer, often represented by the phallus symbol), one of the three Hindu gods, the other two being Brahma, the creator (also the creator of Ayurveda; see Chapter 7) and Vishnu, the protector. It is said that when Ganesh was a small boy, his mother wanted to bathe in the inner courtyard (enclosed bathrooms did not exist in India until modern times). She told her son Ganesh that while she was bathing, no one should be allowed inside the house. So Ganesh obediently stood at the door. While Ganesh's mother was still bathing, his father, Shankar, arrived. Ganesh, aware of his mother's instructions, did not allow him into the house. Shankar got very angry and cut off Ganesh's head. When Ganesh's mother found it out, she was naturally upset and asked her husband to bring her son back to life. In order to soothe her, Lord Shankar cut off the head of an elephant and placed it on the severed neck of Ganesh. Of course, Ganesh became alive and for the rest of his life carried the elephant head on a human body.

7. Bernard, C. *Introduction á l'étude de la médecine expérimentale*. Paris, 1865, quoted by Hudson: Concepts of Disease in the West. In *The Cambridge World History of Human Disease*. Ed. K. F. Kiple (Cambridge: Cambridge University Press, 1993). 45-51.

References

Adams, F. *The Genuine Works of Hippocrates* (Baltimore: William & Wilkins, 1939.

Ibid., 1939a. 32-33.

Bodde, D. *Fung Yu-Lan: A Short History of Chinese Philosophy: A Systematic Account of Chinese Thought From its Origin to the Present Time* (New York: The Free Press, 1948).

Buck, A. H. *The Growth of Medicine from the Earliest Times to About 1800* (New Haven: Yale University Press, 1917).

Bynum, W. *The History of Medicine: A Very Short Introduction* (Oxford: Oxford University Press, 2008).

Conner, C. D. *A People's History of Science: Miners, Midwives, and "Low Mechanicks"* (New York: Nation Books, 2005), 117-160.

Cumston, C. E. *An Introduction to the History of Medicine: From the Time of the Pharaohs to the End of the XVIIIth Century* (New York: Dorset Press [1926], 1987).

Darwin, C. *The Origin of Species* ([1859] New York: Bantam Books, 1999)

Downs, R. B. *Books that Changed the World* (New York: New American Library: Penguin Group, 2004 [1956]).

Duffin, J. *History of Medicine: A Scandalously Short Introduction* (Toronto: University of Toronto Press, 1999).

Edelstein, Ludwig. "The Ethics of the Greek Physician." In *Ancient Medicine: Collected Papers of Ludwig Edelstein*. Ed. Lilian Temkin and Oswei Temkin (Baltimore: Johns Hopkins University Press, 1967).

Entralgo, Lain P. *Doctor and Patient* (New York: McGraw Hill, 1967).

Freeman, E. A. *Comparative Politics* (Danvers, MA: General Books, [1896], 2009).

Garrison, F. H. *An Introduction to the History of Medicine* (Philadelphia: W. B. Saunders, [1913], 1929).

Ibid., 1913a. 96.

Gorton, D. A. *The History of Medicine, Philosophical and Critical: From its Origin to the Twentieth Century* (New York: G. P. Putnam's sons, 1910).

Manyam, B. V. "Epilepsy in Ancient India," *Epilepsia* 33 (1992): 473-475.

Mulay, V. *From Rajahs and Yogis to Gandhi and Beyond* (Calcutta: Seagull Books, 2010) 333-336.

Neuburger, M. *History of Medicine* Vol. 1, Trans. Ernst Playfair (London: Oxford University Press, 1910 [1925]), 38.

Nutton, V. "Galen at the Bedside: Methods of a Medical Detective." In *Medicine and the Five Senses*. Ed. Roy Porter and William F. Bynum (New York: Cambridge University Press, 1993).

Osler, W. *The Evolution of Modern Medicine* (New Haven: Yale University Press, 1921).

Pingree, D. "Hellenophilia versus the History of Science." *ISIS (Journal of the History of Science Society)* 83 (1992): 554-563.

Porter, R. *The Greatest Benefit to Mankind: A Medical History of Humanity* (New York: W. W. Norton, 1997).

Ibid., 1997a. 73-82.

Robinson, V. *The Story of Medicine* (New York: Tudor Publishing, 1931).

Ibid., 1931a. 37-38.

Ibid., 1931b. 151-158.

Ibid., 1931c. 49.

Ibid., 1931d. 54.

Ibid., 1931e. 125-133.

Robinson, V. *Syllabus of Medical History* (New York: Froben Press, 1933), 15-16.

Russell, B. *The History of Western Philosophy* (New York: Simon & Schuster, 1945), 3.

Sarton, G. *Introduction to the History of Science: Vol. 1: From Homer to Omar Khayyam* (New York: Robert E. Krieger, 1927 [1975]), 82-83.

——. "The History of Sciences Versus the History of Medicine," *ISIS* 23 (1935): 315-320.

——. *A History of Science: Hellenic Science and Culture in the Last Three Centuries* (Cambridge: Harvard University Press, 1959), 136.

Sigerist, H. E. *A History of Medicine V.II: Early Greek, Hindu, and Persian Medicine* (Oxford: Oxford University Press, 1961).

Ibid., 1961a. 4.

Ibid., 1961b. 317.

Smith, G. E. *The Ancient Egyptians and the Origin of Civilization* (London: Harper & Brother, 1911).

Spencer, H. *Principles of Biology V.1 and 2* [1864] (Denever, MA: General Books, 2009).

Toynbee, A. *A Study of History* – Abridgement of Vol. I-VI by D. C. Somervell (Oxford: Oxford University Press, 1946a), 1-2.

Ibid., 1946b. 55-56.

Tripathi, M., Maheshwari, M. C., Jain, S., and Padma, M. V. "Ayurvedic Medicine and Epilepsy" *Neurological Journal of Southeast Asia* 5 (2000). 1-4.

Warner, J. H. "The History of Science and the Sciences of Medicine," *OSIRIS* 10 (1995): 164-193.

CHAPTER 9

The Age of Stagnation of Medical Science

To be sure, it is commonplace that birth, flowering and decline constitute the iron circle in which everything human is enclosed, through which it must pass. Thus it would not have been surprising if Greek philosophy, after having reached its zenith in Aristotle, should then have withered. But the death of the hero resembles the setting of the sun, not the bursting of an inflated frog.

Karl Marx[1]

Origen's[2] eloquent argumentation that the teachings of Aristotle and Plato were not incompatible with the teachings of Jesus Christ, acted as a bridge over which antiquity walked into medievalism. Origen's views on the preexistence of the human soul of Christ before he became divine, aroused resentment among his brethren ...he was exiled and excommunicated ...from this time on, a new intolerance ruled the world: the ecclesiastical party which yielded political power was the only orthodox party, and in the name of God destroyed its opponents. Even the crimes of imperial Rome grow pale in comparison with the amount of human blood that was now to be shed over myths.

Victor Robinson[3]

Introduction

The primary objective of this book is to analyze factors responsible for the evolution of medicine as a science. However, because progress is not linear, I feel obliged to discuss factors contributing to the decline and stagnation of medicine as well.

Almost all historians agree that the Christian era, especially from the time of Galen until the Renaissance, could be characterized as the "middle ages" of science in Europe. During this period, Greek philosophy and science not only did not advance but also, in some way, regressed. A similar setback to medicine was also witnessed in India with the decline of Buddhism in about the fourth century AD. On the other hand, during the same period, China had increased its interaction with the outside world, especially Buddhism, and if anything, it was being enriched. Likewise, most of this period registered gigantic progress in Islamic science until the time of Omar Khayyam (1048-1131). In that sense, the period of regression in science from Galen to William Harvey in Europe does not represent a universal phenomenon within that space and time; however, the fact that a regression in medical science occurred in Greece, Italy, and the rest of Europe is of special significance because it is in Europe that rigorous medical science ultimately matured.

The Decline of Civilizations

The decline of civilizations is an aspect of evolution; however, it must not be treated as an incubation period for new advances, although more frequently than not it is so. Toynbee (1946) treats the breakdown and disintegration of civilizations as two different phases where the latter does not necessarily follow the former. In that sense, what happened in Europe was merely a breakdown and not disintegration; the breakdown was followed by rapid growth and later regeneration. Egyptian civilization falls in the other category, where breakdown led to disintegration.

As I revise this book in 2012, we are in an unusual international upheaval, starting with the heinous attack on the World Trade Centre in New York on September 11, 2001, which killed nearly three thousand unsuspecting citizens. Since then, there have been wars in lands far away from the US, relentless terrorist attacks on public places, mindless suicide bombings, extraordinary security measures, arduous air travel restrictions, and a general sense of panic. However, world civilization has substantially advanced and no civilization alive today is likely to disintegrate. In my opinion, this turbulence, which has now persisted for eleven years and is likely to persist for sometime, will resolve into a new situation of peace and tranquillity. If the Taliban are not able to cause irreparable damage to Islam, Islam may well re-enter the golden age that it enjoyed from its birth to Omar Khayyam. This, however, is another subject.

The decline of Hellenic civilization was already apparent in the post-Aristotle period (Bernal 1954a). The Hellenic empire built by Alexander was destined to fall apart; this was not a bad thing in itself. But how and why it happened is important. Feudal expansionism, which both Greece and Rome exercised, by nature, was not sustainable. It had to break and break into pieces. Alexander's empire, which extended from Egypt to Persia, and with ventures like that of the Mongols, to as far as India, broke down into city-states with multiple centres of power. It had no mechanism of sustaining itself other than by a centralized powerful army. The violent feud between generals and other aspirants was natural. The only thing that could bring order within the social conditions existing at that time was religion. And that is what happened. The era of Christianity was inaugurated on the ruins of Greco-Roman empire, but not without a cost.

Compared with the period 700 BC to AD 200 – which nurtured Thales, Pythagoras, Socrates, Plato, Aristotle, Hippocrates, and Galen in Europe; Gautam Buddha, Sushruta, and Charak in India; and Confucius in China – the thousand years that passed between Galen and the Renaissance are a period of quiescence in science and technology. Several factors must have contributed to this interlude, but two deserve special attention.

By the time of Galen, two of the three monotheistic religions – Judaism and Christianity – had already come into being; the third one, Islam, was to arrive in about five hundred years. It too had an impact on science and technology, and this has been presented in Chapter 10. While Judaism, the oldest of the three monotheistic religions, had neither a state nor an army or crusaders and had a democratic tradition, Christianity was gifted with all these without provision for dissent. Rather rapidly, Christianity spread to a large part of Europe. Religion, being an overpowering philosophy, had to and did influence the course of practically all events in Europe, including the development of medical science.

Religion and Science

In its earlier phases, it was the need of Christianity to counter, forbid, and create fear of science in order to establish the authority of the Church; its expansion was aggressive and its assertion forceful. Since the base of Christianity was primarily Europe, it was there that the principal conflict between religion and science manifested itself. According to Mahner and Bunge (1996): "Science and religion are not only different but in fact incompatible." Many sociological observations would support this hypothesis but none as forcefully as the scenario in medieval Europe. On one side was the mighty church, and on the other side were the scattered and unorganized scientists, castigated by the church on the one hand and perceived as allies of the church by the oppressed citizenry on the other hand.

For complex socio-political reasons, Christianity and Islam influenced science differently until at least the eleventh century. Religion is an institution and cannot be equated simply with the religious doctrine inscribed in the sacred books. There are definite reasons for the birth of religions within any social framework. In the European context, not only slaves but even ordinary citizens experienced the tyranny of the aristocracy. They could easily perceive the kinship between the aristocracy, the philosophers, the scientists, and the men of medicine. Bernal (1954b) writes:

> To the religious it was not only idolatry but all that went with the hated, upper-class State that was abominable; the luxury, the art, the philosophy, the sciences were all signposts on the way to hell. Augustine (354-430) and Ambrose (339-397), turning from the wicked learning to holy nonsense, were just as much part of the movement as the monk-led mob who stoned (to death) Hypatia (370-415), one of the last Greek (woman) mathematicians.

While ordinary citizens, oppressed by Roman tyranny, were eager to find respite in Christianity, it is ultimately the church, especially from the fourth century on, that stood as an independent body challenging the empire. A new culture emerged, which asserted that everything is known and written in the holy books; what was demanded of humanity was to imbibe the truth as revealed by the messengers of God and follow rather than dispute and discover new things, or create doubt about the old.

Similar developments were taking place in far-off India as well. Buddhism, which had engulfed most of India without the use of the sword and had spread as far as China, especially through the efforts of Emperor Asoka, faced its own crisis. The Hindu zealot king *Pusyamitra Sunga* (185-151 BC) launched a ruthless persecution of Buddhists. Adi Shankara (788-820) from Kerala undertook the task of re-establishing Vedantic Hinduism in south India. The Hun invasion in North Western India in the sixth century, followed by the Turkish invasion, practically destroyed Buddhism in the place of its birth. Along with the decline of Buddhism, Ayurveda, the Indian art and science of healing, too became a holy dictum with roots in the Vedas; it began to fossilize.

There was yet another factor contributing to the stalemate in sciences in Europe. Science and technology are not the same, but they are twins. They do not spring on their own – rather, from the need to create productive forces. Evolution in productive forces needs renovation in technology.

Technology needs science, which, in turn, advances technology. Although health care is needed all the time, the state of public health is greatly determined by the availability of goods and services on the one hand and the physical effort needed to procure them on the other hand. The feudal social order presents the worst possible scenario for the progress of and accessibility to the overall health care system, which necessarily involves innovations in medical science. The period with which we are concerned here is when Europe was going through a transition to feudalism.

Bernal (1954c) writes:

> *The conditions of feudal production reduced the demand for useful science to a minimum. It was not to increase till trade and navigation created new needs in the later Middle Ages. Intellectual effort was to go in another direction and largely in the service of a radically new feature of civilization – organized religious faiths* [emphasis in original].

Thus post-Galenic Europe was either not conducive or positively hostile to advances in the sciences and philosophy. It had to wait for the Industrial Revolution to make a new beginning. The post-Charaka status of medicine in India is a different story because feudalism reigned supreme till the 20th century. As happens too often, august personalities inadvertently generate followers more than innovators, and this also acts as a roadblock. In this way, the towering personalities of Hippocrates (Temkin, 1991) and Galen (Mattern, 2008) in Greece, Italy and the continent in general became a deterrent rather than a stimulus for research and renovation in medicine. The stalemate lasted for one thousand years.

The book *De Medicina Praecepta* by Serenus Sammonicus (c. – 211), who was murdered in 211 by Caracalla, appeared in Europe at the time. *De Medicina Praecepta* wound out to nine thousand metrical feet; in it, charms and amulets replaced diagnosis and medicine. Sammonicus's famed recipe ABRACADABRA, if stripped of a letter in all succeeding lines and then hung around the neck, was a sure way of forcing the demon to release its grip on the victim. In his book *The Story of Medicine*, Robinson (1931) gives numerous examples of absurdities to which medicine had sunk in Europe in the immediate post-Galenic period. In a way, it was a dark age for sciences, especially for medicine. The Greek language begins to disappear from Europe, and by the fourth century, Rome again becomes a Latin city. In this process, Greek knowledge becomes generally inaccessible.

The New Beginning

In a chapter titled "Ascendancy of the Modern Western Civilization," Toynbee (1956) writes:

> The spread of the Modern Western Civilization over the face of the planet has been the most prominent single feature in the history of the Mankind during the last four or five centuries. The Modern Western sailing-ship was the instrument and the symbol of the West's ascendancy in the World during the Modern Age of Western history . . . .

The discovery of the New World required new tools. Elements for the Industrial Revolution were gradually coming into being. Precisely for these reasons, the evolution of medicine proceeded in Europe and stagnated, or rather came to a halt, in India, China, Egypt, and elsewhere.

This stage of medicine, indeed, coincides with socio-political developments in the world. Galen's influence was limited to Europe, but it was so immense that experimental physiology and anatomy made no further progress until the end of the Middle Ages. The medical world moved on from Galenism only with the appearance of Andreas Vesalius's (1514-1564) work on anatomy in 1543 and William Harvey's work on blood circulation in 1628.

Notes

1. Marx, K. In the "The Difference between the Democritean and Epicurean Philosophy of Nature," 1841. (http://www.marxists.org.archive/marx/works/1841/dr-theses/inex.htm).

2. Origen Adamantius (AD *c.* 185-254) was born in Egypt and taught in Alexandria. He was a *neo-Pythagorean, neo-Platonist,* and ascetic. He was tortured to death for his nonconformist views.

3. Robinson, V. *The Story of Medicine* (New York: Tudor, 1931), 136.

References

Bernal, J. D. *Science in History* (New York: Cameron Assoc. 1954a), 162.

Ibid., 1954b. 167.

Ibid., 1954c. 180-182.

Mahner, M. and Bunge, M. "Is Religious Education Compatible with Science Education?" *Science & Education* 5 (1996) 101-123.

Mattern, S. P. *Galen & the Rhetoric of Healing* (Baltimore: Johns Hopkins University Press, 2008).

Robinson, V. *The Story of Medicine* (New York: Tudor Publishing, 1931), 193-237.

Temkin, O. *Hippocrates in a World of Pagans and Christians* (Baltimore: Johns Hopkins University Press, 1991).

Toynbee, A. *A Study of History* – Abridgement of Volumes I-VI by D. C. Somervell (Oxford: Oxford University Press, 1946), 360-370.

——. *A Historian's Approach to Religion* (Oxford: Oxford University Press, 1956), 147-148.

CHAPTER 10

Islamic Medicine

After the eleventh century, although there was no spectacular collapse, it is evident that the best days of Islamic science were over. There were still brilliant individual scientists. One of the greatest, Averroes, dates from the twelfth century, and Ibn Khaldun [1332-1406] comes as late as the fourteenth, but they are no longer part of a widely based and living movement. The failure of science is here only one symptom of a general political and economic decay of Islam in its original form. Essentially it was the delayed effect of the same social forces that had brought about the decay of classical culture.

John Desmond Bernal[1]

Muslim scholars were not simply translators and copyists; they added extensive critical commentaries, sometimes based on their own original scientific investigations, to the corpus of Greek science. When scholarship in Europe began to revive in the twelfth century, the works of Aristotle and Galen recovered from Arabic sources had been refracted through the interpretive lenses of Ibn Rushd (Averroës), Ibn Sina (Avicenna), al-Razi (Rhazes), and many others.

Clifford Conner[2]

Introduction

Lucien Leclerc (1876) published the first comprehensive documentation of Islamic science and medicine – specifically in Egypt, Persia, and Spain. In subsequent years, most, but not all, books on history of science or medicine have dealt specifically with Islamic medicine. The book *Introduction to the History of Science* by Sarton (1927) is a chronological narrative of sciences, a bit like Toynbee's presentation of the rise and fall of civilizations (Toynbee, 1946). Sarton refers to major Islamic contributions to sciences, with extreme sensitivity to the role of the eleventh century's Sufi Omar Khayyam as a distinguished mathematician, astronomer and philosopher, besides being the author of the Rubaiyat. Subsequent to Omar Khayyam, no noteworthy scholastic contribution of Islam has been documented; the reasons for this are complex and discussed later in this chapter.

In contrast to Sarton's approach, most other books on the history of science are organized thematically or according to their national roots. Sigerist (1961) has a chapter titled "Medicine in Ancient Persia," but it only covers the period before the arrival of Islam. Robinson (1931) titles a chapter of his book as "Arabian Medicine in the Middle Ages" and not as "Islamic Medicine;" he does not compliment Islam in the least for advancing medicine. Like Robinson, Osler (1921) only talks about Arabian medicine and primarily refers to the contribution of Islamic scholars as translators. Porter (1997a) gives the historical context of Islam, as well as the rise and fall of Islamic science and medicine. Cumston (1926) has a chapter "Islamic Medicine" in which he, like Conner (2005a) but unlike Osler (1921), stresses that Islamic scientists were more than just translators. O'Leary (1980) details how Greek knowledge reached Arabic scholars. Garrison (1929) has a chapter titled "The Mohammedan and Jewish Period"; he gives significant details about some of the great scientists and physicians of that period. The diplomat Michael Hamilton Morgan (2007) provides in an admiring tone an outline of Islam's history and many of the accomplishments of Islamic scientists.

My effort is to place Islamic science in a historic context, specifically because of the incorporation of two great civilizations, Persia and Mesopotamia, within the fold of Islam. The books *Science & Islam* by Ehsan Masood (2009) and *Islam and Science* by Pervez Hoodbhoy (1991) are excellent texts on Islamic contribution to science, including medical science, and prominently raise the same question about Islam as Needham raised about China. More recently, Dr. Sharif Kaf Al-Ghazal (2007) wrote a series of five articles on Islamic medicine, one of which makes a strong case for crediting Ibn al-Nafis (1213-1288) for the discovery of pulmonary circulation nearly four hundred years before William Harvey.

The Rise of Islam

Islam originated in Makkah (Latinized as Mecca), the birthplace of Prophet Muhammad. Even in the Prophet's lifetime (c.570-632), and especially after he had to flee from Makkah to Madinah (Medina) in 622, Islam had several thousand followers, including some Jewish rabbis, Christian bishops and clergymen, and even a Hindu king of south India. By the time of the birth of Islam, Christianity had already spread to a large part of Europe; Islam put a halt to it. Consequently, the expansion of Christianity had to wait for several centuries until advances in navigation, the development of slavery, missionaries, and colonization were put in place. In the intervening period, Islam spread from Sindh (now in Pakistan) to Egypt and to Spain, covering almost all the area within this triangle.

Reverend George Bush (1796-1859) opines: "No revolution recorded in history, if we except that effected by the religion of the Gospel, has introduced greater changes into the state of the civilized world, than that which has grown out of the rise, progress, and permanence of Mohammedanism" (Bush, 1833). Religion is a vast subject, and I do not intend to comment on it except on one aspect.

It is understandable that people somehow feel that the religion they acquired at birth is better than others, or at least as good. What is less understandable is that even religions imposed upon them become as much a part of their life, often more, as it would be had they acquired it by birth. In this sense, it is different from all other loyalties, including nationality. Virtually none of the immigrants from the South to the Western countries get fully integrated in the cultural and national ethos of the country they have adopted. With religion, it is different. Consequently, the loyalty of the new adherents to Islam, regardless of how they became Muslims, was supreme, and they made all the sacrifices needed for its further expansion.

While Christianity spread in areas that already had nation or city-states (the remnants of the Greco-Roman empire), and a history of organized governance, the demography of areas that accepted Islam in the very beginning was markedly different, as aptly described by Maxime Rodinson (1915-2004); he writes (Rodinson, 1971):

> What the Christian Church – like the community of Buddhist monks or even the laity – demands of the state is at least to afford it such aid and protection as will allow it to accomplish, as best as it can, its own mission. In contrast, the Muslim community ...originated in a stateless tribal society and was more or less compelled by circumstances to organize itself into a state almost from the beginning. The community of the faithful was at the same time a political structure, a state.[3]

The Impact of Islam on Civic and Political Life

The expansion of Islam and the birth of Islamic science is an accomplishment of a political state with an army and loyal followers. Islam changed the political profile of the tribal and primitive land of its birth and became a civilizing force with definite guidelines on personal, interpersonal, and sociological conduct. This is best illustrated by an episode in the Islamic conquest of Persia.

Chosroes (Khosrau, 501-579) ruled Persia from AD 531-579; he was a powerful despot with a love for science, a bit like Alexander the Great. Robinson (1931a) writes that during his rule, "Greek, Hindu, Jewish, Nestorians,[4] Syrian and Persian physicians mingled at Jundishapur[5] and Chosroes himself ordered Plato and Aristotle to be translated into Persian." Porter (1997b) opines that while physicians of different faiths gathered at Jundishapur, no medical academy existed there. Soon after Chosroes's death, Persia was invaded by Saracens,[6] turned Muslims.

Robinson (1931a) writes:

> The Iranian monarch was amazed. "Who are you to attack an empire?" he asked. "You, of all peoples the poorest, most disunited, most ignorant." The messenger of the Saracens was unabashed: "All that you say was once true. The Arabians were clothed in the hair garments of beasts; their food was green lizards; they buried their infant daughters alive; they feasted on dead carcasses and drank warm blood; they slew their relatives and boasted of the property they stole; we knew not good from evil, nor could we tell what was lawful and what was unlawful. All this is true no longer. God in his mercy has sent us a holy prophet who has given us the only true faith."

The two most important scriptures of Islam are the holy Qur'an and *Hadith*. Although there is some dispute on the origin of Qur'an (Spencer, 2012), the Holy Qur'an remains the undisputed supreme book of all Muslims; this is not the case with *Hadith* (Kamali, 2009). *Hadith* contains words spoken by the Prophet and were passed on orally and inscribed over centuries. There are many categories of *Haidth*. As well, the *Hadiths* of Sunni and Shiite Muslims are not identical. Because *Hadith* is subject to belief and interpretation, it is also a source of differences among Islamic clerics themselves and among Muslim scholars and intellectuals on issues such as dress, music, alcohol, rights of women, attitude toward infidels, and so on.

What we are witnessing in the Islamic world in the beginning of the twenty-first century, principally suicide bombings, of which Muslims themselves are the main target, emanates from one interpretation of Islam and is condemned by followers of another interpretation. However, I am raising this issue not for theological reasons but because this accounts for the decline of Islamic science in the post-Omar Khayyam period.

In the beginning, scientific endeavour became an integral part of Islamic culture of which there were two major expressions. One aspect comprised the assimilation of the existing scientific knowledge of Greco-Roman, Persian, and Indian origin and its translation into Arabic (O'Leary, 1980). The second aspect was to make original and independent discoveries, created partly by local needs and partly in the process of the analysis and interpretation of what they translated.

Background to Islamic Science

Christianity had been filling the vacuum caused by the collapse of the Roman Empire. Islam was to instil order into a tribal society. Two factors contributed to Islamic science. First, as mentioned above, was the rapid increase in the followers of Islam eager to start a cultured civilized life. Second, was the spread of Islam to Persia, Mesopotamia, and Egypt, which were already endowed with advanced civilizations and the culture of science. Hypothetically speaking, if Islam had remained confined to its birthplace and had not engulfed the great civilizations of Persia and

Mesopotamia in its fold, there may have been no reason to include the theme 'Islamic science'.

I have described the science and civilization of Egypt and Mesopotamia in Chapter 5. Persia is equally important, as a civilization, as a rival of Greece and as a conduit to the East, especially India. Prior to the arrival of Islam, the national religion of Persia was Zoroastrianism (Dhalla, 1938) and Persia had a rich civilization.[7]

Islamic Science on Two Legs

As I mentioned above, most historians only emphasize the role of Islamic scholars as translators of Greek knowledge into Arabic. The book *Aladdin's Lamp* by John Freely (2009) has the subtitle: *How Greek Science Came to Europe through the Islamic World*. If translating Greek science into Arabic was the only, or the main contribution of Islam, there would be no such a thing as Islamic science. After all, Arabic texts were retranslated into Latin by Christian monks, and that did not constitute a monk science. As several historians (Conner, 2005a; Cumston, 1926; Sarton, 1927) point out, Islamic scholars were more than just translators and copyists.

Moreover, Muslim scholars were not paid professional translators. The translators were intellectuals, and they translated what they deemed scientifically relevant. This in itself is an important aspect. Not only were they popularizing science by translating Greek texts into Arabic, they were also simultaneously grasping the scientific information contained therein. A lazier version of this venture is a serious and critical study of books. There has never been a historian, philosopher, scientist, and litterateur without an extensive study of books. If reading books enriches intellectual capacity, translating them surely does more. So if a certain Islamic scholar did nothing more than just translate important books, it can be taken that he simultaneously enhanced the pool of knowledge for himself and for society.

By the time of the birth of Islam, Greek science had stagnated or degenerated into magic. Early Greek science would practically be lost to the world had it not been rescued by the followers of Islam. According to Cumston (1926), Muslims earnestly believed that Islam favoured knowledge and science and they did their utmost to fulfil this mission. Nestorian physicians who had access to Greek literature and who faced persecution by the Christian establishments gathered in Baghdad (founded in AD 762) and were welcomed by Muslim rulers. The first tragedy of Greek science and philosophy was that by the second century BC, it had come under Roman control. Almost every Greek scientist and philosopher sought a shelter in Rome either for life or for prolonged periods. Even when Romans moved their capital to the Greek city of Byzantium in the fourth century AD, there was little of Greece there. Saint Augustine of Hippo had already announced, everything is done by God, at God's will, which ought not be tampered with by mortals and scientists. By the time Justinian (527-565) took control of the Byzantine Empire, Greek science had severely deteriorated and the Platonic Academy in Athens was closed.

It is at this critical juncture in the history of science that the Islamic scholars intervened. Baghdad was to emerge as the centre of learning, where the famous Bayt Al-Hikma, literally the House of Wisdom, came into existence. This is when the Abbasid caliph Al-Ma'mun (786-833) organised the translation of foreign books, not just classical Greek, but also Byzantine Greek, Pahlavi, Neo-Persian, and Syriac, into Arabic. He also wanted the Byzantine mathematician Leo (c. 790-869), who had the largest collection of the works of Archimedes of Syracuse (287-212 BC), to come to Baghdad, but the Byzantine emperor did not let that happen. The mathematician Al-Hajjaj Ibn Matar (786-833) translated Euclid of Alexandria's (325-265 BC) *Elements*. Aristotle's *Topics* and *Physics* were translated about the same time. Hunayn Ibn Ishaq (808-873), born a Nestorian, and Thabit Ibn Qurra (c. 836-901) translated the works of Hippocrates and Galen, Euclid's *Elements, De Materia Medica* by Dioscorides, and *Introduction to Arithmetic* by Nichomachus (c. 60-120). The programme of translation continued until about the eleventh century.

Freely (2009a) writes:

> Thus the diaspora of classical learning brought Greek thought from Athens to Rome, Constantinople, and Jundishapur. It took root in the new civilization that emerged in Western Europe, Byzantium, and the Islamic world,

three streams of culture whose eventual confluence would produce a renaissance of science.

Islamic Contribution to Science

Both Mesopotamia and Persia emerged as centres of Islamic science. Major contributions of Islam were in the area of astronomy, mathematics, philosophy, and medicine. Although the contribution in medical science was not as original or significant as in mathematics and astronomy, it is this that is alive today and exists in many parts of the world as Unani-Tibb medicine.

Baghdad caliph al-Mansur (712-775), also known as Abu Ja'far Abdulah ibn al-Masur, not only had Greek books translated but also employed three astrologers/astronomers in his court. More importantly, Al-Khwarizmi (c. 780-850) wrote his treatise *Kitab al-jabr wa'l-Muqabalah* (algebra). He used the Hindu numerals that eventually became the digits that we now use. The three Banu Musa brothers, Banu Musa Jafar Muhammad (800-after 873), Banu Musa Ahmad (805-after 873),[8] and Banu Musa Al-Hasan (810-after 873) were orphaned; they were adopted by the Baghdad caliph al-Ma'mun; all three brothers were mathematicians.

Freely (2009b) gives the following description of one of the mathematical feats of Banu Musa:

> *Al-Ma'mun (caliph of Baghdad) directed the Banu Musa to measure the circumference of the earth, to verify the measurements made by Eratosthenes (c. 276-196 B.C.) and other Greek scientists. The method used by the Banu Musa was to measure the north-south distance between two points in the Sinjar desert where the elevation of the polestar differed by one degree, whereupon they multiplied this by 360 to obtain the circumferences of the earth. The value they obtained, according to ibn Khallikan* [1211-1282], *was 8,000 farsakhs, or 24,000 miles; the presently accepted value is 24,092 miles.*

As in Baghdad, mathematics, medicine, and philosophy also excelled in Persia. The most important Persian of relevance to medical science was Abu Bakr Muhammad ibn Zakaria al-Razi, more commonly known in the West by its Latin equivalent Rhazes. Although a Persian, he is often addressed as the Arab Galen. Rhazes later moved to Baghdad where he attracted students from all over the world. He wrote extensively in Arabic on medicine and philosophy although most of his manuscripts are lost. Of Rhazes' surviving works, *Al-Hawi* (Latin, *Continens*) is significant. Rhazes also wrote on smallpox and measles and this treatise, named *De Peste* in Latin, went through almost forty editions. The notable feature of Rhazes' medical writings is the emphasis on diagnosis and treatment rather than on the mechanisms of diseases.

Rhazes was the first to address the question posed by me in this book – *Why People Prefer Quacks and Charlatans to Skilled Physicians?* Rhazes, like Charaka and Hippocrates before him also addressed the question of medical ethics in his treatise *On The Fact That Even Skillful Physicians Cannot Heal All Diseases.*

More than one thousand years before the national best seller *Perfect Health* of Deepak Chopra (1991), Rhazes wrote in *Tibb ar-Ruhani* (Spiritual Physick), a superb treatise (see Arberry, 1950), on the treatment of ailments involving both the body and the soul. Rhazes also wrote extensively on pharmaceuticals and commented on exorcism and incantations. Many eminent physicians followed Rhazes, including one notable Ali ibn al-Abbas al-Majusi (c. 925-994), whose main writing *Kitab al-Maliki* (Latin, *Liber Regius*) assesses the medical writings of his predecessors including Rhazes. Al-Majusi also wrote about poisons and antidotes and started the discipline of toxicology.

In addition to medicine, Islamic Persia also produced notable figures in astronomy, philosophy, and mathematics. The Persian astronomer Abd al-Rahman al-Sufi (903-986), also known as Azophi, is recognized for his *Treatise on the Constellation of the Fixed Stars*, which critically examines the works of the Egyptian astronomer and mathematician Ptolemy (c. 90-168); his manuscripts show forty-eight constellations along with positions, magnitude, and colours of all stars (Freely, 2009c).

Abu Rayhan al-Biruni (973-1050) was an eminent astronomer, mathematician, and geographer; he wrote on almost every subject of human interest including arithmetic, trigonometry, geometry, medicine, pharmacology, mechanics, philosophy, etc. It so happens that al-Biruni lived at the same time as the Persian despot Sultan Mahmud al-Ghazni (971-1030), who raided India no less than seventeen times between the years 1000 and 1026 to plunder especially Hindu temples for their riches; the most important attack was on Somnath in 1025. It seems that whenever he ran out of treasure, he attacked India and, in the process, destroyed the idols of 'infidels'. Al-Biruni accompanied Ghazni during his raids of India. However, being a scientist and not a religious fanatic, al-Biruni wrote *The Description of India* in which he details India's history, geography, science, religion, and society. Al-Biruni's work introduced Hindu mathematics to the Islamic world. Al-Biruni did much more; he wrote on the customs of various peoples, devised instruments to measure specific gravities of liquids, a mechanical device to measure the width of rivers, height of minarets, the direction of Makkah from any point, rotation and circumference of earth, the existence of gravity in heavenly bodies, to name a few. There have been only a few people in the history of the world with as many talents of excellence as those possessed by al-Biruni.

There were many other talented figures in the Islamic Persia. However, no description would be complete without reference to Ibn Sina (Avicenna: 980-1037) and the venerable Abu'l Fath Umar ibn Ibrahim al-Khayyami, commonly known as Omar Khayyam. Here is a brief description of Omar Khayyam, the mathematician, the physicist, the philosopher, and the litterateur; above all, he was a Sufi, a tradition taken to new heights by Jalaluddin Rumi (1207-1273), which has continued till today and which has certain universal features across religions. I am inclined to think that it is this philosophy of Sufism, which will ultimately save the world rocked by fanaticism not only within Islam but within all religions.

Khayyam's work on algebra is the culmination of Islamic research going beyond that done by al-Khwarizmi mentioned above. Khayyam "used both arithmetic and geometric methods to solve quadratic equations and employed a scheme of intersecting conics to solve cubic equations, an approach first taken by Archimedes" (Freely, 2009d). For better or worse, Omar Khayyam is more known for his Persian Rubaiyat. One might also speculate that within the intolerance prevailing in Persia and Afghanistan of today, Omar Khayyam might have incurred a fatwa for writing certain verses in the *Rubaiyat*, e.g.:

A Book of Verses underneath the Bough,
A Jug of Wine, a Loaf of Bread – and Thou
Beside me Singing in the Wilderness –
Oh, Wilderness were Paradise enow!

Islamic Spain tried to assimilate scientific and philosophical advances made by Muslim scholars in Mesopotamia and Persia. The person of great accomplishment in Spanish Islam was Ibn Rushd (Latin Averroës: 1126-1198), perhaps the last Muslim scholar of distinction. Ibn Rushd wrote commentaries on Aristotle as well as his own philosophical doctrine entitled *Decisive Doctrine about the Concordance between Revelation of Religion, Exposition of the Methods of Demonstration, and the Incoherence of the Philosophers.* He might well be the first philosopher to raise his voice against the discrimination to which women were subjected and which he felt was a serious problem within Muslim society. Ibn Rushd wrote:

> *Our society allows no scope for the development of women's talents. They seem to be destined exclusively to childbirth and the care of children, and this state of servility has destroyed their capacity for larger matters. It is thus that we see no women endowed with moral values, they live their lives like vegetables, devoting themselves to their husbands. From this stems the misery that pervades our cities, for women outnumber men by more than double and cannot procure the necessities of life by their own labors.* (Freely, 2009e)

Unani-Tibb (Hikmat)

Relative to Indian, Chinese, and Greek medicine, Islamic medicine, known by the name *Hikmat* or Unani-Tibb (also written as Yunani-Tibb), covers a shorter period. The Arabic (or Urdu)[9] word for Greece is *Unan*, which correctly identifies the Greek origin of Unani-Tibb, and its roots can be clearly traced to Hippocrates and Galen. Unlike all other known disciplines of medicine discussed in the preceding chapters, Unani-Tibb has no history of magic; this is due to two factors, namely, its roots in Hippocratic and Galenic medicine on the one hand and adherence to the teachings of *Hadith* on the other hand. There are numerous references to health, disease, and therapeutics in *Hadith*, but they are all essentially physical in nature albeit with reference to *Allah*, the Islamic equivalent of the word *God*. However, it still took some time to overcome pre-Islamic beliefs in *Jinni* and the belief that the "water of the well of Zamzam in Makkah had healing properties" (Porter, 1997a).

Unani-Tibb exists in the entire Islamic world as well as in India, which has the second largest Muslim population after Indonesia. The Urdu language (spoken in India and Pakistan) equivalent of Tibb is *Hikmat*, and the physicians practicing this art are known as Hakims. Almost all practitioners of Unani-Tibb medicine (Hakims) in India are Muslims although its recipients come from all religious backgrounds. In recent years, Tibb institutions have been established in Australia, the USA, the UK, South Africa, and countries of South Asia, North Africa, the Persian Gulf, and the Middle East. Tibbia is formally recognized as a medical system in India along with Ayurveda and homeopathy. A major pharmaceutical institution that emerged out of the practice of Unani-Tibb in India and Pakistan is the Hamdard (compassionate) Foundation, a major manufacturer of Unani medicines (Pati and Harrison, 2001). The charitable arm of this company has established Jamia (university) Hamdard, a modern institution based in Delhi, which now enjoys the status of a university.

Although the origin of Unani-Tibb is corpus Hippocraticum and Galen's medicine, it also has substantially new additions. Cumston (1926a) writes:

> Even in the realm of pure theory one meets with more than one manifestation of the philosophical spirit which inspired the learned men of Islam. They made more than one attempt to place in doubt the ideas then current, but they were timid and had no results. When one reads such reflections as those of the Arabian physician Najm ed-Din ibn el-Loboudi to the effect that the existence of the body and its preservation depend exclusively upon the blood and not upon the four humours, as was generally maintained by physicians and philosophers; when we consider the aphorism of the learned Arabian alchemist Geber, that "the various bodies are composed of the same elements, but in different proportions," one is tempted to believe that the great thinkers of this period foresaw many truths that modern discoveries have revealed.

The observation stated above both, with regard to the role of blood as opposed to four humours and the composition of the body, are closer to what modern science has established than is the case with Hippocrates' postulates on these matters. The originality of Islamic scholarship is also apparent if one examines the contribution of Ibn Sina (Avicenna), who wrote *Tibb el Unani* in his medical classic *al-Qanun* as well as Ishaq ibn Ali al-Ruhawi (1200 AD) who wrote *Adab el-Tibb* or medical ethics. Unani-Tibb is an advance over Hippocrates just as is modern medicine. For example, the *materia medica* of the Greek pharmacologist Pedanius Dioscorides had less than a thousand medicaments; Ibn Al-Baytar (AD 1188-1248) had a compendium of "over 3000 items, including 800 botanical drugs, 145 mineral drugs, and 130 animal drugs" (Porter, 1997c). Indeed, it is in the area of chemistry and pharmaceuticals that Muslim scientists were way ahead of anything that the Greeks had accomplished.

Conner (2005b) writes: "The [Islamic] alchemists 'discovered sal ammoniac, they prepared caustic alkalies' (the word *alkali* is a variant transliteration of *al-qili*, the Arabic term for sodium carbonate)." Likewise, Bernal (1954a) concludes that, "it was in chemistry, however, that the Islamic doctors, perfumers, and metallurgists made their greatest contribution to the general advancement of science." Indeed Bernal (1954a) attributes *the beginning of scientific chemistry* to Arab Muslims.

During the last five hundred years, Unani-Tibb flourished in India as one of the two major medical disciplines, the other being Ayurveda. Eminent Hakims (practitioners of Unani-Tibb) have claimed that "the formative influence of Unani-Tibb's history in India was stronger and more relevant to Tibb today than its Greek legacy" (Attewell, 2007). There is a substance to this argument because nearly two hundred million Indian Muslims would either seek modern medicine or Unani medicines or homeopathy, but only rarely Ayurvedic medicine. Ayurvedic medicine almost does not exist in Pakistan and Bangladesh, which were formerly part of one country that is India. On the other hand, Unani-Tibb exists in both these countries. So the population of South Asia that relies on Unani-Tibb is greater than the total population of any single country of the world. Surprisingly, far less literature in English exists on the Unani-Tibb system of medicine than on other medical schools such as homeopathy, Ayurveda, and Chinese medicine. Attewell's book (2007) is also an excellent treatment of the history of Tibb in India during and before British colonial rule but does not deal with the Unani-Tibb medical discipline. The same can be said about other books (Pati and Harrison, 2001; Sivaramakrishnan, 2006; Freely, 2007) that deal with medical systems in colonial India (see Chapter 6).

Since the theoretical foundation of Unani medicine is Corpus Hippocraticum, my own commentary on its merits or demerits is the same as I presented in the chapter on Greek medicine. Since effective therapy for most diseases was rather poor until the middle of the twentieth century by any school of medicine, it is indeed futile to evaluate the relative merit of Unani-Tibb, or for that matter any system of medicine, from the point of view of therapeutic efficacy.

Notwithstanding this limitation, there have been steady advances in rational medical systems through the acquisition of new drugs, mainly natural, over the years. In that sense, Unani medicine is certainly superior to what Hippocrates and Galen did.

Interestingly, all medical systems have discovered something that goes by the general terminology of tonics and health aids. For example, Indian Hakim Abdul Hameed (1908-1999) made products like *Safi, Sharbate Rooh Afza, Sinkara*, gripe water, *Joshina*, all household names; *Sharbate Rooh Afza* enjoys the same popularity in South Asia as Coca-Cola does in America. I have heard several physicians say, and I subscribe to this in my own experience, that *Joshina* (a mixture of herbs) is, by far, the best remedy against the common cold; its efficacy depends not only on what it contains but also because it is boiled and then taken as a hot beverage like tea. My literature search did not find if *Joshina* contains vitamin C despite boiling, which has been strongly advocated by Linus Pauling (1970). I am not aware of any studies comparing the efficacies of Ayurvedic, homeopathic and Unani-Tibb medicine; my guess is that if and when it will be done, Unani-Tibb will be the winner.

The Decline of Islamic Science

It is generally agreed that the Golden Age of Islamic science ended with Omar Khayyam. Science must make progress for it to remain relevant.

In that sense, there might have been some progress in Unani-Tibb, but not enough to make it into modern medical science. In terms of other sciences such as physics, mathematics, and astronomy, as well as in philosophy, the decline in Islamic science in the last seven hundred years has been steady and spectacular. It is also possible that years after the founding of Islam, orthodox clerics misused the Holy Qur'an to suppress philosophical discourse in the Islamic world. Why did physics, mathematics, and astronomy share the same fate is a challenging question, and perhaps sensitive enough to remain unanswered.

The Pakistani physicist Pervez Amirali Hoodbhoy (2007) puts the question in contemporary times in the following words:

> The question I want to pose – perhaps as much to myself as to anyone else – is this: With well over a billion Muslims and extensive material resources, why is the Islamic world disengaged from science and the process of creating new knowledge? To be definite, I am here using the 57 countries of the Organization of the Islamic Conference (OIC) as a proxy for the Islamic world.

After providing data that indeed science is lagging behind in the Islamic world, Hoodbhoy goes on to answer his own question. The reasons, according to Hoodbhoy, are not the marginalization of women in educational institutions, relative lack of democracy in most of the Islamic countries, and religious orthodoxy. When it comes to identifying reasons, Hoodbhoy's arguments are rational but not sufficient. For example, it is true, as Hoodbhoy says, that the West's hostility toward Iranian Mohammad Mossadegh (1882-1967), Indonesian Ahmed Sukarno (1901-1970), and Egyptian Gamal Abdel Nasser and more importantly the arming of Islamic fundamentalists in Afghanistan to counter Soviet presence – all help "to create an extensive globalized jihad network, which became a deterrent to science." However, I do not think that this is sufficient explanation. Indeed Hoodbhoy's call that "Muslims must be introspective and ask what went wrong" contains the answer but is not the answer.

One might also ask why there is so much emphasis on the decline of Islamic science. Is it uniquely an Islamic phenomenon? Is the discriminatory attitude of the West to Muslims the root cause? When we look at all these questions singly, and more importantly together, we find we are not close to the correct answer. Jewish people have a longer history of discrimination even in the USA until the mid-twentieth century, but never lagged behind in science. The current world population is approximately seven billion, of which only approximately one billion reside in the scientifically advanced countries of Europe, England, the USA, Canada, Australia, Japan, and Israel, the centre of science. Muslims, Chinese, Indians, Africans, each are about one billion, and that is where science is in a sad state. One might as well ask why China and India, each with about one billion people, the same as the world population of Muslims, are lagging in science.

If one examines the totality of the state of affairs of science, the first answer is that backwardness in science is not confined to the Muslims. Science is behind in Africa, Latin America, Eastern Europe, and a large part of Asia. Science is behind in Greece as well. It would also appear that replacement of the feudal mode of production by the capitalist mode of production is the minimal but not sufficient precondition for the growth of science. A change in mode of production does not completely change the culture but it does start the process. There ought to be freedom of expression, open discourse, and dissent as the drivers of scientific thought. I feel optimistic that all these issues are being raised in the Islamic world. Persian Gulf countries are beginning to host major international scientific conferences. Democratization of Saudi Arabia, Malaysia, and Indonesia is also necessary for the growth of science in the Islamic world. Ultimately, however, what can change the state of science in the Islamic world is the same as is necessary in other parts as well, including India and China. Capitalism is a powerful system and must force society to espouse liberalism as well as engage in science and technology and bypass religion if it comes in the way. I would rather paraphrase Hoodbhoy's question as follows: Why does feudalism, and particularly feudal culture, reign supreme in the Islamic world?

I would not venture to answer this.

Notes

1. Bernal, J. D. *Science in History, Vol. 1* (New York: Cameron Assoc. 1954), 205.

2. Conner, C. D. *A People's History of Science* (New York: Nation Books, 2005),162.

3. Maxime Rodinson. *Muhammad*. Trans. Anne Carter (New York: The New Press, 1980), xvi-xvii.

4. Nestorianism is akin to Christianity and was founded by *Nestorius*, patriarch of Constantinople from 428-431. Nestorians advocated Jesus to be both human and divine, which led to their persecution and they were forced to flee to Persia, where they were welcomed by Zoroastrian Chosroes. Debarred from political power, they became healers. Robinson, V. *The Story of Medicine* (New York: Tudor, 1931), 138-139.

5. Jundishapur of Persia was like Alexandria. Under Chosroes (531-579), it was the place where "Greek, Hindu, Jewish, Nestorian, Syrian and Persian physicians mingled in Jundishapur." Robinson, V. *The Story of Medicine* (New York: Tudor, 1931), 143.

6. Nomadic barbarian tribe of Arabia who became followers of Islam. See Bush, G. *The Life of Mohammed: Founder of the Religion of Islam, and the Empire of Saracens* (New York: J&J Harper, 1833).

7. It is perhaps the first monotheistic religion founded by the Prophet Zoroaster who lived around 1000 BC. During the period of Zoroastrianism, Persia had a rich civilization. The Persian king Darius I the Great (521-486 BC), a follower of Zoroastrianism, had done a better (or worse) job in extending the Persian Empire from Egypt to India than was accomplished by Alexander the Great. Persian culture was indigenous but was enriched by Egypt, India, and also China. Zoroastrianism was tolerant to Judaism. The Islamic conquest of Persia was followed by persecution of Zoroastrians, who were unwilling to espouse Islam; they had to flee from Persia and most of them settled in and around Bombay (now Mumbai) in India (see Dhalla, 1938). They built an exemplary community life, perhaps reminiscent of their old tradition, which uniquely ensures until today, the well-being of all members of the community, somewhat similar to social life among the Ismailia Muslims. The current population of Zoroastrians is approximately one hundred thousand; and yet their contribution in science, entrepreneurship, literature, music and medicine stands out, which undoubtedly reflects their heritage. The only other community whose contribution to science, philosophy, and literature is disproportionately so great is the Jewish people; the reasons for this are complex and beyond the scope of this book.

8. Dates of deaths of Banu Musa brothers are approximate; they died sometime after AD 873.

9. Urdu language emerged in India from all North Indian languages as well as Arabic and Persian during the rule (1628-1658) of Mughal Emperor Shah Jahan (1592-1666), who built the famous Taj Mahal in Agra as a monument to his favourite wife, Begum Mumtaz Mahal. Urdu is written from right to left in Arabic script. The spoken Urdu, and the other North Indian language *Hindi* or *Hindustani*, written from left to right in the Sanskrit alphabet do not differ much grammatically and share sufficient common words to be understood by speakers of either language.

References

Al-Ghazal, S. K. "The Influence of Islamic Philosophy and Ethics on the Development of Medicine in the Islamic Civilization," *Foundation for Science Technology and Civilization*, http//www.fstc.co.uk. 2007.

——. "The Valuable Contribution of al-Razi (Rhazes) in the History of Pharmacy," *Foundation for Science, Technology, and Civilization*, http//www. fstc.co.uk. 2007.

——. "Ibn al-Nafis and the Discovery of Pulmonary Circulation," *Foundation for Science, Technology, and Civilization*, http//www.fstc.co.uk. 2007.

Ibid., 2007a.

Arberry, A. J. *Rhazes, The Spiritual Physic (Tibb ar-Ruhani)*. Trans. Arthur J. Arberry (London: John Murray (http://oll.libertyfund.org/title/1791/97655).

Attewell, G.N.A. *Refiguring Unani Tibb: Plural Healing in Late Colonial India* (London: Orient Longman, 2007),15.

Bernal, J. D. *Science in History* (New York: Cameron Assoc. 1954), 192-207.

Ibid., 1954a. 202.

Bush, G. *The Life of Mohammed: Founder of the Religion of Islam, and of the Empire of the Saracens* (New York: J & J Harper, 1833),17.

Chopra, D. *Perfect Health: The Complete Mind/Body Guide* (New York: Harmony Books, 1991).

Conner, C. D. *A People's History of Science* (New York: Nation Books, 2005),161-165.

Ibid., 2005b. 164.

Cumston, C. G. *An Introduction to the History of Medicine* (New York: Dorset Press, 1926), 180-211.

Ibid., 1926a. 190-191.

Dhalla, M. N. *History of Zoroastrianism* (New York: Oxford University Press, 1938. Available free online).

Freely, J. *Aladdin's Lamp: How Greek Science Came to Europe through the Islamic World* (New York: Alfred A. Knopf, 2009).

Ibid., 2009a. 71.

Ibid., 2009b. 79.

Ibid., 2009c. 87.

Ibid., 2009d. 91.

Ibid., 2009e. 117-118.

Garrison. F. H. *An Introduction to the History of Medicine* (Philadelphia: W. B. Saunders, 1929), 126-139.

Hoodbhoy, P. A. *Islam and Science: Religious Orthodoxy and the Battle for Rationality* (London: Zed Books, 1991).

——. "Science and the Islamic World – the Quest for Rapprochement," *Physics Today* 60 (2007): 49-55.

Kamali, M. H. *A Textbook of Hadith Studies: Authenticity, Compilation, Classification and Criticism of Hadith* (Leicestershire: The Islamic Foundation, 2009).

Leclerc, L. *Histoire de la médecine Arabe* (New York: Burt Franklin (first published in Paris, 1876; available free on line).

Masood, E. *Science & Islam: A History* (London: Icon Books, 2009).

Morgan, M.H. *Lost History: the Enduring Legacy of Muslim Scientists, Thinkers, and Artists* (Washington DC: National Geographic 2007).

O'Leary, D. E. *How Greek Science Passed to the Arabs* (London: Routledge & Kegan Paul, [1949], 1980).

Osler, W. *The Evolution of Modern Medicine* (New Haven: Yale University Press, 1921), 68-79.

Pati, B. and Harrison, M. *Health, Medicine and Empire: Perspectives on Colonial India* (Hyderabad: Orient Longman, 2001).

Pauling, L. *Vitamin C and the Common Cold* (New York: Bantam Books, 1970).

Porter, R. *The Greatest Benefit to Mankind: A Medical History of Humanity* (New York: W. W. Norton, 1997a), 92-105.

Ibid., 1997b. 94.

Ibid., 1997c. 101.

Robinson, V. *The Story of Medicine* (New York: Tudor Publishing, 1931a), 138.

Rodinson, M. *Muhammad*, Tr. From French into English, Anne Carter in 1971 (New York: The New Press, 2002), pp xvi-xvii.

Sarton, G. *Introduction to the History of Science: Vol. 1, From Homer to Omar Khayyam* (New York: Robert E. Krieger Publishing, 1927).

Sigerist, H. E. *A History of Medicine V. 2: Early Greek, Hindu, and Persian Medicine* (Oxford: Oxford University Press, 1961), 197-207.

Sivaramakrishnan, K. *Old Potions, New Bottles: Recasting Indigenous Medicine in Colonial Punjab* (1850-1945) (New Delhi: Orient Longman, 2006).

Spencer, R. *Did Muhammad Exist? An Inquiry into Islam's Obscure Origins* (Wilmington: ISI Books, 2012).

Toynbee, A. *A Study of History* – Abridgement by D. C. Somervell (Oxford: Oxford University Press, 1946).

CHAPTER 11

The Age of Witch Hunt

It is often attempted to palliate slavery by comparing the state of slaves with our poorer countrymen: if the misery of our poor be caused not by the laws of nature, but by our institutions, great is our sin; but how this bears on slavery, I cannot see; as well might the use of the thumb-screw be defended in one land, by showing that men in another land suffered from some dreadful disease. Those who look tenderly at the slave owner, and with a cold heart at the slave, never seem to put themselves into the position of the latter; what a cheerless prospect, with not even a hope of change! picture to yourself the chance, ever hanging over you, of your wife and your little children – those objects which nature urges even the slave to call his own – being torn from you and sold like beasts to the first bidder! And these deeds are done and palliated by men, who profess to love their neighbours as themselves, who believe in God, and pray that his Will be done on earth! It makes one's blood boil, yet heart tremble, to think that we Englishmen and our American descendants, with their boastful cry of liberty, have been and are so guilty …

Charles Darwin[1]

Because the Medieval Church, with the support of kings, princes and secular authorities, controlled medical education and practice, the Inquisition (witch-hunt] constitutes, among other things, an early instance of the "professional" repudiating the skills and interfering with the rights of the "nonprofessional" to minister to the poor. Contemporary physicians display the same intolerance toward medically untrained therapists; and psychiatrists, toward those not legitimized by their own guild.

Thomas S. Szasz[2]

Introduction

I described in Chapter 4 how medicine originated in the form of witchcraft or spiritual medicine, which were the earliest attempts to explore the causes of illnesses and the methods of healing; this assumption is in accordance with the postulates of Jules Michelet [1798-1874] (1863), Matilda Joslyn Gage [1826-1898] (1893), Sir James George Frazer [1854-1941] (1922), William Henry Davenport Adams [1821–1891] (1889) and numerous other historians.

In contrast to witchcraft, the witch hunt is anti-medicine, anti-science and inhuman.

For a variety of reasons, witch hunting was primarily a European phenomenon and, paradoxically, dawned at the same time as the Renaissance and the Industrial Revolution.

There are many books on this subject but this Chapter is mainly based on the following books or articles: (Cawthorne, 2003; Ehrenreich and English, 1973; Maple, 1962; Maxwell-Stuart, 2001; McGough, 2006; Michelet, 1863). The Salem witch trials in the USA in the late seventeenth century, though small in comparison with the European witch hunt, are subjects of many books (Aronson, 2003; Boyer and Nissenbaum, 1974; Hill, 1995; Karlsen, 1987; Norton, 2002), and the beautiful play *The Crucible* by Arthur Millar [1915-2005] (1952).

The Birth of the Witch Hunt

The practice of witch hunt may have begun soon after the decline in the healing art of witchcraft and the beginning of materialist medicine. The witchcraft practitioners were probably not condemned to death but they and their healing arts were certainly discredited. What is especially significant is that, while miracle healers were central to religions, lay healers were demonized as witches; the elements of this paradox can be easily found in both the Old and New Testament as well as in Hindu religious texts (Saletore, 1981).

The first known persecution of a witch occurred in Egypt about 1300 BC (Fox, 1968). However, the witch hunt, as an organized activity, came much later. Conditions had to be created to garner social approval of witch hunting.

While the Renaissance gave rise to a liberal culture divorced from the authority of the church, it also generated hostility to superstition, magical feats, and unlicensed professionalism. The latter took many forms, one of which translated into witch hunting. The witch hunt also became a justification for the assertion of the "true spirit" of the Bible. Witches were branded heretics deserving the severest and the cruellest possible punishment.

As well, the practice of witch hunting needed the sanction of the Church and the blessings of venerable personalities of the time. It needed mass approval of cruelty; indeed, cruelty had to become a spectacle. Society was made ready to accept the existence of witches. But because witches do not exist, laws and trickeries were invented to find them.

Although allopathy (overdosing) and bloodletting used by doctors of that time cannot be equated with the witch hunt, it perhaps did contribute to the silence of the medical profession with respect to the witch hunt.

Creating a Climate for the Witch Hunt

The idea of the existence of witches and the practice of the witch hunt was the prerogative of great men of philosophy, science, and literature, not of commoners. The witch hunt needed public support and only men of high ranks could accomplish it. Here I present only a few examples of the role of revered men as protagonists of the existence of witches.

King James I of England (James VI of Scotland) was a professed demonologist (author of *Daemonologie*, written in Scottish dialect) and an expert in all maters relating to witches. He gave a great impulse to the persecution of witches in England. Adams (1889a) writes, "Sorcery and witchcraft were made felony, without benefit of clergy," and "For some years the country was witch-ridden, and it is appalling to think of the hundreds of hapless, ignorant, and innocent creatures who were cruelly done to death under the influence of this extraordinary mania." During the reins of Henry VIII (1491-1547), Elizabeth I (1533–1603), and James I, statutes against witchcraft were enacted by parliament.

King James I was also a great admirer of William Shakespeare, and so was the bard of the king. It was to please King James I that Shakespeare wrote *Macbeth* and staged it for the first time before him.

This is how *The Tragedy of Macbeth* starts:

> Act I, Scene I [An open place.]
> Thunder and lightning. Enter three witches

> First Witch: When shall we three meet again?
> In thunder, lightning, or in rain?
> Second Witch: When the hurly-burly's done,
> When the battle's lost and won.
> Third Witch: That will be ere the set of sun.
> First Witch: Where the place?
> Second Witch: Upon the heath.
> Third Witch: There to meet with Macbeth.
> First Witch: I come, Graymalkin!
> Second Witch: Paddock calls.
> Third Witch: Anon.
>
> ALL:
> Fair is foul, and foul is fair:
> Hover through the fog and filthy air.

Shakespeare retained his fascination with witches and returned to them in his penultimate play, *The Tempest* (1611).

Joseph Glanvill (1636–1681) was a noted philosopher and a member of the Royal Society, the highest academic distinction in England; in 1668, he wrote *A Philosophical Endeavour towards the Defence of Being Witches and Apparitions*. The treatise was printed under different names (*Sadducismus Triumphatus; Blow at Modern Sadducism in Some Philosophical Considerations About Witchcraft*, etc.) and more recently reviewed by Moody E. Prior [1901-1996] (1932). This book not only reinforced the concept of the existence of evil-doing witches, but also disarmed people with opposite views. This book was used as a justification for the Salem Witch Trials in America.

The *Malleus Maleficarum* (The Hammer of Witches), the 1486 treatise on witches challenged all opponents who expressed doubt on the existence of witches, and instructed state authorities to identify, interrogate, and convict witches; it was granted approval by Pope Innocent VIII (1432-1492), who in 1484, had already issued a bull enjoining the detection, trial, and punishment (by burning) of witches.

The jurist and educationist Sir William Blackstone (1723–1780) wrote:

> To deny the possibility, nay, the actual existence of witchcraft and sorcery, is at once flatly to contradict the revealed Word of God in various passages

> of the Old and New testament, and the thing itself is a truth to which every nation in the world hath, in its turn, borne testimony, either by example seemingly well attested, or by prohibitory laws, which at least suppose the possibility of a commerce with evil spirits. (Adams, 1889b)

George Bartisch (1535-1606) wrote the text *Ophthalmodouleia*, which was published in 1583. From his high position as the court ophthalmologist, Bartisch "felt that the devil was an active force in the world, and the devil had his evil spirits working among the population. The humans who did the devil's will were mostly witches …the governmental punishment was for them to be burned at the stake until their bodies were totally consumed by fire" (Blanchard, 2005).

Political factors also contributed to the witch hunt. Africans were captured and exported like animals to far off places, and, if they survived the journey, were treated worse than animals. Colonization created a culture of dividing people and nations into two groups – those fit to rule and those only good enough to be ruled. The indigenous people of America became intruders and were named Indians as a tribute to Columbus. In almost every case of the Salem witch hunt there was some American Indian victim. The Body of Liberties was adopted in 1641 in Massachusetts, according to which "if any man or woman be a witch (that is hath or consulteth with a familiar spirit) they shall be put to death."

The Industrial Revolution had a shady side as well. While the peasants were liberated from the shackles of feudalism, they had to labour under extremely harsh working conditions in the cities, almost like robots as depicted in Charlie Chaplin's (1840-1902) 1936 film *Modern* Times and in the book *Germinal* by Emile Zola (1840-1902).[3]

I described in Chapter 3 how the acceptance of cruelty delayed the discovery of anaesthesia (Greene, 1971); likewise, similar factors allowed the practice of witch hunt, which delayed the blossoming of the science of medicine and allowed unlimited use of Galenic medicine, allopathy (overdosing) and bloodletting.

Opponents of the Witch Hunt

As is to be expected, numerous persons of science and philosophy did what they could to put an end to the practice of witch hunting. Foremost among them was Darwin. Charles Darwin vented his disgust in his historic *The Voyage of the Beagle*, from which the first quote is taken. It is interesting, that among the popular quotes of Darwin, only the portion "if the misery of our poor be caused not by the laws of nature, but by our institutions, great is our sin" is highlighted, leaving out its direct link to slavery. Even Stephen Jay Gould (1941–2002), a great opponent of the genetic theory of intelligence based on Alfred Binet's (1857–1911) *Intelligence Quotient* (IQ), mentions only this abbreviated version of Darwin's narrative in his book *The Mismeasure of Man* (Gould, 1966).

The prestigious journal *Nature* (Editorial, 2009) drew a parallel between Darwin's stand on the issue of slavery and that of Abraham Lincoln (1809–1865), using the identical birth dates of both (February 12, 1809) as the context. However, Darwin's opposition was humanist and not out of political necessity. This fact becomes obvious from another passage in the same book, *The Voyage of the Beagle*; here Darwin (1839[2006]) cites an episode while at Lagoa Marica in Brazil:

> This spot is notorious from having been, for a long time, the residence of some runaway slaves, who, by cultivating a little ground near the top, contrived to eke out a subsistence. At length they were discovered, and a party of soldiers being sent, the whole were seized with the exception of one old woman, who, sooner than again be led into slavery, dashed herself to pieces from the summit of the mountain. *In a Roman matron this would have been called the noble love of freedom: in a poor Negress it is mere brutal obstinacy* [emphasis added].

In 1584, Reginald Scot (1538-1599) wrote in the *Discovery of Witchcraft*:

> That lawful favour and Christian compassion be rather used towards these poor souls than rigour and extremity. Because they which are commonly accused of witchcraft are the least sufficient of all other persons to speak for themselves, as having the most base and simple education of all others; the extremity of their age giving them leave to dote, their poverty to beg, their wrongs to chide and threaten.

Scot did not have much success; instead, he exposed himself to the charges of atheism and sadduceeism.

The "Wonderful Teacher" Roger Bacon (1214–1294) of England was imprisoned for several years for insistence on the value of experimental science, which had no room for superstition. The philosopher Francis Bacon (1561–1626) discusses the ingredients of "witches' ointment" and accepts that they should all be of a soporiferous character, such as henbane, hemlock, moon shade, mandrake, opium, tobacco, and saffron. American physician John Weyer (1515–1588) disputed the existence of witches; his contention was that there are people with mental problems but there are no witches.

The Witch Hunt in Operation

France became the first nation to commence witch hunts, with their persecution peaking in the last decade of the sixteenth century when one prosecutor, Nicholas Rémy (1530-1616), shamelessly boasted that he burned nine hundred witches in about ten years. French Lawyer Jean Bodin (1530-1596) attributed fifteen vices to witches, of which the denial of God was number one. However, France was also the first country to deplore the mania and Louis XIV (1638-1715), *le Roi-Soleil* (the Sun King) abolished the witch hunt in a 1682 edict.

Michelet (1863) narrates how even the sadist Holy Roman Emperor Ferdinand II (1578-1637) reacted to the witch hunt:

> Even Ferdinand II, the savage Emperor of the Thirty Years' War, was driven, bigot as he was, to keep a watch on these worthy bishops, else they would have burned all their subjects. In the Wurtzburg list I find one Wizard a schoolboy, eleven years old; a Witch of fifteen: and at Bayonne two, infernally beautiful, of seventeen years.

Gage (1893b) comments:

> Burning a witch, probably because of its greater frequency, cost, but little over one-half as much as boiling in oil. The battle of gladiators with wild beasts in the Coliseum at Rome in the reign of Nero [AD 37-68], had in it an element of hope. Not the priesthood but the populace were the arbiters of the gladiator's destiny, giving always a chance for life in cases of great personal bravery. But in France and England the ecclesiastical code was so closely united with the civil as to be one with it; compassion equally with justice was forgotten, despair taking their place.

Ehrenreich and English (1973) write:

> The witch-hunts were well-organized campaigns, initiated, financed and executed by Church and State. To Catholic and Protestant witch-hunters alike, the unquestioned authority on how to conduct a witch hunt was the Malleus Maleficarum, or Hammer of Witches, written in 1484 by the Reverends Kramer and Sprenger (the "beloved sons" of Pope Innocent VIII).

This sadistic book lay on the bench of every judge and every witch-hunter for three centuries.

Adams (1889c) also supported the thesis that the victims of witch hunt were mainly women:

> Both (magician and the witch) could blight the promise of the harvest, baffle the plans of their enemies, or wither the health of their victims. But while the magician was frequently a man of ability and learning, and belonged to the cultured classes, the witch was almost always a woman of the lower orders, ignorant and uneducated, though occasionally ladies of high rank, and even ecclesiastics, have been accused of practising witchcraft.

Maple (1968) writes:

> The witch hunters spared neither age nor sex and little children were actually flogged while their mothers were burned alive before their eyes. The implements of torture ranged from thumb screw, eye gougers, branding irons, and rack to apparatus known as The Question, which could dislocate every bone in the body. The foulest cruelties were reserved for those who had the courage to recant their enforced confessions, and these prisoners were made to suffer the worst deaths.
>
> Witch hunting became an industry employing vast number of inquisitors who had vested interest in preserving their institution and privileges and were determined that their factories of death should never want for raw material.

Cawthorne (2003) gives examples of witch hunts in the United States, France, Germany, Scandinavia, Italy, Scotland, and Ireland. He opens the first chapter, "The Crucible" as follows:

> The devil is abroad in New England in 1692. The colonial powers England and France were at war. The Indians were on the warpath. Pirates were hindering trade. Smallpox was raging. The winter was cruel and taxes were

crippling. To the Puritans of New England, such litany could only be the work of the devil and his agents on Earth – witches.

The numbers persecuted or put to death during the festivity of the witch hunt are astounding; Maxwell-Stuart (2001a) comments:

> How many witches were arrested, and of those how many were found guilty and put to death? How many died in prison awaiting trials? How many committed suicide while they were in prison, or succumbed to the hardships and insanitary conditions of confinement? How many were lynched? ...Projected number of executions range from 40,000 (regarded by a majority of witchcraft scholars as a credible estimate) to a million (undoubtedly much exaggerated), . . .

In the Salem (Massachusetts, USA) trials, 185 persons were tried, 27 convicted, and 19 executed between 1692 and 1693 (Maxwell-Stuart, 2001b). Although the Salem trials were much smaller in magnitude than the ones in Europe, they are significant for another reason. They were held less than a 100 years before the American Revolution, of which Massachusetts was the epicentre. There should have been an enlightened atmosphere and not a witch hunt. From the published accounts of the Salem trials, one could infer that the prevalence of poverty, the shortage of arable land, and the presence of a sizable population of Indians generated the necessity and enthusiasm for witch hunt among the ruling elite of that time. In most cases of the Salem trials some American Indian was involved, and in almost each case, there is evidence of the confiscation of the property of some poor woman. Arthur Miller's play *The Crucible* centres around the land issue in Salem trials but one cannot fail to see its connection with McCarthyism.

The Witch Hunt in Modern Times

The mania of the witch hunt has passed. However, isolated incidents continue. Mishra (2003) documents the execution of 61 female, 13 male, and 2 children between 1991 and 1997 in the state of Jharkhand, one of the poorest states of India, with a substantial population of adivasis (forest dwellers). Mishra also gives data on deaths, mainly by burning, of hapless victims of witch hunt in the twentieth century in Hungary,

Pennsylvania (USA), Germany (WW II, the era of the Third Reich), France, Mexico, Congo, Kenya (a total of 300), and North Africa.

The phenomenon of witch hunt is need-based – the need of the privileged and the powerful. With time it took another form, more subtle, political, and discriminatory. Of course, the most horrendous of these was the Holocaust in which nearly 6 million innocent Jews perished. But this was not all. Black Americans were being lynched for being in the wrong place. During the years of the Wisconsin Senator Joseph McCarthy (1908-1957) in the United States in the 1940s and early 1950s, many a distinguished artist and academic had to suffer. My friend and colleague, distinguished Professor Mark Nickerson (1916-1998), had to leave his tenured position in the United States and seek a job in Canada. Julius Rosenberg (1918-1953) and his wife, Ethel Rosenberg (1915-1953), were executed on the fateful June 19, 1953, on unproven charges of spying (Wexley, 1955). Paul Robeson (1898-1976), the internationally acclaimed black American singer, had his passport revoked in 1950. The distinguished scientist Linus Pauling was denied a US passport for a while; had that not been the case, he would have gone to the UK and perhaps discovered the double helical structure of DNA.

The notorious 1937-1938 Moscow trials under Joseph Stalin resulted in the execution of the brilliant political scientist Nikolai Ivanovich Bukharin (1888-1938) and many other important leaders in the now nonexistent Soviet Union; being a supporter or sympathizer of Leon Trotsky (1879-1940) was judged a crime punishable by a bullet in the head (Schapiro, 1960).

Most academic institutions practiced some form of discrimination against women, Jews, sexual minorities, and people of colour. Even in modern times, we occasionally witness civil wars of attrition as in Rwanda and Somalia, atrocities against religious minorities such as in India and Pakistan, and bloody foreign intrusion as in the Middle East. These are all modern forms of witch hunts.

The Socio-political Dimension of the Witch Hunt

There has been considerable debate as to the reasons for witch hunting. Some scholars have developed theories, ten of them, on the genesis of the witch hunt, which Pavlac (2006) summarizes as follows: "due to illnesses of different types, location in specific areas such as mountainous regions, greed in order to confiscate property of others, suppression of religious rebellion, conflicts between different Christian denominations, unexpected natural disasters and so on."

Most likely, all these elements were present to a varying degree in each case of a witch hunt. In the final analysis, however, the genesis of the brutal practice of witch hunt is in the ignorance, insolence, and malice on the part of the witch hunters. It has been a revenge of the evil against the innocent, of the powerful against the powerless, of men against women. That is why its domain has extended to political dissent.

The Role of the Medical Profession

Ever since the emergence of the formal profession of medicine, some of the unwelcome intruders have been traditional healers whose source of medical knowledge was rooted in folklore, tradition, or sheer communal necessity. For example, some women with experience of their own childbirth had become experts in helping other women in birthing, successfully in uncomplicated cases, and less successful than trained obstetricians in a small number of complicated cases. These women healers also administered remedies for other ailments, and it is doubtful that even Hippocrates treated every patient better than a lay practitioner of witchcraft. However, with advancing civilization and the establishment of institutions to train healers, those without formal training became an obstacle for the lucrative medical profession. Traditional healers became witches whose profession was declared to bring disease and not health.

In this endeavour of the witch hunt, physicians found some kind of protection from the church because both were threatened by witches, sorcerers, and magicians. Consequently, the challenge for physicians was not the church but the witches, the traditional healers without a medical degree. So an alliance of the church and the body of physicians came into existence to punish the aberrant, the so-called witches, most of whom were poor old women.

Notes

1. Darwin, C. *The Voyage of the Beagle* [1839] (Vercelli, Italy: White Star, 2006), 676-677.

2. Szasz,T. S. *The Manufacture of Madness* (London: Routledge & Kegan Paul, 1971), 91.

3. Emile Zola. *Germinal* (1885) (English translation 2004, London: Penguin books). The novel gives vivid descriptions of the terrible working conditions of the miners in Italy.

References

Adams, W.H.D (1828-1891). *Witch, Warlock, and Magician: Historical Sketches of Magic and Witchcraft in England and Scotland* (London: Chatto & Windus, 1889).

Ibid., 1889a. 240.

Ibid., 1889b. 209.

Ibid., 1889c. 204.

Aronson, M. *Witch Hunt: Mysteries of the Salem Witch Trials* (New York: Atheneum, 2003).

Blanchard, D. E. "Superstitions of George Bartisch," *Survey of Ophthalmology* 50 (2005): 490-494.

Boyer, P. and Nissenbaum, S. *Salem Possessed: The Social Origin of Witchcraft* (Cambridge: Harvard University Press, 1974).

Cawthorne, N. *Witch Hunt: History of a Persecution* (Toronto: Arcturus Publishing, 2003).

Darwin, C. *The Voyage of the Beagle* [1839] (Vercelli, Italy: White Star 2006), 38.

Editorial. "Humanity and Evolution," *Nature* 451 (2009): 463-464.

Ehrenreich, B. and English, D. *Witches, Midwives, and Nurses: A History of Women Healers* (Old Westbury, NY: Feminist Press, 1973), 8.

Fox S. J. *Science and Justice: The Massachusetts Witchcraft Trials* (Baltimore: Johns Hopkins Press, 1968), 121.

Frazer, J. G. *The Golden Bough* (1922) (New York: Simon & Schuster, 1996).

Gage, M. J. *Woman, Church and State: A Historical Account of the Status of Women Through the Christian Ages; With Reminiscences of the Matriarchate.* 2nd Ed. (New York: The Truth Seeker Co., 1893).

Ibid., 1893a. 241.

Ibid., 1893b. 268-269.

Gould, S. J. *The Mismeasure of Man* (New York: W. W. Norton, 1966), 19.

Greene, N. M. "A Consideration of Factors in the Discovery of Anesthesia and their Effects on Its Development," *Anesthesiology* 35 (1971): 515-522.

Hill, F. *A Delusion of Satan: The Full Story of the Salem Witchcraft Trials* (New York: Doubleday, 1995).

Karlsen, C. F. *The Devil in the Shape of a Woman: Witchcraft in Colonial New England* (New York: Vintage, 1987).

Maple, E. *The Dark World of Witches* (New York: Pegasus, 1962).

Maxwell-Stuart, P. G. *Witchcraft in Europe and the New World, 1400-1800* (New York: Palgrave, 2001).

Ibid., 2001a. 56.

Ibid., 2001b. 95.

McGough, L. J. "Demons, Nature, or God? Witchcraft Accusations and the French Disease in Early Modern Venice," *Bulletin of the History of Medicine*, 80 (2006): 219-246.

Michelet, J. *La Sorciere. The Witch of the Middle Ages*, Trans. L. J. Trotter (London: Simpkin, Marshall, 1863).

Mishra, A. *Casting the Evil Eye* (New Delhi: Roli Book, 2003).

Norton, M. B. *In the Devil's Snare: The Salem Witchcraft Crisis of 1692* (New York: Random House, 2002).

Pavlac, B. A. "Ten General Historical Theories about the Origins and Causes of the Witch Hunts," *Women's History Resource Site*, June 6, 2006 (URL).

Prior, M. E. *Joseph Glanvill, Witchcraft, and Seventeenth-Century Science: Modern Philosophy* (Chicago: University of Chicago Press, 1932), 167.

Saletore, R. N. *Indian Witchcraft* (New Delhi: Abhinav Publications, 1981).

Schapiro, L. *The Communist Party of the Soviet Union* (New York: Random House, 1960), 361-473.

Wexley, J. *The Judgment of Julius and Ethel Rosenberg* (New York: Cameron & Kahn, 1955).

CHAPTER 12

The Age of Allopathy [overdosing][1] and Homeopathy

Hahnemann's system of homoeopathy rapidly drifted into absurdities. From 1829 onwards he recommended the administration of all drugs at the thirtieth potency, which corresponds to a concentration of 1 part in 10^{60} parts. This works out at a content of 1 molecule of drug in a sphere with a circumference equal to the orbit of Neptune.

A. J. Clark[2]

No, no. Human beings do not die so easily of such trifling ailments. No, I say! Could those crumbling bones and ghastly relics speak, they would tell you in deep sepulchral but in thunder tones: "This infant died of antimony and ipecac. This child was destroyed with calomel and opium. This youth was killed with nitre and digitalis. This man was slain with bleeding and blisters. This woman perished of henbane and strychnine, and all victims to 'medical science.'"

R. T. Trall[3]

Two Hundred Years of Homeopathy

Homeopathy started at the dawn of the nineteenth century; its use is now second only to that of modern medicine. Soon after its inception, there were twenty-two homeopathic medical schools, one hundred homeopathic hospitals, and over one thousand homeopathic pharmacies in the United States. Boston University, Stanford University, and New York Medical College were teaching homeopathy. At the present, homeopathy has a large following in Russia, India, Switzerland, Mexico, Germany, Netherlands, Italy, England, and South America.

Homeopathic therapy is frequently used on the advice of friends who vouch for its efficacy. The scepticism about modern medicine in general and the culture of love for natural foods and drugs has had a profound effect on the medical profession. MDs write popular books, as was also the case of Sir Arthur Ignatius Conan Doyle (1859-1930), who started creating Sherlock Holmes while eagerly waiting for patients.

Homeopathic doses are minute; consequently, there is a good chance that they do no harm. Since there are not as many regulations governing the practice of homeopathy as there are about modern medicine, the number of practicing homeopaths is quite substantial. Sometimes, one becomes a homeopath by just reading a small book; Homeopath Dr. Andrew Lockie (1993) lists 135 books for further reading besides his own. There is a provision for an online homeopathic degree.

Samuel Hahnemann

Samuel Hahnemann (1810) announced the founding of homeopathy by publishing his book *Organon of Medicine* in 1810. Since then, several editions have appeared, and all are available online. I did not find Hahnemann's book enlightening, but I assume the interpretation of this book by homeopaths like Andrew Lockie (1993), Morrell (1999), and Chris Kurz (2005) to be appropriate; they view Hahnemann, and appropriately so, as the father of homeopathy.

Hahnemann was born and raised in Germany and moved to Paris late in his life. His parents were not rich, but that did not stop him from pursuing an academic career. He was a brilliant student, fluent in Greek, Latin, English, and all other European languages. He received his MD degree from the University of Erlangen in Germany in 1779. Hahnemann had educated himself rather well in chemistry and philosophy. Some scholars (Handley, 1990; Morrell, 2004a, 2004b) suggest that Hahnemann was influenced by the philosophies of Rene Descartes, Baruch Spinoza (1632-1677), Gottfrie Wilhelm Leibnitz, Jean-Jacques Rousseau (1712-1778), and especially Immanuel Kant (1724-1804), as well as great scientists like Michael Faraday (1791-1867), Joseph Priestley, John Dalton (1766-1844), Antoine Lavoisier (1743-1794), Carolus Linnaeus (1707-1708), and Jean-Baptiste Lamarck (1744-1829). I am unable to connect Hahnemann's medical thesis with the philosophic and scientific works of those mentioned above.

Hahnemann practiced as a small-town physician for some time but made a living mainly as translator. Finding the existing practice of medicine rather useless or harmful, he gave up his practice as an MD. If one examines the state of therapeutics up to the time of Hahnemann, as described in Chapter 13, one must conclude that Hahnemann's disgust with modern medicine was more than justified.

What seems to have greatly influenced Hahnemann to found the discipline of homeopathy was Cullen's *Materia Medica.* William Cullen (1710-1790) was a distinguished Edinburgh physician and also a chemist and a gifted lecturer. His three main publications are the following: *Institutions of Medicine, Practice of Physic,* and *Synopsis Nosologiae.* His lectures were immensely popular and are published as *Lectures on the Materia Medica as Delivered by William Cullen, MD* (1781). The book by Cullen is fascinating and vastly different from, and in my opinion better than, the *Materia Medica*[4] by Horatio C. Wood [1841-1920] (1887), and Sir William Whitla [1851-1933] (1881); the latter two were used as textbooks in medical schools in the late nineteenth century.

Cullen developed his own classification of diseases; according to him, diseases fall in four groups: (1) pyrexiae (febrile); (2) neuroses (nervous); (3) cachexiae (due to bad habits); and (4) locales (cancer, etc.). Unlike Wood and Whitla, both of whom list a number of drugs for a variety of conditions, hardly any of which are currently used, Cullen goes into excruciating details about almost all possible foods, and of course, all available medicaments of his time.

Cullen devotes 15 of the 452 pages in the book on *Materia Medica* to a description of Peruvian bark. He discusses the effectiveness of the Peruvian bark against intermittent fever, advises against overdose, and says that its antipyretic effect is neither due to its odour nor to its flavour. The cause of intermittent fever was not known by the time of Cullen; he suggested the usefulness of the Peruvian bark against fevers in general but stresses its importance in intermittent fevers, which is characteristic of malaria.

It is during the translation of Cullen's treatise from English into German that Hahnemann was particularly perplexed by the complexity of the effectiveness of the Peruvian bark against intermittent fever. This was to play a big role in the life of Hahnemann and in the origin of homeopathy. Smith (1976) gives a lucid historical description of the use of quinine in fever since antiquity; he mentions the name of Hahnemann but does not talk about Hahnemann's experiments with the Peruvian bark. Others, engaged in the practice of homeopathy, exaggerate Hahnemann's aptitude for scientific research (Morrell, 1999, 2004a; Lockie, 1993).

Homeopathy Versus Allopathy

Allopathy is the opposite of homeopathy, both in theory and in dosage formulations. Essentially allopathy resorts to producing too much effect. I am not using the term *allopathy* as synonymous with *modern medicine* although the identity of the two terms is a popular misconception. In the presentation below, the origins of allopathy and homeopathy are not discussed separately because the former paved the way for the latter; rather, both are presented in relation to each other. Suffice it to say that allopathy, that is overdosing, was already there at the time of Galen in the third century, if not earlier. On the other hand, homeopathy came into being nearly 1,600 years later, between 1803 and 1810.

Why did homeopathy originate, and particularly at a time when the Industrial Revolution had stirred Europe, especially England and Germany, a time, which Russell (1945) defines as the period of "the diminishing authority of church, and the increasing authority of science"? This is also the period when the traditions of materialistic medicine started by Hippocrates, Galen, Ibn Sina (author of the Canon of Avicenna), Paracelsus[5] (1493-1541) and Indian and Chinese medicine were being refined.

Between 1700 and 1900, gigantic progress had been made in natural sciences and technology. Medical science also advanced, but mainly in areas of physiology, anatomy, and details of the symptomatology of diseases. On the other hand, the knowledge of the pathology of disease, according to Henry Jacob Bigelow (1818-1890), son of Dr. Jacob Bigelow

(1787-1879), was rudimentary (Bigelow, 1849), and the state of therapeutics, dismal (Trall, 1880b). Russell T. Trall, an advocate of drug-free hygiene but not a scientist by modern standards, refers to the opinion of other distinguished physicians to support his disgust with the therapeutics of his time, three of whom are quoted below (Trall, 1880b).

> There has been a great increase of medical men of late, *but*, upon my life, *diseases have increased in proportion* (John Abernethy, MD [1763-1831]).

> Some patients get well with the aid of medicines; more without it; and still more in *spite of it* (Sir John Forbes, MD, FRS [1787-1861]).

> All medicines which enter the circulation *poison the blood* in the same manner as do poisons that produce disease (Joseph M. Smith, MD [1789-1866]).

It is during this state of dismal therapeutics that Samuel Hahnemann introduced the homeopathic system of medicine. That it was an appropriate period to show disdain for Hippocratic medicine – scientific or non-scientific – is besides the point. Paul H. De Kruif (1890-1971) made a similar argument one hundred years ago in his book *Our Medicine Men* (De Kruif, 1922); I am trying to present a similar argument now.

During the times of Hahnemann, the medical profession harboured two extremes. On the positive side, medical science had kept pace with advances in physics, chemistry, mathematics, philosophy, and political economy. William Harvey had already discovered the physiology of blood circulation in 1628; Edward Jenner had developed the smallpox vaccination in 1796; Humphrey Davy had announced the anaesthetic properties of nitrous oxide. James Lind (1716-1799) had discovered the cure for scurvy by citrus fruits in 1747 though unaware that these fruits were a rich source of vitamin C; William Withering (1714-1799) had taken the advice of an old woman and begun using foxglove (source of digitalis) to treat dropsy (fluid accumulation due to heart failure) by 1785.

However, the state of therapeutics was no better than it was at the time of Hippocrates and Galen and may have been worse than that offered by other medical systems. However, the scientific upheaval was so great that physicians felt obliged to prove they could treat every disease only if they dared to. But the enthusiasm of physicians does not confer therapeutic properties to poisons.

Medical science differs from physics and chemistry. In the case of the latter two, the link between science and technology is often obvious. Knowledge of physiology has increased but the nature of disease cannot be predicted by an understanding of physiology (Darby, 1880) nor does an understanding of the physiology invariably lead to therapeutics. Harvey elaborated the physiology of blood circulation in 1628 but an effective treatment of hypertension was not discovered until the 1960s or even later.

However, the poor state of meaningful therapeutics did not restrain men with MD degrees from the same universities that produced Galileo, Boyle, Pascal, Newton, and Priestley from resorting to quackery. They unleashed an enthusiastic program of allopathy (overdosing) and bloodletting with no indications for their use and no proof of their efficacy. Medical schools had opened all over Europe and the United States and in some colonies as well; these institutions started producing certified doctors in numbers with hardly any medicaments to treat patients with. The medical profession promised to do no harm but then went on to do precisely the opposite.

Alfred Joseph Clark (1885-1941), who is quoted at the beginning of this chapter, was a physician and the leading pharmacologist of his time. Clark (1933) pointed out the absurdities of drug use by Hippocratic physicians; and it is this absurdity that gave birth to Hahnemann's homeopathy, Russell T. Trall's drug-free hygiene, and Daniel David Palmer's (1845-1913) chiropractic system.

Clark wrote (1933a):

> The dominating personality of James Gregory (1753-1821),[6] helped greatly to spread over the world the system of heroic symptomatic treatment which was termed allopathy. The favourite remedies were bloodletting, emetics and purgatives, and these were used until the dominant symptoms of the disease were suppressed. The scale on which these procedures were practised is illustrated by the following example. Malaria and dysentery were treated by purging with 20-grain (1.3 gram) doses of calomel (mercury preparation) until collapse was produced. In the year 1827, 32 million leeches were used in France, and, since blood-letting was practiced on a corresponding scale, opponents of the system dubbed it "vampirism." In a

> large proportion of cases the suppression of the symptoms by collapse was followed shortly by death, and it was in connection with such an event that the phrase was used "il est mort guéri" [He died cured.]

Bloodletting as a therapeutic manoeuvre was started by Greek physicians as an extension of Hippocrates' theory of black bile, which was considered obnoxious; the tradition was taken to absurd levels by Galen, who advocated "letting blood until the patient faints (and may be difficult to awaken), or removing several pounds of blood"[7] (Mattern, 2008). George Washington, the first president of the United States, was killed by bloodletting (Abel, 1970); Prince Albert, the husband of Queen Victoria, succumbed to alcohol-based stimulants (Trall, 1880). If this could happen to the American president and British royalty, who would care to count the common folks succumbing to the allopathy of physicians?

In short, it is this enthusiasm of physicians of the eighteenth and nineteenth century to administer nonsensical drugs in overdoses, which paved the way for the introduction of ultra minute-drug therapy called homeopathy.

The Doctrine of Homeopathy

Homeopathy (Greek *homeos* means "similar" and *pathos* means "suffering") is based on the principle of *Similia Similibus Curantur* (like cures like). Homeopathic medicine is based on symptomlogy, although this is not where it differs fundamentally from the medical system advocated by Hippocrates, Galen, and Paracelsus, as well as by Chinese and Hindu medicines. They all rely on symptoms.

In *Organon of Medicine*, Hahnemann (1810) states this law:

> A weaker dynamic affection is permanently extinguished in the living organism by a stronger one, if the latter (whilst differing in kind) is very similar to the former in its manifestations.

Hahnemann also postulated that the efficacy of a drug increases with dilutions.

Conceptually, homeopathy is unrelated to any other medical school; it is also the youngest medical system unless one treats chiropractic as a medical discipline. On the other hand, one comes across assertions about homeopathy that are exactly what people like Deepak Chopra say about Ayurveda (see Chapter 6). For example, Kurz (2005a) says, "Homeopathy is a holistic approach to healing which rightly puts the whole human being at the heart of its practice. Without acknowledging the indivisibility of body, mind, soul, and spirit, perceiving the totality of the individual disease will remain an elusive goal."

Homeopathic enthusiasts such as Andrew Lockie (1993) claim that what is unique about their system is that it only helps nature to cure. However, helping nature to cure is the underlying principle of all medical disciplines and had been held so for a very long time. If there is a skin burn, there is no application of antiseptics and bandages, and even antibiotocs are only applied on the site of the burn. Application of antibiotics, antiseptics, or bandages is aimed at eliminating the microorganism and not at the formation of new skin; nature takes care of that.

There are three basic theoretical postulates of homeopathy, which are described below as "Like Cures Like," "The Inverse Relationship between Dilution and Potency," and "Miasm."

Like Cures Like

While translating William Cullen's *Materia Medica* from English to German, Hahnemann came up with the principle of Similars, primarily because of Cullen's description of Peruvian bark, which cured intermittent and other fevers. According to the homeopath Lockie[8]:

> Why, Hahnemann wondered, should quinine have an effect on malaria when, other, more powerful, astringents did not? He decided to investigate. For several days he dosed himself with quinine and noted down his reactions in great detail. It seemed that in a healthy person, himself, quinine produced all the symptoms of malaria – fever, sweating, shivering, weakness. Was this why it also cured malaria?

Lockie (1993) goes on to say that Hahnemann repeated the tests on his acquaintances as well as tested arsenic, belladonna (the source of atropine), and mercury. I am not sure why Hahnemann did all that in the first place and how these tests constitute "provings" (proofs) as Lockie asserts. I do, however, wish to add that in the quote above, many statements of Lockie are false – at least in their detail. To begin with, Cullen talks about intermittent fever and not malaria because by the time of Cullen and Hahnemann, malaria was not known as the cause of intermittent fever for another hundred years. Second, Hahnemann could not have taken quinine because it was not until 1820, ten years after Hahnemann had already formulated his homeopathic theory, that quinine was isolated from Peruvian bark. Hahnemann talks about Cinchona[9] but not quinine. However, these errors of Lockie (1993) may be technical and not conceptual.

The most important point is that fever is not a common effect of quinine; my search of the literature found only one reference to fever due to quinine and that too only in rare cases of idiosyncrasy (Goodman and Gilman, 1941). The *Materia Medica* by Wood (1887) devotes seventeen pages on Cinchona but does not say it produces fever nor does the book by Torald Sollmann [1874-1965] (1948). Quinine is bitter and used to be added to soft drinks, and there are no reports of mass affliction with fever. It is possible that Hahnemann was a special case of idiosyncrasy to quinine or something like that, but it is unlikely that all his associates, on whom Hahnemann conducted experiments, were idiosyncratic.

Finally, while Cullen (1781) does attribute astringent properties to the Peruvian bark, quinine is not an astringent. Astringents are chemicals that can protect the mucosa of the gut either by coating the mucosa or by precipitating protein, which thereby provide a covering on the intestinal linings and relieve intestinal irritation. Kaolin, bismuth oxychloride, and magnesium oxide belong to the first category; tannin acid belongs to the second (Clark, 1923). In contrast, quinine is a well-known protoplasmic poison and, if anything, an irritant and by no stretch of imagination an astringent.

I quote below Hahnemann's[10] experiments with Peruvian bark in his own words:

> By combining the strongest bitters and the strongest astringents, one can obtain a compound which, in small doses, possesses much more of both these properties, than the bark, and yet no specific fever will ever come of such a compound.
>
> Substances which excite a kind of fever, as very strong coffee, pepper, Aconite, Ignatia, Arsenic, extinguish the types of the fever. I took by way of

> experiment, twice a day, four drachms of good China. My feet, finger ends, etc., at first became cold; I grew languid and drowsy; then my heart began to palpitate, and my pulse grew hard and small; intolerable anxiety, trembling (but without cold rigor), prostration throughout all my limbs then pulsation in my head, redness of my cheeks, thirst, and, in short, all these symptoms, which are ordinarily characteristic of intermittent fever, made their appearance, one after the other, yet without the peculiar chilly, shivering rigor.
>
> Briefly, even those symptoms which are of regular occurrence and especially characteristic – as the stupidity of mind, the kind of rigidity in all the limbs, but, above all the numb, disagreeable sensation, which seems to have its seat in the periosteum, over every bone in the body – all these make their appearance.
>
> This paroxysm lasted two or three hours each time, and recurred if I repeated this dose, not otherwise; I discontinued it, and was in good health.
>
> How comes it that the effects of bark are so short lived, as is indeed the case, if it be not true that bark, besides the astringent and tonic bitter propensities ascribed to it by writers, especially by the author, possesses another power (that of exciting fever of a peculiar kind)?

A comment on Hahnemann's self-exposure to the Peruvian bark: Hahnemann does not specifically mention fever as one of the symptoms, and he says he had no "cold rigor." On the other hand, the characteristic of malaria is the cold rigor or chill and shivering. Patients try to cover themselves with a blanket, but because the source of cold is not external, the blanket does not help. There is no such thing as malaria without fever and cold rigor. Hahnemann ingested "four drachms of good China"; this would amount to minimum of six grams of Cinchona, which would contain approximately three hundred milligrams quinine and would be about half the standard dose used in the treatment of malaria. In short it is a high and not a low dose. By the term *paroxysm*, Hahnemann must be implying all the symptoms he described he got.

Clark (1933a) says Hahnemann "had previously suffered from malaria and the gastric irritation excited the paroxysm." Clark was a distinguished pharmacologist so he talks about the ability of quinine to cause gastric irritation as opposed to acting as an astringent.

Because of the relevance of malaria, fever, and quinine in the genesis of homeopathy, I would dwell as briefly as possible on all these three subjects. In passing, I might add that there have been many other researchers who have experimented upon themselves; it would be out of place to go into that except for the outstanding contribution of Professor John Scott Haldane, who worked out every detail of carbon monoxide poisoning by experiments on himself to save the lives of coal miners (see Varma et al., 2009).

Fever

Fever is produced by *pyrogens*, which could enter the body from outside (exogenous) or be produced in the body (endogenous). Intermittent fever with definite regularity is characteristic of malaria. In most infections, fever is invariably present although usually less in the morning than in the evening because of less physical activity during the night than during the day. Moreover, the severity of the fever is unrelated to the virulence of the infection. A patient of active tuberculosis carries fever until cured or dead. A patient of malaria looks absolutely normal between the episodes of fever at least until the repeated destruction of red blood cells causes severe anaemia. The intermittency of fever at fixed intervals, mostly two to three days, is how village folks in India diagnose themselves as suffering from malaria without the help of physicians; the diagnosis is sometimes confirmed by microscopic visualization of the parasite in blood slides.

Many diseases produce fever. However, whatever be the cause of fever, its severity is fixed by the heat centres in the brain (hypothalamus), which, like a thermostat, allow the persistence of a certain body temperature. Ordinarily, more heat is produced by metabolism than is needed for core body temperature so that the brain controls temperature by mechanisms of heat loss. Shivering and fever are related. Here is how Wilson and Schild (1959) who revised Clark's book put it:

> The fever is initiated by some toxin exciting the heat centres, either directly or indirectly, and this causes the centres to set the body temperature above normal. The patient feels cold and the heat production is increased by shivering, and the temperature rises until it reaches a new level, which is determined by the severity of the fever; at the same time the heat loss is reduced

> by vasoconstriction. The amount of heat required to be retained to produce a rise of temperature of 3°C, is quite small, only about 200 calories, which is less than 10 percent of the normal daily heat production of the healthy body at rest.
>
> When the crisis of a fever occurs, heat loss is increased by sweating and the temperature may fall rapidly and return to normal in a few hours. The heat centres during fever, therefore, balances the heat production and heat loss of the body in an almost normal manner. The total exchange is greater, for the basal metabolism of the body is increased. This rise in metabolism is to be expected for, according to the law of Van't Hoff, the velocity of any chemical reaction is increased two – or three-fold by a rise of 10°C. Du Bois calculated from extensive observations of the basal metabolism in fever that the rises observed in basal metabolism corresponded fairly exactly with a temperature coefficient of 2.3. This rule implies that when a patient's temperature rises from normal to 104°F., his basal metabolism increases 28 per cent.

Since the discovery of *Plasmodia* as the cause of malaria in the1880s, it is known that the intermittency of fever is determined by the time it takes for the parasites to grow sufficient in number inside the red blood cells to cause their rupture, leading to fever and chill; the interval is usually two to three days depending upon the type of *Plasmodium*. The existence of intermittent fever has been known for thousands of years, but its cause was not known by the time of Cullen, and he does not talk about the fever-producing property of quinine.

Quinine

The description below is mainly based on two textbooks (Clark, 1923; Goodman and Gilman, 1941) and two historical reviews (Smith, 1976; McTavish, 1982). Because of the declining importance of quinine, the later the edition of a textbook, the less is said about it.

Peruvian bark contains many alkaloids, the most important being quinine and its dextrorotatory isomer quinidine; both share properties, but quinine is mainly used against fever and as a bitter in many tonics while quinidine is primarily a heart drug, the use of which is becoming less frequent. The most important effect of quinine is its ability to reduce malarial fever by eliminating the cause of malaria, namely the *Plasmodium*; the next important effect is its general antipyretic action. Indeed, quinine was the only drug against fever until Charles Frédéric Gerhardt (1816-1856) synthesized aspirin in 1853 and the antipyretic activity of sodium salicylate was demonstrated by Carl Emil Buss (1849-1878) in 1875 (McTavish, 1987).

There is a phenomenon called hypersensitivity or idiosyncrasy to drugs. Unlike allergic or anaphylactic reactions that require prior exposure to the drug, as is the case with penicillin, hypersensitivity to a drug can manifest itself on first contact. Hypersensitivity to quinine and related compounds is much more common than is the case for other drugs (Dawson and Garbade, 1930; Goodman and Gilman, 1941; Wilson and Schild, 1959) so that it is advisable to do a hypersensitivity test before using quinine. In any case, only Goodman and Gilman textbooks (all editions from the first in 1941 to the eleventh in 2006) mention fever as one of the manifestations of hypersensitivity to quinine. A paper (Dawson and Garbade, 1930), which describes actual case reports of quinine hypersensitivity, does not mention fever as one of the signs. Whatever be the case, it is obvious that although quinine can produce multiple toxic effects, fever is not a common side effect. It is quite possible that Hahnemann was hypersensitive to quinine; but his thesis of like cures like would require the fever-producing property of quinine to be a universal phenomenon, which it certainly is not.

The Relation Between Symptoms and Therapy

It is said that homeopathy is based on symptoms; the cause of the disease is not critical. However, while diseases are many, symptoms are finite in number, and many diseases produce the same symptoms. Why then is the same homeopathic powder not a cure for many diseases producing similar symptoms? Moreover, some diseases, even serious ones – such as cancer, AIDS, syphilis, hypertension, diabetes, heart failure, et cetera – produce no symptoms or negligible ones until it is too late to cure them or until some complication sets in; at what stage of the disease, then, does homeopathy become useful, if at all?

The Inverse Relationship between Dilution and Effect

The second major component of homeopathy is that the dilution of a medicament increases its potency by activating vital energy of the diluted substance. Hahnemann developed this principle after he noticed that "trituration of mercury" increased its pharmacological action. However, according to Clark (1933a) mercury was first converted to mercurous and then to mercuric oxide in this process. Whatever be the case, Hahnemann diluted solids like quartz and oyster shells by grinding them with lactose. Hahnemann created the centesimal or "C" scale, diluting a substance by a factor of 100 at each stage; accordingly, a 6C dilution repeats this process six times, ending up with the original material diluted by a factor of 10^{12} and a 200C dilution will be 10^{400}, that is the dilution of the homeopathic influenza remedy *Oscillococcinum* made from duck liver.

Because homeopathic potions are infinitesimally small, it has bewildered the imagination of many because at this concentration the probability of any molecule of administered drug reaching the system of the patient is remote, if not impossible. On the other hand, there is a contention that the effect of the homeopathic potion is transmitted to all substances of contact so the effect can be produced whether or not the original substance reaches into the patient.

Dr. Jacob Bigelow served at the Massachusetts General Hospital and the Harvard Medical School. He was also a botanist, a poet, and was the president of the American Academy of Arts and Sciences from 1847 to 1863. He was opposed to overdosing and bloodletting as therapeutic measures. His book *Nature in Disease* (Bigelow, 1859) includes the following passage on homeopathy:

> Its (homeopathy) character is, that, while in reality it waits on the natural course of events, it commends itself to the ignorant and credulous by a professed introduction into the body inappreciable quantities of medicinal substances. Now the nugatory effect of such quantities is demonstrated by the fact that in civilized life every person is exposed to the daily reception, in the form of solutions, dust or vapour, of homeopathic quantities of almost every common substance in nature and art, without any appreciable consequences being found to follow. And the pretended exactness with which such nominal doses are administered by homeopathic practitioners is doubtless a fallacy, capable of producing in the living body no other effects than those which charlatanry has in all ages produced in the minds of imaginative patients.

A relatively recent academically charged debate on the effects of excessively high dilution followed the publication of an article by a team of researchers at the INSERM laboratory at the University of Paris in collaboration with scientists from Italy, Israel, and Canada, in the world's most prestigious journal *Nature* (Davenas et al., 1988).

Human blood cells belong to two basic categories, red and white. White blood cells belong to different groups, one of which is called polymorphonuclear basophils. These basophils contain immunoglobin E (IgE) type antibodies on their surface. Authors of the *Nature* paper (Davenas et al., 1988) reported that when these basophils were exposed to anti-IgE antibodies at dilutions as high as 10^{130}(zillions), an effect was observed. Since the authors could not detect any molecule of the antibody at this dilution, they concluded that the "biological information could be related to the molecular organization of water." A journalist termed it as the water memory theory. This paper was published when Sir John Maddox (1925-2009) was the editor of *Nature*. He agreed to have the paper published after demanding independent verification of the data. Maddox, with two colleagues, visited the INSERM laboratory to observe replication of the data and then wrote, (Maddox et al., 1988) "that the claims made by Davenas et al. are not to be believed." The senior author of the high dilution paper, Dr. Jacques Benveniste (1935-2004) defended his paper in reply (Benveniste, 1988).

Recently researchers at the Indian Institute of Technology (IIT, Bombay) went a step further. Unlike Davenas et al. (1988), they claim to have successfully detected, using highly sophisticated tools, metal-derived medicine as nanoparticles following as much as 10^{400} –fold dilution (Chikramane et al. 2010). However, the technique used by Indian scientists to produce such high dilutions is suspect. Perhaps a better method of dilution would have been to throw a small sample of their metal-based homeopathic medicine into the nearby Indian ocean on the shores of Bombay and collect a water sample near Port Elizabeth (South Africa) or better still from the Pacific Ocean near San Francisco USA); if the conjecture of the researchers is valid, they should be able to detect their molecules in water samples from these places. There is not enough water in the oceans to dilute their homeopathic medicine more than 10^{400}.

In terms of the therapeutic claims of homeopathy, I reach the conclusion stated above in the passage from Bigelow's book that if such infinitesimally small dilutions produce an effect, then we are being constantly drugged and nothing is drug-free in its normal state. We are constantly being treated by most, if not all, homeopathic drugs, and there should be no need for further homeopathic treatment.

Miasm (Miasma)

The third relevant aspect of homeopathy is its philosophy of health and disease; it is the concept of miasm, which Hahnemann proposed several years after founding the doctrine of homeopathy. According to Kurz (2005b), what led Hahnemann to advance the theory of miasm was "his increasing frustration with not being able to cure deep-seated chronic diseases with the hitherto practiced homeopathic wisdom."

The concept of miasm is most probably borrowed from Hippocrates, who believed the source of disease to be dirty water or air. The concept is also present in Ayurvedic texts. Undoubtedly, there is much truth in the postulate that dirty water or air can cause disease. However, it was the genius of Louis Pasteur, from whom the word *pasteurization* is derived, who provided experimental verifiable evidence for the germ theory of disease, along with Robert Koch in about 1900, years after Hahnemann's homeopathy came into existence.

Hahnemann's miasm is not, and could not be, identical to Pasteur-Koch's germ theory. Hahnemann had to spice and mystify it. "To him [Hahnemann] a miasm denoted a constitutional weakness contracted by parasitic infection which is somehow hereditary and can be transmitted over generations. What actually is inherited by the next generation is not the infection per se but the constitutionally weakened vital force" (Kurz 2005c).

In a way, the miasm concept is similar to early spiritual medicine, which postulated that disease was a curse of the heavens. Homeopathy, too opines that diseases and sickness are caused by disturbances in a hypothetical vital force or life force and sees these disturbances as manifesting themselves in unique symptoms. Homeopathy maintains that the vital force has the ability to react and adapt to internal and external causes, which homeopaths refer to as the law of susceptibility.

The law of susceptibility states that a negative state of mind can attract hypothetical disease entities called miasms to invade the body and produce symptoms of diseases. Hahnemann treated disease as an integral part of the life process.

In my opinion, if the theoretical foundations of any phenomenon are faulty, and for some reason not subject to correction, the postulate has no choice but to become mystic and spiritual. So is the case with homeopathy.

The Homeopathic Patient

The clients of homeopathic medicine are educated citizens rather than common folks. There is a great merit to the idea of "do no harm" with drugs. Homeopathy was least likely to harm. Since in the majority of ailments nature succeeds over disease, any harmless intervention would and should get the credit.

Given the popularity of homeopathy in both the North and the South, its therapeutic efficacy has been evaluated using a modern approach. Almost all such studies show that homeopathic medicines are no better than placebos. However, if patients feel that they have benefited from homeopathic therapy, they will seek out homeopathic doctors. Indeed, the drug is only one element and may be the least important one, in the placebo effect, which is the sum total of the confidence of the patient in the doctor and the rapport between the patient and the physician.

Conclusion

What I have tried to show in this chapter is the scientific hollowness of homeopathy. In my opinion, the basic premise of homeopathy is fundamentally wrong. In the meantime, there is plenty of room for homeopathy, as for Ayurveda, acupuncture, and chiropractic since the overwhelming majority of ailments are self-limiting.

Notes

1. The term "allopathy" is often considered synonymous with modern medicine. Some private medical schools in India use this term to distinguish themselves from Ayurvedic medical schools. However, in the strict sense, allopathy means the admin-

istration of huge doses of drugs, which became a norm with practitioners of modern medicine especially in 18th Century Europe. In this book the term allopathy is used not to indicate modern medicine but rather the practice of administering massive doses of drugs, almost always in toxic amounts.

2. Alfred Joseph Clark, *Applied Pharmacology* 5th ed. (Philadelphia: P. Blakiston's Son & Co. 1933), 3.

3. Russell T. Trall (1812-1877) *True Healing Art or Hygienic vs. Drug Medication* 1880. *WWW.Kessinger.net*. ISBN 1-56459-808-X. 20-21. Antimony is effective against some parasitic infections which do not exist in the United States; ipecac (emetine) is a plant product that causes vomiting and is effective against amebiasis, which is also rare in the United States except in the South; calomel is a mercury preparation and can act as a purgative but is of no therapeutic value; opium is of value only against pain and will stop diarrhea, but an overdose kills by suppressing breathing; nitre is potassium nitrate, which has no therapeutic value; digitalis is a heart drug and, if not administered carefully, is invariably fatal; bloodletting came out of Hippocrates' theory of black bile and has killed many, but saved, perhaps, none; strychnine causes convulsions and is used as a rat poison; all these drugs were indeed used at the time of Dr. Trall.

4. There are many editions of these books. I have used Wood, H. C. *Treatise on Therapeutics Comprising Materia Medica and Toxicology With Special Reference to the Application of the Physiological Action of Drugs to Clinical Medicine.* (Philadelphia: J. B. Lippincott & Co., 1874; digitalized by Google).

5. Paracelsus introduced minerals (mercury, sulphur, potassium, antimony) to replace traditional herbs and publically set afire the books of Ibn Sina and Galen to show his contempt for them.

6. Dr. Gregory was not alone; Dr. Benjamin Rush of the United States, being one of them, advocated mega doses of poisonous drugs or dangerous bloodletting to treat such diverse diseases as pneumonia and typhoid.

7. The total volume of blood in an adult male is approximately five litres; a pound of blood would be approximately 500 ml.

8. http://www.enotalone.com/article/5794.html

9. The name cinchona, was given by botanist Carolus Linnaeus; cinchona is the source of quinine, but quinine was not isolated until 1820.

10. *The Life and Letters of Dr. Samuel Hahnemann* By Thomas Lindsley Bradford, MD, Presented by Dr Robert Séror.

References

Abel, A. L. "Blood Letting: Barber-Surgeon's Shaving and Bleeding Bowls," *Journal of American Medical Association* 214 (1970): 900-901.

Benveniste, J. "Dr. Jacques Benveniste Replies, " *Nature* 334 (1988) : 291.

Bigelow, J. *Nature in Disease* (Boston: Phillips, Sampson & Co. 1859), 107.

Bigelow, H. J. *Introductory Lecture Delivered at the Massachusetts Medical College*, November 6th 1849 (Boston: David Clapp, 1850), 4.

Chikramane, P.S., Suresh, A.K., Bellare, J.R. and Kane, S.G. "Extreme Homeopathic Dilutions Retain Starting Materials: A Nanoparticulate Perspective". *Homeopathy* 99 (2010), 231-242.

Clark, A. J. *Applied Pharmacology* (London: J. & A. Churchill, 1923), 211.

——, *Applied Pharmacology* (Philadelphia: P. Blakiston's Sons, 1933).

Ibid., 1933a. 3.

Cullen, W. *Lectures on the Materia Medica as Delivered by William Cullen, MD* (Dublin: W. & H. Whitestone, 1781.243-256 [Google books]).

Darby, J. C. *Science and the Healing Art: Or a New Book on Old Facts* (Louisvile: John P. Morton, 1880).14-37.

Davenas, E., Beauvais, F., Amara, J. et al. "Human Basophil Degranulation Triggered by Very Dilute Antiserum against IgE," *Nature* 333 (1988): 816-818.

Dawson, W. T. and Garbade, F. A. "Idiosyncrasy to Quinine, Cinchodine and Ethylhydrocupreine," *Journal of American Medical Association* 94 (1930), 704-705.

De Kruif, P. H., *Our Medicine Men* (New York: The Century Co., 1922).

Goodman, L. S. and Gilman, A. *The Pharmacological Basis of Therapeutics* (New York: Macmillan, 1941), 903-915.

Hahnemann, S. *Organon of Medicine*, 1810 (New York: General Books, 2009).

Handley, R. *A Homeopathic Love Story* (Berkley: North Atlantic Books, 1990).

Kurz, C. *Imagine Homeopathy: A Book of Experiments, Images, and Metaphors* (Stuttgart: Georg Thieme Verlag, 2005a), 7.

Ibid., 2005b. 110.

Ibid., 2005c. 111.

Lockie, A. *Family Guide to Homeopathy: Symptoms and Natural Solutions* (New York: Simon & Schuster, 1993).

MacTavish, J. R. "Antipyretic Treatment and Typhoid Fever: 1860-1900," *The Journal of the History of Medicine and Allied Sciences*, 42 (1987): 486-506.

Maddox, J. Randi, J. and Stewart, W. W. "High-Dilution Experiments a Delusion," *Nature*,

334 (1988): 287-290.

Mattern, S. P. *Galen & the Rhetoric of Healing* (Baltimore: The Johns Hopkins University Press, 2008), 142.

Morrell, P. *Some Reflections on the Origin of Hahnemann's Ideas* (http://w.w.w.homeoint.org/morrell/articles/pm -origin.htm, 1999).

——. *Hahnemann's Good Reputation and Empirical Stance* (http://w.w.w.homeoint.org/morrell/articles/empiricalstance.htm, 2004a).

——. *Hahnemann and Homeopathy* (New Delhi: B. Jain Pub., 2004b).

Russell, B. *The History of Western Philosophy* (New York: Simon & Schuster, 1945), 491.

Smith, D. C. "Quinine and Fever: The Development of Effective Dosage," *Journal of History of Medicine and Allied Sciences* 31 (1976): 343-367.

Sollmann, T. *A Manual of Pharmacology and its Application to Therapeutics and Toxicology* (Philadelphia: W. B. Saunders, 1948).

Trall, R. T. *True Healing Art or Hygienic vs Drug Medication* (1880 wwwKessinger.net [ISBN 1-56459-808-X]).

Ibid., 1880b. 86-88.

Varma, D. R., Mulay, S., and Chemtob, S. "Carbon Monoxide: Public Health Risk to Painless Killer" in *Handbook of the Toxicology of Chemical Warfare Agents.* Ed. R. C. Gupta (San Diego: Elsevier 2009), 271-292.

Whitla, W. *Whitla's Pharmacy, Materia Medica and Therapeutics* (London: Henry Renshaw 1881).

Wilson, A. and Schild, H. O. *Applied Pharmacology* (Clark) 9th Ed. (London: J. & A. Churchill, 1959), 320-321.

Wood, H. C. *Treatise on Therapeutics Comprising Materia Medica and Toxicology with Especial Reference to the Application of the Physiological Action of Drugs to Clinical Medicine* 6th Ed. (Washington: Lippincott, 1887).

CHAPTER 13

Therapeutics Since Antiquity

Thus science must begin with myths, and with the criticism of myths; neither with the collection of observations, nor with the invention of experiments, but with the critical discussion of myths, and of magical techniques and practices. The scientific tradition is distinguished from the pre-scientific tradition in having two layers. Like the latter, it passes on its theories; but it also passes on a critical attitude towards them. The theories are passed on, not as dogma, but rather with the challenge to discuss them and improve upon them.

Karl Popper (1902-1994)[1]

Theocracy is the alliance of religion with the state. Pharmacracy is the alliance of medicine with the state.

Thomas S. Szasz[2]

Introduction

In the preceding chapters 1 have commented on different schools of medicine. All these systems have their specific medicaments. However, I have not listed drugs used by other schools of medicine nor am I planning to list all the drugs of modern medicine. Rather, I am dealing with drugs that denote significant conceptual advances in therapeutics.

Unlike diagnosis and prognosis, which can be ascertained by means of careful observation, use of modern tools such as x-rays, CAT (computer-assisted tomography) scan, NMR (nuclear magnetic resonance) spectroscopy, and PET (positron emission tomography), biochemical tests, as well as professional experience in differential diagnosis, there are no clear guidelines, even today, for discovering an effective and appropriate therapy.

Since antiquity, the efficacy of therapeutics was based on a trial and error approach. Not much has changed. Even the blind studies to differentiate between the efficacy of a treatment from the placebo effect is not as modern as many think. As early as the eighteenth century, the American politician-scientist Benjamin Franklin (1706-1790) used a blind study and concluded against the therapeutic efficacy of Friedrich Anton Mesmer's (1734-1815)[3] magnetized rods.

Problems in Drug Discovery

In earlier times, the problem of drug discovery was compounded by an erroneous understanding of diseases. Even in the nineteenth century, there were wild speculations about disease and treatment as described by Humphrey Thomas Pledge (1903-1960):

> In every age medical ideas with a certain undoubted scope and certain ingenuity about them have been erected into panaceas. In the 18th century this tendency reached its climax so far as qualified professional doctors go, being thereafter increasingly the province of quacks. One of these ideas was the very simple one of John Brown of Edinburgh, that all ills are either depressions or excitements; to be treated, respectively, with alcohol or opium. His own ills were depression and he died of the cure. ... Far more interesting was another of these ideas, that what kills cures – in extremely small doses. (Pledge, 1939)

It is very possible that in the above quote, Pledge (1939) is referring to allopathy (massive doses), which the pharmacologist Clark (1933) characterized by referring to French saying *il est mort guéri* (Died cured) and homeopathic therapeutics (the potency of a drug increases with dilution).

Advances in physiology, pathology, biochemistry, and genetics have been ahead of therapeutics since the beginning of medical science. A scientific way of discovering medicines is very recent and still limited in scope (Maxwell and Eckhardt, 1990; Sneader, 2005; Brunton et al., 2006). Successes of this approach depend upon the availability of unequivocal sufficient facts. Otherwise, end with problems as described by the philosopher Immanuel Kant in his treatise *Critique of Pure Reason* (Kant, 1787):

> *The apagogic method of proof is, however, permissible only in those sciences where it is impossible mistakenly to substitute* [emphasis in the original] what is subjective in our representation or what is objective, that is, for the knowledge of that which is in the object. Where such substitution tends to occur, it must often happen that the opposite of a given proposition contradicts only the subjective conditions of thought, and not the object, or that the two propositions contradict each other only under a subjective condition which is falsely treated as being objective; the condition being false, both can be false, without it being possible to infer from the falsity of one to the truth of the other.

Physiology of the body and pathology of a disease have not changed substantially with time. Therapeutics is a human intervention and naturally subject to errors. Therapeutics is qualitatively different from other human needs. A drug must exert its intended effect or else it is, perhaps, worse than no drug at all.

Ancient drugs, still in use – such as quinine, quinidine, morphine, aspirin, digitalis, artemisinin, emetine, and so on – were discovered by communal effort using trial and error approach and not by physicians. In the ensuing period, the trial and error method has become a bit more sophisticated, often first tried on animal models before venturing into humans.

Until the mid-nineteenth century, only two therapies of significance were based on the knowledge of the cause of the disease and the postulated effect of the intervention: these were the anti-smallpox vaccine and the disinfectant carbolic acid.

The Unpredictability of Drug Effects

The clinical usefulness of a drug can neither be predicted with certainty by the knowledge of its effects determined in the laboratory or even controlled clinical trials, nor by an understanding of the mechanisms of these effects. Rather, the true usefulness of a drug is established by epidemiological studies, once a drug has gone into popular usage, by which time it might have helped or harmed thousands of patients. The thalidomide tragedy was noted only when nearly ten thousand babies without limbs were born to mothers who consumed this wonder drug to treat morning sickness; it was unpredictable toxicity. In the meantime, thalidomide is proving of value in the treatment of leprosy, cancer and inflammatory diseases (Franks et al. 2004); this too was unpredictable.

The beta-blocker propranolol was introduced against ischemic cardiac diseases on the basis of rational pharmacology; that a sudden cessation of therapy can cause fatal cardiac complication was found only when it did occur. Aspirin has been in use for more than a hundred years before it was introduced as a prophylactic agent in individuals with risk of cardiovascular diseases. Smoking in one form or another has been going on since antiquity and yet its association with lung cancer was noted only in the late twentieth century. Sigmund Freud was a great scientist but he could not associate his throat cancer with his cigars.

Metformin, which almost never lowers blood sugar to unacceptable levels has been in use for a long time to treat type II diabetes; reports are now appearing that it might be useful against cancer. Many more examples of unpredictable consequences of drug usage can be cited. The description that follows would provide a glimpse of some of them.

Therapeutics During the Last Five Thousand Years

I have divided this long span of five thousand years to coincide with the evolution of medicine from spiritualism to modern medicine. The first period extends from antiquity to approximately 700 BC, that is, before the beginning of Hindu, Chinese, and Greek medicine; this is essentially the time frame designated as the period of spiritual medicine or witchcraft. The second period spans from the beginning of Hindu, Chinese, and Greek medicine to the end of the nineteenth century; during these two thousand years, many medicines were introduced, but the introduction of very few can be justified by modern standards. The third period covers the twentieth century, during which major therapeutic advances have been made on a rational basis; however, the progression from less rational to more rational therapeutics had its own time frame so that I have divided this period into the first, second, third, and fourth quarter of the twentieth century.

Therapeutics during the Age of Witchcraft: From Antiquity to 700 BC

The period of witchcraft, in my opinion, is the golden age of therapeutics. The three greatest medicines of all times – poppy plant (*Papaver somniferum*) seeds (source of morphine; opium) against pain; Peruvian bark (source of quinine) against fevers, especially malaria; and willow bark (source of salicin, the mother of aspirin) against pain and fever – were introduced during this period by a community of unknown and untrained physicians. Unfortunately, historians of drug discovery emphasize only the individuals and the period when their discovery became known to the Western World (Sneader, 2005). Julius Lips has a chapter titled "Having a Good Time" in his classic *The Origin of Things*; here he describes the discovery of salt, tobacco, alcohol, cacao, areca, coca (cocaine), opium, marijuana, toxicant mushrooms, and so on – all by the primitive civilization and most of them intoxicants (Lips, 1947).

Morphine remains till today the drug of choice against pain and often the last drug that patients of many terminal cancers receive. Even Paracelsus, who burned the books of Galen and Avicenna to show his disgust with their herbal drugs, found opium useful; he prepared a tincture of opium, which he named laudanum and which remained in use until the twentieth century.

Besides morphine, the poppy plant also contains codeine and papaverine. Codeine is a weak form of morphine; it is still used as a cough suppressant and a combination of codeine and acetaminophen (Tylenol), or aspirin is a favourite analgesic of dental surgeons. However, codeine can get converted into morphine in the body and in some subjects this conversion is very efficient, so that the dose of codeine equals that of morphine and can be fatal in children. Papaverine remained in use to relax blood vessels until the twentieth century; indeed, the efficacy of papaverine injection into blood vessels supplying the penis to overcome erectile dysfunction predates and might even be the basis of the discovery of sildenafil (Viagra) in late twentieth century.

Aspirin (acetyl salicylic acid) and aspirin-like compounds not only remain drugs par excellence against inflammatory pain, numerous new uses of this drug have also been discovered. The other agents effective against inflammation are steroids, discovered thousands of years later. In a gross injustice to history, most textbooks, describe *aspirin and related drugs* as non-steroidal anti-inflammatory agents, giving primacy to steroids. The term aspirin-like drugs would have been appropriate, as used by Sir John Vane in his classical paper describing the mechanism of their action (Vane, 1971). Aspirin is now an important cardiovascular drug and many people over the age of fifty take a little aspirin as if it were a vitamin.

I have said enough about quinine in Chapters 3 and 12. Quinine was the first and the only drug which could cure a disease until the discovery of sulphonamides in mid-1930. Although quinine got pushed to a secondary place by chloroquine since World War II, it still remains a valuable drug in the treatment of malaria.

Andean natives knew the stimulant properties of the leaves of *Erythroxylon coca* (source of cocaine), which they chewed during travails on mountain terrains; most probably they also knew of the numbing effect of these leaves on the tongue. However, the possibility of the use of cocaine as a local anaesthetic was conceived by Sigmund Freud on whose advice cocaine was used as the first local anaesthetic in eye surgery by his ophthalmologist friends, Dr. Leopold Königstein (1850-1924) and Carl Köller (1857-1944).

An accurate history of other useful drugs like artemisinin against chloroquine-resistant malaria, emetine against amebiasis, digitalis against heart failure, *Ephedra* plants (source of ephedrine) against asthma, caffeine as a stimulant, *Atropa belladonna* (source of atropine) to suppress excessive secretions and colic pains is not known.

Life Span of Drugs

The life span of most drugs discovered in the twentieth century is relatively short. William Heberden (1710-1801) quipped, "New medicines and new methods of cure always work miracles for a while" (Alpert (2006). William Osler remarked, "One should treat as many patients as possible with a new drug while it still has the power to heal." Interestingly, Heberden and Osler expressed their cynicism with new drugs in the eighteenth and late nineteenth century when not many new drugs were being introduced; imagine the implications of their statements in the twentieth and twenty-first centuries when the Food and Drug Administrations in most countries work overtime to deal with applications for the approval of new molecules.

Drugs are discarded after use for two reasons. One reason for this is the discovery of a superior drug with fewer side effects. For example, streptomycin was replaced by rifampin in the treatment of tuberculosis; indomethacin was replaced by ibuprofen against arthritis; acetazolamide was replaced by thiazide diuretics, and so on. A second reason is the identification of toxicity, which could not be detected during the process of evaluation by double-blind clinical trials, but got known during what is called observational studies (Oates, 2006) when the drug is marketed for general use; this is because the drug is now used in a larger population than was the case during clinical trials, and its effects are observed over a longer period. There are many examples of drugs being discarded for this reason; the sedative thalidomide is a glaring example. Cycloxygenase-2 (COX-2) inhibitor rofecoxib was introduced by Merck Pharmaceutical company in 1999 and withdrawn in 2004 because of increased cardiovascular risk (Graham, 2006). Giant pharmaceuticals are aware of the potential short life span of new drugs and therefore aim at profiting from their new formulations within a few years after their release. In stark contrast to this is the list of drugs mentioned above, discovered by our ancestors of antiquity and still in use.

Certain problems of therapeutics are integral to how drugs are discovered and then marketed. In an editorial in the *Journal of American Medical Association* titled "The Influence of Money on Medical Science," DeAngelis (2006) writes,

> In some instances, the marketing goal of a company dominates the scientific aspect of the company-funded research. There have been a number of high-profile examples of such irregularities involving for-profit companies, such as the refusal to provide all study data to the study team, reporting only 6 months of data in a trial designed to have 12 months of data as the primary outcome; incomplete reporting of serious adverse events; and concealing clinical trial data showing harm.

DeAngelis is really reinforcing what Johann Wolfgang von Goethe (1749-1832) said to Johann Peter Eckermann (1792-1854) on December

21, 1823 (Hobsbawm, 1962): "Questions of science," remarked Goethe, "are very frequently career questions. A single discovery may make a man famous and lay the foundation of his fortunes as a citizen ...Every new observed phenomenon is a discovery, every discovery is property. Touch a man's property and his passions are immediately aroused."

Therapeutics from 700 BC to AD 1900

This long span of over 2,500 years had been a dismal period for therapeutics. With the exception of anaesthetics diethyl ether (or ether), chloroform, nitrous oxide (laughing gas), and the antiseptic carbolic acid, not many useful drugs were introduced during the entire period spanning from Hippocrates to the end of the nineteenth century.

Since textbooks of *Materia Medica* or pharmacology do not differ in their list of drugs, I am going to rely on references made by Hippocrates, Galen, and Paracelsus and the books on *Materia Medica* by William Cullen and Horatio C. Wood – the latter was the recommended textbook on *Materia Medica* at McGill Medical School and most probably at other medical schools (Cullen, 1781; Wood, 1874).

Hippocrates did not introduce any drug of therapeutic value; his four humour theory of disease gave rise to bloodletting taken to absurd levels by Galen (Mattern, 2008) and his followers like the famous American physician Benjamin Rush of the eighteenth century (Abel, 1970; Mattern, 2008); on the other hand, rational use of slow blood removal by leeches has a place in plastic surgery (Gross and Apesos, 1992). Galen used willow bark and opium but did not discover them. What he introduced was a broth containing, among other things, goat dung, pieces of mummy and adder's heads; this potion was manufactured on a large scale and used until the end of the eighteenth century although it could not have helped anyone.

Paracelsus introduced metals (antimony, mercury, sulphur, bismuth, etc.) in place of herbal medicines; yet he admired opium and had a rather positive attitude towards St. John's wort. Some of the metals introduced by Paracelsus remained in use for a long time, although not necessarily as recommended by him; some are still used at present. For example, mercurials were important diuretics until the discovery of thiazide diuretics in the late 1950s. Mercury is not used anymore in modern medicine. Mercury was also used for the treatment of syphilis, but without much benefit, until it was replaced by arsenic in late nineteenth century. Antimony preparations are still used in the treatment of schistosomaiasis (bilharzia[4]) caused by parasites. Since the disease is not endemic in Europe, Paracelsus could not have used antimony to treat bilharzia. Bismuth still has a place as an astringent and in the management of peptic ulcers.

The physicians who followed Paracelsus, especially Cullen and Wood, whose textbooks I have used, merely describe therapeutics during their times. Cullen (1781) talks mainly about the quality of foods and very little about drugs; a hundred years later, Wood published his *Materia Medica*, which describes the pharmacology and toxicology of many drugs and toxic substances. The poverty of therapeutics by the end of the nineteenth century is apparent from a paragraph in the preface of Wood's book; he writes (Wood, 1874):

> This is so well known that it seems superfluous to cite examples of the therapeutic discord; and only shall be mentioned, namely, rheumatism. In this disease, bleeding, nitrate of potassium, quinine, mercurials, flying blisters, purgation, opium, the bromides, veratria, and a host of other remedies, all have their advocates clamorous for a hearing; and above all the tumult are to be heard the trumpet tone of a Chambers, "Wrap your patients in blankets and let them alone."

Wood names all the drugs (or poisons) known by his time and extensively quotes published data or clinical opinions of physicians. However, it is difficult to know from his book whether there is much difference between turpentine and digitalis as "cardiac stimulants," between veratrum alkaloids and potassium cyanide as "cardiac sedatives," and bismuth and lead as "astringents." A careful study of Wood's scholarly book clearly reveals that he was reflecting the poor state of therapeutics of his time and not any lack of expertise on his part. Nonetheless, what Wood and other physicians advised was neither then, nor is now, of any value, and many are harmful. For example, Wood dwells on the therapeutic value of lead, but we know now that lead has no therapeutic value and even lead pipes in homes are illegal. Interestingly, wrapping the patient in a blanket and leaving him/her alone was probably the best treatment despite Wood's scorn for this method.

Besides the drugs that were already in use before the time of Hippocrates, Wood describes only a few new agents, such as ether, chloroform, cod liver oil, colchicine (for acute gout), sodium bicarbonate, iron preparations, many disinfectants, ergot, chloral hydrate (a hypnotic), nitrates (used in cardiac pain, angina), numerous tinctures, and syrups. Very few of these molecules are used now and for indications not identified by Wood's time; nitrates against anginal pain are the exception.

In the unabridged version of this book, I reproduced an Examination Paper in Pharmacology administered to medical students at McGill University, Montreal, Canada, in 1872, 1884 and 1955 with a statement that no current professor of pharmacology could get a passing grade in the 1872 and 1884 papers. The names of drugs in 1872 and 1884 papers were Latinized; they are all now obsolete and were obsolete then. I feel it is not necessary to reproduce these examination papers, which can neither be understood by physicians nor by others.

Prophylaxis

The three significant advances during this period were in prophylaxis – anti-smallpox vaccine, antiseptic carbolic acid, and handwashing by surgeons. I have mentioned all these in previous chapters.

Therapeutics from 1900-2000

Major advances had taken place in physics, chemistry, mathematics, and astronomy by the end of the nineteenth century but had exerted little influence on therapeutics. Things began to change in the following century. The two important aspects of therapeutics from 1900 to 2000 are the rejection of the obsolete remedies of the past and the introduction of therapeutically relevant drugs. This is apparent from the size of *The Merck Manual*, which contained only 192 pages in 1899 but the thirteenth edition published one hundred years later in 2001, contains 2,564 pages; this increase in the size of the manual is a good indication of the advances in therapeutics in the course of the twentieth century.

The enumeration of drugs below is based on four textbooks: *Applied Pharmacology* by A. J. Clark (1923); Goodman and Gilman's *The Pharmacological Basis of Therapeutics* – Edition 1, 1941; edition 5, 1975; and edition 11, 2006, edited by Brunton et al. (2006). I also consulted the *A Manual of Pharmacology and Its Application to Therapeutics and Toxicology* by Torald Sollmann (1948); although this text is far more elaborate on pharmacy and *Materia Medica* aspects than the book by Goodman and Gilman, it does not contain any additional drugs. These books are published twenty to thirty years apart and reflect the rapidly changing discipline of pharmacology in two respects – the replacement of old drugs by new and better drugs and the emphasis on drugs of clinical relevance.

Therapeutics during the First Quarter of the Twentieth Century

Disinfectants are a part of cleaning supplies in many households and hardly any one thinks of them as therapeutic agents. Yet the state of therapeutics was so dismal in the beginning of the 20th century that the first chapter of the first edition of A. J. Clark's *Applied Pharmacology* published in 1923 dealt with disinfectants; the second chapter was on mercury and the third on arsenic and antimony. By 1941, disinfectants become the thirteenth of the sixteen chapters in the first edition of Goodman and Gilman's book and the eleventh edition published in 2006 contains no such chapter. The progressive decline in the emphasis on disinfectants merely reflects its place among the newly acquired drugs over eighty years.

The first barbiturate, barbitonum (Veronal), was introduced in 1903 and this drug, along with chloral hydrate, paraldehyde, urethane, and alcohol, is mentioned in Chapter X of Clark's book under the title "Depressants of the Central Nervous System." None of these drugs are used now. Clark provides a detailed description of the pharmacology of cocaine, which was already known as a local anaesthetic since 1884; he makes the following significant comment (Clark, 1923a): "The cocaine habit is easily established, and produces more rapidly deleterious effects than any other drug."

Clark's chapters on the autonomic nervous system, alimentary canal, heart, blood circulation, respiration, kidneys, uterus, temperature regulation, and endocrine system are noteworthy from the viewpoints of physiology and pathology but do not add anything new to therapeutics. Clark, however, presents a more scientific description of all known drugs, along with their toxicity, than can be found in Wood's *Materia Medica*. Clark has a Chapter (XXIII) on radiation and introduces its antitumor actions, which has evolved as an important adjuvant in current cancer chemotherapy. Additionally, Clark gives a sound description of the basis of allergy, treatment of toxins, and the mechanism of action of certain venoms. In summary, therapeutics had not made significant advances by the end of the first quarter of the twentieth century. This is illustrated by a prescription dated c.1922 in Newfoundland by Crellin (2004) in which Mrs. Bennett is prescribed tincture (Tr.) camphor, Chlorodine, Tr. Scillae, Potassium acetate, Solution of Strychnine Hydrochloride, Spirit of Chloroform, Syrup, Solution of Cochineal and Water; this prescription has no therapeutic value whatsoever.

Therapeutics during the Second Quarter of the Twentieth Century

By the year 1941, when the first edition of Goodman and Gilman's classic book *The Pharmacological Basis of Therapeutics* appeared, many new and better drugs had been introduced. Compared with Clark's 1923 book, which had 390 pages, Goodman and Gilman's 1941 book contains 1,383 pages. The book starts with a discussion of the general principles of drug action. The currently used inhalation anaesthetics like halothane and enflurane were not yet discovered. Ultra short-acting barbiturates for the induction of anaesthesia were known. Curiously, nitrous oxide, which failed to produce anaesthesia when first tried in 1845 by Horace Wells (1815-1848) at the Massachusetts General Hospital, is still in use while ether, which passed the first test, is not permitted even to anaesthetize laboratory rats.

Major advances had been made in the area of hypnotics and sedatives, and Goodman and Gilman list seventeen barbiturates. As well, the use of barbiturates against epilepsy was discovered. But a very significant advance was the discovery in 1938 of the anti-epilepsy drug, Dilantin (diphenyl hydantoin), by H. Houston Merritt (1902-1979) and Tracy Jackson Putnam (1894-1975) (Merritt and Putnam, 1938). It was the very first demonstration that tonic-clonic convulsions (grand mal epilepsy) can be suppressed without causing general sedation. We now know that through the use of more selective drugs discreet functions of the brain can be modulated. Dilantin is still used seventy years later.

Several substitutes of cocaine for use as local anaesthetics were discovered by the 1940s. Many substitutes of the endogenous transmitter acetylcholine[5] were discovered although these have not been a major breakthrough in therapeutics. In contrast, inhibitors of acetylcholine, the oldest being an alkaloid atropine derived from *Atropa belladonna* and known since antiquity, is much more useful in suppressing excessive secretions and relieving certain colic pains. Many adrenaline substitutes were also discovered, which proved effective against asthma, and one of them, albuterol (Ventolin), discovered much later and mainly administered by inhalation, remains the primary agent for the treatment of asthma.

It is a pity that atropine and adrenaline are treated as "molecules of murder" (Emsley, 2008) because some unseasoned criminals used them for homicide.

The next major group of compounds after Dilantin introduced during this period is sulphonamides. Germany was the most advanced country in chemistry, and it was there that experiments with azo dyestuffs started. Gerhard Domagk (1895-1964) reported in 1935 that mice with streptococcal septicaemia could be protected by prontosil. A new era of chemotherapy started for the first time. Domagk was honoured with the Nobel Prize in medicine in 1939, and many Nobel Prizes were to follow for contributions in this area. The discovery of prontosil is a significant advance for other reasons as well. Synthesis of new molecules based on the structure of prontosil generated many sulphonamides and firmly established the sub-discipline of chemical structure-biological activity relationship. Fortunately, Domagk tested prontosil in mice with septicaemia; had he done the test in a dish, the results would have been negative because prontosil needs to be metabolized into its active moïety sulphanilamide in the body in order to act as an antibacterial agent.

Sulphonamides could cure – not merely relieve – symptoms; thus began the era of chemotherapy and the supremacy of modern medicine over all other schools of medicine. Until the discovery of sulphonamides, quinine, discovered in antiquity, was the only drug that could cure. No wonder Goodman and Gilman (1941) devote 100 out of 1,300 pages of their first edition of the book to a description of sulphonamides.

So far, I have listed two major developments in therapeutics – Dilantin against epilepsy and sulphonamides against bacterial infections.

The third major breakthrough placed Canada on the map of therapeutic innovations. Frederick Banting (1891-1941), Charles Herbert Best (1899-1978), James Bertram Collip (1892-1965), and John James Rickard Macleod (1876-1935) announced in 1922 that a purified extract of the pancreas saved the life of the nineteen-year-old patient Leonard Thompson, and the effect could be noticed in a single day. That miracle extract contained insulin, which remains the backbone of the control of diabetes and is destined to remain so until a cure is discovered. Just one year later, unprecedented in the history of Nobel Prizes in any discipline, Banting and Macleod were awarded the Nobel Prize in medicine in 1923, which they shared with their other two colleagues, Best and Collip. This generosity on the part of Banting and Macleod is significant because if many subsequent winners of this coveted honour had followed this practice, many of them would have landed with just a few thousand dollars rather than more than one million. For sure, Salvador Moncada, now Sir Salvador, who identified nitric oxide and the pathway of its synthesis, would have had a share in the Nobel Prize for nitric oxide awarded in 1998 to Robert F. Furchgott (1916-2009), Louis J. Ignarro and Ferid Murad; he might also have shared the 1982 Nobel Prize for prostaglandins awarded to Sune K. Bergstrom (1916-2004), Bengt I. Samuelsson, and Sir John R. Vane.

Therapeutics during the Third Quarter of the Twentieth Century

All chemicals are potentially toxic. Therefore, a great deal of effort gone into finding out how much and how often a particular drug should be given. Precisely for that reason, pharmacology books necessarily contain an introductory chapter on the methods of drug administration, the kinetics of absorption and excretion of drugs, drug metabolism, the relationship between the doses producing therapeutic and toxic effects, and how the effects of drugs are modified by gender, age, and disease. The section covering these aspects has increased over the years from zero pages in Clark's 1923 book to 136 pages in the eleventh edition of Goodman and Gilman (Brunton et al., 2006). This fact by itself points to progress in therapeutics.

Besides the remarkable progress in the understanding of drug metabolism, excretion and dosing regimen, noteworthy additions to therapeutics were also made during this period.

Modern inhalation anaesthetics such as halothane and enflurane were introduced, which are neither flammable like ether nor explosive like cyclopropane, nor cardiotoxic like chloroform. By and large, inhalation anaesthetics are both administered and excreted by the lungs; if they do not undergo metabolism in the body, so much the better. Enflurane, more or less, meets this criterion as well. Techniques for local and regional anaesthesia were also perfected. On the other hand, anaesthetics are an unusual kind of drugs. They are not used to treat any diseases but merely to anaesthetize a patient needing surgery.

Certain kinds of sedatives have been used since antiquity, and these found a substitute in the early 1900s in the form of barbiturates, which was replaced by safer benzodiazepines (e.g., diazepam, Valium) (see Chapter 2).

By 1975, the field of psychopharmacology had made its appearance in a big way. Many factors triggered this development, but perhaps the article "Rauwolfia Serpentina, a New Indian Drug for Insanity and High Blood Pressure" (Sen and Bose, 1931) and two other articles (Bhatia, 1942; Vakil, 1949) describing *Rauwolfia's* anti-hypertensive property played an important role. It was soon found that reserpine, one of the alkaloids of *Rauwolfia*, is the main active molecule (Siddiqui and Siddiqui, 1931) and that it interferes with the storage of noradrenaline in nerve terminals, which underlies its effects on blood pressure as well as on mood.[6]

These seminal contributions by Indian scientists did not draw attention for some time. However, by the 1960s, interest in reserpine was so high that practically every pharmacology establishment all over the world had somebody on staff experimenting with this drug.

Also around the same time, another chemical, chlorpromazine, was discovered. Chlorpromazine belongs to the phenothiazine group of chemicals, which were known since 1883. However, it was the publication of the effects of chlorpromazine on mood (Lehmann and Hanrahan, 1954) that gave additional impetus to the field of psychopharmacology.

A third significant contribution in the area of psychopharmacology made at the same time as the discovery of chlorpromazine was the discovery of inhibitors of monoamine oxidases.[7] Isoniazid (isonicotinic acid hydrazide) was known since 1912. It was first used to treat tuberculosis in 1952. It was noted by nurses that patients receiving isoniazid appeared cheerful, and it was soon found that this mood elevation was the result of the inhibition of the enzyme monoamine oxidase (MAO), which metabolizes several amines like serotonin, adrenaline, et cetera. Iproniazid, a drug similar to isoniazid but with no anti-tubercular activity was then synthesized specifically to inhibit MAO, and it did have a mood-elevating effect; many and better MAO inhibitors were soon synthesized.

Thus the drugs reserpine, chlorpromazine, and iproniazid, each with their characteristic pharmacology but all psychoactive in their own specific ways, ushered in the era of psychopharmacology, a very broad and complex area of therapeutics. When I was a medical student in Lucknow between 1950 and 1955, we were required to travel a distance of two hundred kilometres to observe patients at a mental asylum in Agra, the city of the architectural marvel Taj Mahal. This mental asylum was worse than any prison. The Taj Mahal is still there, but not the mental asylum. This is the contribution of psychopharmacology.

However, much more was accomplished in the field of psychopharmacology than just getting rid of mental asylums. At the same time, psychopharmacology is greatly influenced by societal factors in which the subject, parents, school teachers, physicians, researchers, and pharmaceutical industries play a role; and the probability of misuse of psychotherapeutic drugs is quite high (Szasz, 1971, 1974).

Approaches to Drug Discovery

In most cases, therapeutically useful drugs are discovered through one of the following approaches.

Modification of the structure of an active moiety

No one knows exactly how opium, quinine, and aspirin were discovered. But once they were discovered, modifications in the molecule led to the discovery of many other drugs, including the morphine-substitute heroin and its antidote naloxone, as well as a host of aspirin substitutes like the superior anti-inflammatory drug ibuprofen. Numerous examples can be cited.

Mimicry of endogenous molecules

I mentioned earlier that the discovery of the adrenaline-substitute albuterol (Ventolin) was an important advance in the control of asthmatic attacks. However, antagonists of adrenaline proved just as useful. How they were discovered and how their usefulness was identified is fascinating in its own right – somewhat like Christopher Columbus (1451-1506) discovering America while on his way to India.

Many compounds have been developed on the basis of mimicry of chemical structure; but perhaps the most important among them is propranolol, discovered by Sir James Black (1924-2010). The structure of adrenaline and noradrenaline through which sympathetic nerves increase the blood pressure or stimulate the heart was known. As early as 1947, Mark Nickerson (1916-1998) had already reported that a chemical dibenamine blocked the effects of noradrenaline and adrenaline on blood pressure (Nickerson and Goodman, 1947). It was already known that the compound dichloroisoproterenol (DCI) could be used to block the effects of adrenaline on the heart (Slater and Powell, 1957). Using all these leads, Black et al. (1964) succeeded in developing the pure antagonist of the effects of adrenaline-like compounds on the heart. Although originally expected to modify the harmful effects of adrenaline-like chemicals on the heart only, as, for example, in the case of angina, propranolol was also found to lower blood pressure. Sir James Black was awarded the Nobel Prize in medicine 24 years later in 1988.

By the time of his death in 2010, Black was trying to solve the problem of heart failure, albeit, in my opinion, using an erroneous premise. He was trying to find a molecule that could increase the contractile force of the heart.[8]

Many pharmacologists think that heart failure is due to the inability of adrenaline-like agents to increase the heart's contractions. The noted pharmacologist Robert J. Lefkowitz (Lefkowitz et al., 2000; Koch et al., 1995) put this idea forward. In my opinion, the kind of heart failure, which is a major clinical problem and which almost always results in death, is not due to a deficiency in the contractile property of the heart; strong evidence in support of this suggestion came from the studies of Yue et al. (1992). Beta adrenergic receptor blockers like propranolol can produce heart failure on their own. However, Yue et al. (1992) showed in experimental models that carvedilol, a beta adrenergic receptor blocker, actually corrected heart failure by acting as an antioxidant. While clinical studies have found that carvedilol and some other beta adrenoceptor blockers reduced mortality in patients with heart failure (Braunwald, 2001), the exact mechanism is unlikely to be the one postulated by Yue et al. (1992, 1999). I had the privilege of having Tian-Li Yue as my PhD student at McGill University.

A recent study has demonstrated that experimental heart failure in rats leads to redistribution of the two types of beta receptors within and outside the myocardial cells (Nikolaev et al., 2010; Dorn, 2010); however, this to me seems to be an effect rather than the cause of heart failure because the primary event in their study was induction of heart failure and the reverse was not tested.

Discoveries based on basic science

Advances in physiology and biochemistry have also contributed to drug discovery. Biochemical research had led to an understanding of the necessary constituents in the development of cells. An antimetabolite is a substance that resembles one of the essential compounds in cell functioning but cannot be used by the cells; instead, through its chemical similarity, the antimetabolite interferes with the utilization of the essential molecule. In a sense, sulphonamides act as an antimetabolite.

Para-aminobenzoic acid (PABA) is essential for the growth of bacteria. Because sulphonamides resemble PABA, they interfere with its utilization by bacteria and therefore act as antibacterial agents. Many molecules, such as purines and pyrimidines, are essential for cell growth. The faster the cell growth, the greater is the need for purines and pyrimidines. This understanding of the biochemistry of cell functioning was brilliantly utilized by Gertrude B. Elion and George H. Hitchings to discover 6-mercaptopurine and azathioprine, the first major breakthrough in anticancer and immunosuppressant therapy, and both shared the Nobel Prize with Sir James Black in 1988.

Inquisitiveness and insight into one's data

"A discovery is said to be an accident meeting a prepared mind," said Albert von Szent-Gyorgyi (Hager, 2006). Developments in science also enhance the ability of scientists to draw rational inferences from chance observation. The discovery of penicillin by Sir Alexander Fleming is a case in point. Fleming noticed that his agar plates, which were contaminated by moulds, interfered with the growth of bacteria; all he needed to do, as perhaps many had done before him, was to use properly sterilized plates. But not Fleming; he pondered over this mishap and inferred that these fungal moulds might contain some antibacterial activity. They indeed did, and soon after, we had penicillin.

World War II was going on. While Fleming was struggling with his bacterial plates and the mould, Hitler's Luftwaffe were pounding London and other industrial cities. Soldiers and civilians alike needed penicillin, of which the supply at that time was so limited that it had to be scavenged from patients' urine. Penicillin was, and remains, a miracle drug. It started the era of antibiotics, and many drugs were to follow soon after so that many infections, which almost always had been fatal, could now be tamed. Fleming was awarded the Nobel Prize in 1945 along with Ernst B. Chain and Sir Howard Florey.

Sulphonamides were already known and being used; these drugs are given orally. It was noted by the French clinicians (Janbon et al., 1942) that patients with typhoid fever receiving certain sulphonamides developed hypoglycaemia. The significance of this observation did not remain unnoticed. They reasoned that, on the basis of the basic chemical structure of sulphonamides, drugs could be tailored to be given orally for the management of diabetes. Insulin was until then the only anti-diabetic agent, but it cannot be given orally because, being a protein, it gets destroyed in the gut. Soon thereafter, Auguste-Louis Loubatière (1912-1977) showed that the hypoglycaemic effects of sulphonamides required a functioning pancreas (see Loubatière, 1957), which is the case in type 2 diabetes, the most common form of the disease. Thus started the era of oral hypoglycaemic drugs, of which many are now available.

Improvement upon existing drugs

Most drugs introduced in the third quarter of the twentieth century were discovered by mimicry of other drugs. That is why they are often referred to as first generation, second generation, and so on, simply to denote improvement in any specific area; many oral hypoglycaemic drugs and antibiotics are denoted in this fashion. Other ways of improving drugs could simply be by replacing a drug that could only be given by injection by a substitute that can be taken orally (replacement of the anti-tuberculosis drug streptomycin by rifampin), prolonging the duration of action such as crystalline insulin by protamine zinc insulin, finding a less toxic substitute (many drugs found their way in this manner).

The kidney is a very important organ. The American physiologist Homer William Smith (1895-1962) titled his textbook on kidney physiology as *From Fish to Philosopher* (Smith, 1962) to emphasize the point that the kidney was central to the evolution from aquatic to terrestrial life. The kidney also plays a critical role in maintaining acid-base balance. No matter what we eat and drink, the pH of the blood does not change much. Bicarbonate (HCO_3^-) is the principal ion involved in maintaining this balance; it is formed by a combination of water (H_2O) and carbon dioxide (CO_2) and is regulated by an enzyme called carbonic anhydrase. The body store of bicarbonate is preserved by its reabsorption in the kidney. If the carbonic anhydrase enzyme is inhibited, the urinary excretion of bicarbonate as well as sodium is increased.

Consequently, taking advantage of the structure of sulphonamides, drugs were synthesized to act as diuretics; acetazolamide is an example. However, the diuretic effect of acetazolamide does not last for a long period because it starts to cause the depletion of bicarbonate and acidosis begins to set in, which the kidney does not allow to happen. After a while, acetazolamide ceases to act as a diuretic. Paracelsus introduced mercury as a drug. It is a very powerful diuretic. However, mercury produces diuresis by increasing the excretion of chloride ions (Cl-); the depletion of chloride ions causes alkalosis, and again, the kidney terminates the diuretic effect of mercury. What scientists did was to make a drug that has elements of both acetazolamide and mercury and synthesized an entirely new compound, which proved to be a powerful diuretic; the first compound was ethacrynic acid, which was soon replaced by the less toxic and more effective furosemide (Lasix).

In summary, almost all drugs that are currently used were discovered between 1950 and 1975 by one of the approaches described above.

Therapeutics in the Fourth Quarter of the Twentieth Century

The remarkable feature of the final quarter of the twentieth century is not so much the discovery of new drugs but, rather, a refinement in therapeutics on the basis of a better understanding of the pharmacology of drugs, the pathology of diseases, and lessons learned from epidemiological studies. I will give a few examples of groups of drugs either because they are widely used or because their discovery is ingenious.

The 5-hydroxytryptamine (5-HT) or serotonin is one of the many endogenous amines. The 5-HT produces many effects, but its role in depression and migraine is clinically very relevant. Both are common conditions. The chemical 5-HT is released in many tissues, including the brain, and it exerts its effects by activating specific receptors, of which at least four distinct types have been identified. Once 5-HT is released by nerve endings, it produces its effects through its receptors but is also taken back into nerve terminals. If somehow this reuptake is inhibited, its concentration in the vicinity of the receptor increases and so does its effect. Such drugs have been developed, and fluoxetine (Prozac) is one such drug. It is widely used to treat depression; many people claim that it helped them quit smoking. It has also been misused. St John's wort, mentioned earlier, supposedly also acts by inhibiting the uptake of 5-HT.

In most cases, migraine attacks occur usually one to four times a year, but when they do, they can be quite debilitating. Exactly why these periodic attacks of migraine occur is still not clearly known, but there is evidence that, for some reason, blood vessels on the brain surface dilate so that blood accumulates in these vessels and less blood becomes available for nervous tissues of the brain; the resulting relative deprivation of blood to the brain causes migraine. If these blood vessels on the surface of the brain could be constricted, they would not be able to act as a sink for the blood and would not be able to deprive the brain of an adequate blood supply. The 5-HT can do this job. By acting on its specific receptors on blood vessels, 5-HT causes their constriction and allows blood flow to brain tissue, which terminates or prevents migraine attacks. Many drugs, collectively known as *triptans*, simulate the effects of 5-HT and constrict the brain surface blood vessels; these are favourite drugs against migraine. Ergot alkaloids do not act at the same receptor sites as 5-HT but still produce the same effect.

Parkinson's disease is another common ailment. Most of us have watched somebody having trouble holding a cup of coffee or worse. The disease does not discriminate between its victims on the basis of gender and ethnicity; it occurs in all ages, but more commonly in people older than sixty-five years whose numbers are gradually increasing. Researchers have identified that the disease is caused by a deficiency in functional dopaminergic neurons in the brain area called substantia nigra, which is a bit darker than surrounding tissues. The function of these nerve cells is performed by releasing dopamine. The biochemical process of synthesizing adrenaline from the amino acid tyrosine involves its conversion first to L-DOPA, then to dopamine, then to noradrenaline, and finally to adrenaline. All these three amines can act as transmitter, but Parkinson's disease is a result of deficiency in dopamine. The normal treatment would be, therefore, to give dopamine, but dopamine, like adrenaline and noradrenaline, would get destroyed in the gut or the liver; and even if they were not destroyed, they would be prevented from reaching the brain by what is known as the blood-brain barrier, which nature has developed to protect the brain from a multitude of undesirable chemicals. This barrier does not let everything that we ingest by mouth reach the brain. Dopamine is one such chemical that cannot defy the blood-brain barrier. Scientists, however, found a solution to this problem. Although dopamine cannot reach the brain, its precursor DOPA, which is an amino acid and not an amine, can. Consequently, tremors and rigidity and associated disability of Parkinson's patients can be controlled by oral administration of the levorotatory form of DOPA, that is: L-DOPA. Once L-DOPA is in the brain, it gets converted into dopamine and relieves the symptoms of Parkinson's disease.

Willow bark has been used since antiquity, and its active constituent salicin had eventually led to the synthesis of aspirin by the late nineteenth century. Because it was such a common household remedy and was often stored in easy-to-open containers, aspirin remained the most common cause of drug poisoning in children until child-proof containers were introduced in the 1970s. While the analgesic activity of aspirin was universally known, no one knew exactly how it worked. It was left to Sir John Robert Vane to solve the puzzle; he reported in 1971 that aspirin acted by inhibiting the synthesis of prostaglandins (PG). A necessary by-product of this discovery, for which John Vane was awarded the Nobel Prize in 1982, was an intensive study of prostaglandins, the discovery of which can be traced to a 1930 observation (Kurzrok and Lieb, 1930) that uterine tissue contracted when exposed to human semen. Because the active substance was present in semen and must have come from the prostate gland, it got named prostaglandin. Following Vane's paper on the mechanism of the action of aspirin-like drugs, the biochemical mechanisms in the synthesis, storage, and metabolism of different forms of prostaglandins as well as their numerous actions were identified. An offshoot of these studies was the finding that two different enzymes are involved in the synthesis of prostaglandins – cyclooxygenase I (COX-I), and cyclooxygenase II (COX II). COX-I produces most of the PGs, including the PGs of the E series, which protect the stomach lining. In contrast, COX-II produces PGs that are involved in inflammation. Because aspirin inhibits both COX-I and COX-II, it causes gastric toxicity while being used to suppress pain and inflammation. Therefore, an aspirin-like drug that selectively inhibits COX-II but not COX-I could be a good anti-inflammatory drug devoid of gastric toxicity. Such drugs were eventually synthesized; celecoxib is one such compound.

However, celecoxib is a recent drug, and despite every information that could be gathered in the laboratory or during clinical trials, the full spectrum of the beneficial and harmful effects are actually revealed only when a drug enters the retail market and is used on a mass scale. Nonetheless, the discovery of celecoxib demonstrates the role of basic knowledge in drug discovery.

Just as drugs were discovered after a knowledge of the synthesis of PGs, so also angiotensin-converting-enzyme (ACE) inhibitors were discovered after it became known that it is this enzyme that converts angiotensin I (the inactive molecule) to angiotensin II (the active molecule), a potent vasoconstrictor. ACE inhibitors are among the commonly used drugs in the treatment of hypertension and systolic heart failure.

Sometimes, a clearer understanding in the pathology of a disease leads to the use of a drug that already exists but was not known to have any potential benefit. Gastric ulcer or peptic ulcer is a common disease; it can progress to rupture of the stomach or cancer. Gastric ulcer is an ancient disease, and it has been known that it is caused by acidity and that acid secretion is increased by histamine. However, usual antihistamine drugs were not beneficial in the treatment of peptic ulcer. The first question was, why not? The answer was that histamine acts through two different types of receptors, termed H1 and H2. Activation of H1 receptors produces symptoms which patients experience during hay fever and allergies but is not involved in gastric acid secretion. It is the H2 receptors through which histamine increases gastric acid secretion. Once this fact became known, antagonists of H2 histamine receptors such a cimetidine were synthesized. It proved very useful but could not eradicate gastric ulcer.

However, the story of gastric ulcer seems more complex than the role of H2 histamine receptors. In the early 1980s, Australian scientists revived the century-old story that peptic ulcer may be due to an infection by the bacteria *Helicobacter pylori* (Warren and Marshall, 1983); although this news was initially received with due scepticism, their suggestion eventually got recognition in the form of the 2005 Nobel Prize. A new approach to peptic ulcer therapy was initiated that comprised of, among other things, a course of cimetidine with an antibiotic (amoxicillin or clarithromycin) and maybe bismuth as an astringent.

But I am not sure this is the end of the saga of peptic ulcer. *H. pylori* are commonly present in the stomach. Usually, when bacteria make the human (or animal) body a place of their routine residence, they develop some symbiotic relationship. That is why when broad-spectrum antibiotics are used people develop diarrhea, because bacterial flora of the large bowel get disturbed. It would take some time before we know if *H. pylori* reach the stomach just to produce ulcer or they also do something else.

Evidence-Based Medicine

Simon Singh is a renowned science journalist whose books, like *Fermat's Enigma*, the *Code Book*, and the *Big Bang* can be found at most bookshops. Singh's latest book *Trick or Treatment?: Alternative Medicine on Trial* co-authored with Edzard Ernst (Singh and Ernst, 2008) starts with premises that the book *Trick or Treatment?* is guided by Hippocrates' dictum and the principles of *evidence-based medicine*. However, Hippocrates did not say anything that can be used to test the efficacy of drugs. The phrase, though not the idea of, evidence-based medicine is recent. Scientific medicine was always evidence-based or else it would have remained where it was at the time of Hippocrates or even earlier. The current implication of evidence-based medicine involves the entire discipline of clinical medicine (Straus et al., 2005); but what is relevant here is its emphasis on controlled clinical trials, elegantly described in epidemiology texts (Fletcher and Fletcher, 2005; Lilienfeld and Lilienfeld, 1980). These clinical trials compare two or more existing therapies for a given ailment or assess the merit of a new drug. Evidence-based medicine is unsuited to evaluate alternate systems of medicine just as the laws of physics cannot scrutinize the merits of a religion.

The hype about evidence-based medicine is examined in a hilarious article by Smith and Pell (2003) in the *British Medical Journal.* The authors tried to investigate whether there are any randomized controlled trials to examine the efficacy of parachutes in minimizing injuries during a free fall. They could not find any studies that satisfied their objective criteria. Does it imply that parachutes should not be used when the pilot jumps out of a plane until such trials have been done? Would throwing animals or just a big pumpkin from a flying helicopter with or without the aid of a parachute and examining the injury after the fall satisfy Smith and Pell (2003), or would they remain unsatisfied until these tests are done on humans?

The paper by Smith and Pell, indeed, points to the absurdity inherent in mechanical rules to judge efficacy of medicines or, for that matter, anything. A correct scientific inference itself dictates how it should be arrived. Darwin examined hundreds of plants and animals to conclude how species arose; yet he would have been dismissed if the rule of evidence-based medicine were applied because he missed visiting the Tundra. The concept of evidence-based medicine is recent and was introduced by a group of physicians in 1992.[9] Would that imply that quinine, penicillin, and insulin were introduced on false grounds? Insulin was tested only on one person as was the anti-smallpox vaccine.

What I have just said does not mean that there is no merit to randomized clinical trials, double-blind studies, and meta analysis of available data.[10] And yet, controlled randomized blind trials often give an equivocal answer. Since all drugs produce placebo and toxic effects without guaranteeing a therapeutic effect, physicians are no nearer to a clear guideline than they were at the start. Many randomized trials were needed to find out whether to give tamoxifen as a prophylactic against breast cancer or hormone (oestrogen) replacement therapy to overcome postmenopausal changes. Likewise, the question as to what public measure to take against the herbal home remedy St John's wort remains evasive.

St. John's wort, which has been known for a long time, was rediscovered in twentieth century, perhaps as a result of the growing popularity of other schools of medicine. It is an extract from the plant *Hypericum perforatum* and is an immensely popular remedy in Europe and the USA against depression, which is often self-diagnosed. St John's wort has received endorsement from the popular media and even by Singh and Ernst (2008), albeit with some reservations. It took many trials and many meta-analyses to detect a slightly improved effect of St. John's wort over that of placebos and only against mild depression. However, St John's wort is not a single molecule; it contains almost eleven different chemicals, like most herbal preparations. Most importantly, St. John's wort induces liver drug metabolizing enzymes as summarized by one of the authors of the book (Ernst, 1999). Whenever any drug inhibits or induces liver drug metabolizing enzymes, it is bound to decrease or increase the activity of many other drugs taken simultaneously because most drugs are metabolized by these enzymes. Since St. John's wort is not a prescription drug, often the physician who is prescribing other drugs is unaware of the patient's drug history.

Moreover, a rational treatment of depression and selection of the best drug is very complex, and the placebo effect is as high as 30 to 40 percent. It will thus take a long time before St. John's wort gets accepted or rejected by modern science.

Stem Cell Research and Gene Therapy

Both stem cell and gene therapy, especially the former, are politically charged issues. Both have the potential for therapeutic marvels as well as for gross misuse, like the atomic theory of Ernest Rutherford (1871-1937). The quest for the therapeutic use of stem cells and gene substitution is still an emerging field, and I prefer not to go into great detail in this area at this time. Many centres are researching into gene therapy. Perhaps stem cell therapy is also in operation, though not as openly.[11] Here I will indicate very briefly the underlying principles of both stem cell and gene therapy.

The story of Stem Cell can be traced to the seminal observation made by Canadian scientists Ernst A. McCulloch (1926-2011) and James Edgar Till and their student Andy J. Becker (Becker et al., 1963) that certain cells from the bone marrow when injected into a mouse whose immune system has been suppressed by radiation can form discreet colonies in the spleen. As happens with many fundamental observations the significance of these studies of the Canadian scientists did not receive due recognition until the beginning of 21st Century.

Since the dawn of the 21st century, the use and misuse of stem cells is hotly debated and governments take a position whether or not to allow stem cell research, which opens the possibility of taking any group of cells, preferably embryonic and transforming them into any type of cells. These cells can then be used for the repair and replacement of damaged cells, be it in the brain of an Alzheimer patient or in cancer. According to a news item in the *Economist* (February 25, 2012), researchers are aiming to replace meat from cattle by meat raised from cattle's muscle in Petri dishes. While stem cells offer all these possibilities, they can also be perilous (Cyranoski, 2010).

Gene therapy involves the insertion of a specified gene using an appropriate vector to replace a defective gene underlying a disease (Panno, 2011). However, neither of these areas has been, thus far, sufficiently studied to forecast what good or harm they can do, but the potential for both exists. On the other hand, using chemical genetics strategy, Gao et al. (2010) recently reported a chemical (iminothiazolidinone BMS-790052) with promising results against viral hepatitis, which affects nearly two hundred million people. Whether or not this or a similar compound proves clinically effective cannot be stated with certainty, but they do show that even complex diseases can be eventually tamed.

Usually, the forward march of science cannot be stopped on ethical grounds, nor can unethical use be universally prevented. The world, as it exists today, is wrought with violence and injustice but also with a movement to end all this. It is very possible that in a world saner than it is today, both stem cell and gene therapies might offer cures for diseases that can hardly be controlled today, much less cured.

Conclusion

In the final analysis, the history of medicine revolves around human effort to eradicate a disease or, at the very least, to alleviate suffering. Drugs occupy a central position in this endeavour. However, while human achievement is historically determined, the most appropriate therapy for a disease often lags behind. Consequently, a host of medicaments have been tried. Although the communal quest had yielded some excellent remedies in antiquity, the period from Hippocrates to the beginning of the twentieth century has little to show in terms of therapeutics. The picture changed since the beginning of the twentieth century. We are now at a stage where one can foresee not only further refinements of medicines we already have but also acquisition of much-needed medicine for diseases that have been elusive, like cancer; "*The Emperor of All Maladies*" (Mukherjee, 2010) can be dethroned. It is very possible that advances in therapeutics propelled by scientific medicine can usher in an era in which an individual lives a disease-free life until death; as a by-product, the science of medicine can bury unscientific alternative medicine.

Notes

1. Popper, K. *Conjectures and Refutations: The Growth of Scientific Knowledge* (London: Routledge & Kegan Paul, 1963), 66-67. Sir Karl Raimund Popper (1902-1994) was one of the greatest science philosophers of the twentieth century who introduced the concept of critical rationalism. He was born in Vienna; being of Jewish origin, he had to move, with the advent of Nazism, first to New Zealand and then to England, where he was knighted. He was based at the London School of Economics.

2. Szasz, Thomas S. *The Myth of Mental Illness* (New York: Harper-Perennial, 1974), 300.

3. King Louis XVI (1754-1793) had commissioned Benjamin Franklin (1706-1790), the first US ambassador to France, to find out if Mesmer's magnetized iron rod therapy had any merit. Franklin blindfolded patients so they did not know whether or not they were being subjected to a magnetized rod; he concluded that magnetized rods were no better than non-magnetized rods. King Louis XVI and his queen, Marie Antoinette (1755-1793), were executed on January 21, 1793, during the French Revolution. Marie Antoinette was both attractive and indulgent, and what is popularly known is that when she was told that the crowd outside the palace were demanding bread, she asked ushers to tell them to eat cake instead; most probably this metaphor is not true and has been manufactured to make the queen appear foolish. It is very possible that she was well aware of what was going on in France.

4. Bilharzia is prevalent in Asia, Africa, and Northern Brazil; it is caused by three different kinds of *Schistosomes* (haematobium, mansoni, and japonicum) and carried by freshwater snails. Antimony salts are still used to treat the disease.

5. Nerves communicate with organs they supply by releasing chemicals known as neu-

rotransmitters. The peripheral nervous system can be divided into voluntary and involuntary; the former is used to move arms and legs, etc., while the involuntary comprises of the parasympathetic and sympathetic division; the former acts by releasing acetylcholine and the latter by releasing noradrenaline, which is slightly different from adrenaline.

6. The plant Rauwolfia contains many alkaloids but one, reserpine, possesses unusual pharmacological activity, which somehow explains such diverse effects as reduction of blood pressure and effects on mental disorder. The sympathetic system (syn. adrenergic system) exerts its effects by releasing the chemical noradrenaline (similar to but not identical with popularly known adrenaline) from the nerve endings. Somehow, reserpine prevents the storage of noradrenaline (and a few other molecules) in nerve endings so that the sympathetic system is essentially non-functional. Because noradrenaline increases blood pressure, its decrease lowers the blood pressure. Noradrenaline is also a transmitter in the brain, which underlies the effects of reserpine on mood.

7. Monoamine oxidases (MAO) are enzymes inside nerve terminals. There are different forms of this enzyme. Amines are safely stored inside the vesicles in nerve terminals or anywhere else; once they are released, they come in contact with MAO and can get destroyed. If MAOs are inhibited by drugs, the concentration of these amines increases and so does their effects, one of which is the elevation of mood.

8. Sir James Black mentioned his attempt to treat heart failure by increasing cardiac contractions during the Nickerson Memorial Lecture titled "Beta-Adrenoceptors in the Heart" on September 24, 2004, delivered at the Department of Pharmacology and Therapeutics, McGill University, Montreal, Canada. He died in 2010.

9. "Evidence-Based Medicine: A New Approach to Teaching the Practice of Medicine," *Journal of American Medical Association* 268 (1992): 2420-2425. This paper is authored by different specialists from all over the world and led by McMaster University, Hamilton, Canada, Professor Gordon Guyatt. The Health Science Division of McMaster University is relatively recent (1968-1969) and pioneered innovative integrated case-based teaching in contrast to teaching by didactic lectures in different subspecialties like anatomy, physiology, pharmacology, etc.

10. Meta analysis is a statistical method and involves using existing data from a number of trials to re-evaluate the merit of certain claims.

11. On March 20, 2010, the Canadian newspaper *Globe and Mail* published a lengthy article with a photograph of one Dr. Geeta Shroff. According to the article, Dr. Shroff runs a multimillion-dollar stem-cell treatment from her posh private hospital in Delhi and treats patients from all over the world at an average cost of $21,000 per patient.

References

Abel, A. L. "Blood Letting: Barber-Surgeon's Shaving and Bleeding Bowls," *Journal of American Medical Association* 214 (1970): 900-901.

Alpert, J. S. "Commentary: The Triumph of Hope Over Experience," *The American Journal of Medicine* 119 (2006): 1003-1004.

Becker, A.J., McCulloch, E.A. and Till, J.E. "Cytological Demonstration of the Clonal Nature of Spleen Colonies Derived From Translanted Mouse Marrow Cells," *Nature* 197 (1963): 452-454.

Bhatia, B. B. "On the Use of Rauwolfia Serpentina in High Blood Pressure," *Journal of Indian Medical Association* 11 (1942): 262-267.

Black, J. W., Crowther, A. F., Shanks, R. G., Smith, L. H., and Dornhorst, A. C. "A New Adrenergic Beta-Receptor Antagonist," *The Lancet* 283 (1964): 1080-1081.

Braunwald, E. "Editorial: Expanding Indications for Beta-Blockers in Heart Failure," *New England Journal of Medicine* 344 (2001): 1711-1712.

Brunton, L. L., Lazo, J. S. and Parker, K. L. *Goodman & Gilman's The Pharmacological Basis of Therapeutics*, 11th Ed. (New York: McGraw Hill, 2006).

Clark, A. J. *Applied Pharmacology* (London: J & A. Churchill, 1923).

Ibid., 1923a. 148.

——. *Applied Pharmacology* (Philadelphia: P. Blakiston's Son, 1933), 3.

Crellin, J. K. *A Social History of Medicines in the Twentieth Century: To Be Taken Three Times a Day* (New York: Pharmaceutical Products Press, 2004), 110.

Cullen, W. *Lectures on the Materia Medica as Delivered by William Cullen, M.D.* (Dublin: W. & H. Whitestone, 1781. Google books).

Cyranoski, D. "Strange Lesions After Stem-Cell Therapy," *Nature* 465 (2010): 997.

DeAngelis, C. D. "The Influence of Money on Medical Science," *The Journal of American Medical Association* 296 (2006): 996-998.

Dorn, G. W. "Refugee Receptors Switch Sides," *Science* 327 (2010): 1,586-1,587.

Emsley, J. *Molecules of Murder: Criminal Molecules and Classic Cases* (Cambridge: The Royal Society of Chemistry, 2008).

Ernst, E. "Second Thoughts about Safety of St. John's Wort," *Lancet* 354 (1999): 2014-2016.

Fletcher, R. H. and Fletcher, S. W. *Clinical Epidemiology: The Essentials* (Philadelphia: Lippincott Williams & Wilkins, 2005).

Franks, M. E., Macpherson, G. R. and Figg, W. D. "Thalidomide," *Lancet* 363 (204): 1,802-1,811.

Gao, M., Nettles, R. E., Belema, M. et al. "Chemical Genetics Strategy Identifies an HCV NS5A Inhibitor with a Potent Clinical Effect," *Nature* 465 (2010): 96-100.

Goodman, L. S. and Gilman, A. *The Pharmacological Basis of Therapeutics* (New York: Macmillan, 1941).

Ibid., Fifth edition, 1975.

Graham, D. J. "Cox-2 Inhibitors, Other NSAIDs, and Cardiovascular Risk," *Journal of American Medical Association* 296 (2006): doi:10.1001/jama.296.13. jed60058.

Gross, M. P. and Apesos, J. "The Use of Leeches for Treatment of Venous Congestion of the Nipple Following Breast Surgery," *Aesthetic Plastic Surgery* 16 (1992): 343-348.

Hager, T. *The Demon under the Microscope* (New York: Harmony Books, 2006), 139.

Hobsbawm, E. J. *The Age of Revolution 1789-1848.* (London [1962]: ABACUS, 1977), 336.

Janbon, M., Chaptal, J., Vedel, A., and Schaap, J. "Accidents Hypoglycemiques Graves par un Sulfamidothiadiazol (le VK57 ou 2254RP)," *Montpellier Medicines, 1942* (Quoted in Goodman and Gilman, 1975, 1530).

Kant, I. *Critique of Pure Reason* [1787] Trans. Norman K. Smith (New York: St. Martin's Press, 1965).

Koch, W. J., Rockman, H. A., Samama, P. et al. "Cardiac Function in Mice Overexpressing the Beta-Adrenergic Receptor Kinase or a Beta ARK Inhibitor," *Science* 268 (1995): 1350-1353.

Kurzrok, R. and Lieb, C. C. "Biochemical Studies of Human Semen II. The Action of Semen on Human Uterus," *Proceedings of the Society of Experimental Biology and Medicine* 28 (1930): 268-272.

Lefkowitz, R. J., Rockman, H. A. and Koch, W. J. "Catecholamines, Cardiac ß-Adrenergic Receptors and Heart Failure," *Circulation* 101 (2000): 1,634-1,637.

Lehmann, H. E. and Hanrahan, G. E. "Chlorpromazine, a New Inhibiting Agent for Psychomotor Excitement and Manic States," *American Medical Association Archives of Neurology and Psychiatry*, 71 (1954): 227-237.

Lilienfeld, A. M. and Lilienfeld, D. E. *Foundations of Epidemiology* 2nd ed. (Oxford: Oxford University Press,1980).

Lips, J. *The Origin of Things* (New York: AA WYN 1947).

Loubatière, A. "The hypoglycaemic Sulphonamides: History and Development of the Problem from 1942 to 1955," *Annals of the New York Academy of Sciences*, 71 (1957):

4-11.

Mattern, S. P. *Galen & the Rhetoric of Healing* (Baltimore: Johns Hopkins Press, 2008).

Maxwell, R. A. and Eckhardt, S. B. *Drug Discovery: A Casebook and Analysis* (Clifton, NJ: Humana Press, 1990).

Merritt, H. H. and Putnam, T. J. "Sodium Diphenyl Hydantoinate in Treatment of Convulsive Disorders," *Journal of American Medical Association* 111 (1938): 1,068-1,073.

Mukherjee, S. *The Emperor of All Maladies: A Biography of Cancer* (New York: Scribner, 2010).

Nickerson, M. and Goodman, L. S. "Pharmacological Properties of a New Adrenergic Blocking Agent: N.N-Dibenzyl-ß-chloroethylamine (dibenamine)," *Journal of Pharmacology and Experimental Therapeutics*, 89 (1947): 167-185.

Nickolaev, V. O., Moshkov, A., Lyon, A. R. et al. "ß2-Adrenergic Receptor Redistribution in Heart Failure Changes cAMP Compartmentation," *Science* 327 (2010):1,653-1,657.

Oates, J. A. "The Science of Drug Therapy." In *Goodman & Gilman's The Pharmacological Basis of Therapeutics.* Eds. L. L. Brunton, J. S.Lazo, and K. L. Parker, 11th Ed. (New York: McGraw Hill, 2006), 117-136.

Panno, J. *Gene Therapy: Treatment and Cures for Genetic Diseases* (New York: Facts on Life, Inc. 2011).

Pledge, H. T. *Science Since 1500: A Short History of Mathematics, Physics, Chemistry, and Biology* (London: His Majesty's Stationery Office. 1939),100-101.

Sen, G. and Bose, K. C. "*Rauwolfia serpentina*, a New Indian Drug for Insanity and High Blood Pressure," *Indian Medical World* 2 (1931): 194-201.

Siddiqui, S. and Siddiqui, R. H. "Chemical Examination of the Roots of *Rauwolfia serpentina Benth*," *Journal of Indian Chemical Society* 8 (1931): 667-680.

Singh, S. and Ernst, E. *Trick or Treatment?: Alternative Medicine on Trial* (London: Transworld Publishers, 2008), 241-244 and 345-346.

Slater, I. H. and Powell, C. E. "Blockade of Adrenergic Inhibitory Receptor Sites by 1-(3',4'-Dichlorophenyl)-2-Isopropylaminoethanol Hydrochloride," *Federation Proceedings*, 16 (1957): 336.

Smith, G.C.S. and Pell, J. P. "Parachute Use to Prevent Death and Major Trauma Related to Gravitational Challenge: Systematic Review of Randomised Controlled Trials," *British Medical Journal* 327 (2003): 1459-1461.

Smith, H.W. *From Fish to Philosopher* (New York: Doubleday, 1962).

Sneader, W. *Drug Discover: A History* (Chichester, West Sussex: John Wiley & Sons, 2005).

Sollmann, T. *A Manual of Pharmacology and its Application to Therapeutics and Toxicology* (Philadelphia: W. B. Saunders, 1948).

Szasz, T. S. *The Manufacture of Madness: A Comparative Study of the Inquisition and the Mental Health Movement* (London: Rutledge & Kegan Paul, 1971).

——. *The Myth of Mental Illness: Foundations of a Theory of Personal Conduct* (New York: Harmer-Perennial, 1974).

Straus, S. E., Richardson, W. S., Glasziou, P., and Haynes, R. B. *Evidence-Based Medicine: How to Practice and Teach EBM.* 3rd ed. (Edinburgh: Elsevier Churchill Livingstone, 2005).

Vakil, R. J. "A Clinical Trial of *Rauwolfia serpentina* in Essential Hypertension," *British Heart Journal* 11 (1949): 350-355.

Vane, J. R. "Inhibition of Prostaglandin Synthesis as a Mechanism of Action of Aspirin-Like Drugs," *Nature-New Biology* 231 (1971): 232-235.

Yue, T-L., Cheng, H-Y., Lysko, P. G. et al. "Carvedilol, a New Vasodilator and Beta Adrenoceptor Antagonist, Is an Antioxidant and Free Radical Scavenger," *Journal of Pharmacology and Experimental Therapeutics* 263 (1992): 92-98.

Yue, T. L., Ruffolo, R. R., and Feuerstein, G. "Antioxidant Action of Carvedilol: A Potential Role in the Treatment of Heart Failure," *Heart Failure Reviews* 4 (1999): 39-51.

Warren J. R., Marshall B. "Unidentified Curved Bacilli on Gastric Epithelium in Active Chronic Gastritis," *Lancet*, 321 (1983): 1273-1275.

Wood, H. C. *Treatise on Therapeutics Comprising Materia Medica and Toxicology With Special Reference to the Application of the Physiological Action of Drugs to Clinical Medicine* (Philadelphia: J. B. Lippincott & Co., 1874; digitalized by Google).

CHAPTER 14

Modern Medicine Comes of Age

> The latest investigations respecting the early condition of the human race are tending to the conclusion that mankind commenced their career at the bottom of the scale and worked their way up from savagery to civilization through the slow accumulation of experimental knowledge.
>
> Lewis Henry Morgan[1]

> The supernational character of scientific concepts and scientific language is due to the fact that they have been set up by the best brains of all countries and all times. In solitude, and yet in cooperative effort as regards the final effect, they created the spiritual tools for the technical revolution which have transformed the life of mankind in the last centuries. Their system of concepts has served as a guide in the bewildering chaos of perceptions so that we learned to grasp general truths from particular observations.
>
> Albert Einstein[2]

Introduction

Medicine is both science and art (Warner, 1995). Conceptual advances in both aspects have been the singular feature of modern medicine as distinct from all other schools of medicine. On the other hand, precisely because medicine has both a basic and an applied aspect, both its merits (Porter, 1997) and its faults (Illich, 1976) have been exaggerated.

In this Chapter, I will attempt to point out salient conceptual advances in the domain of medicine.

Changing Time Frame of Discoveries

Modern medical science has sufficiently advanced to find the answer or to correct errors more speedily and accurately than it did in the past. This is largely because of advances in other sciences, notably physics and chemistry, which provide newer and better tools for investigation than ever before.

Take, for example, the case of AIDS (acquired immune deficiency syndrome). The US Surgeon General Dr. William H. Stewart declared in 1969 that nothing more needed to be known about infectious diseases (Porter, 1997a). Not too long after, there was an increase in the incidence of Kaposi's Sarcoma in the United States and in cases of the rare lung infection by *Pneumocystis carinii;* why was it happening?

By 1981, a task force on Kaposi's Sarcoma and Opportunistic Infections (KSOI) was announced by the Center for Disease Control (CDC), USA. No one knew exactly what was happening. The situation was reminiscent of mysterious cholera until Dr. Snow had solved the problem in the mid nineteenth century. The CDC predicted that the disease posed no threat to non-homosexuals or women and terms like *gay compromise syndrome, gay-related immune deficiency, gay cancer*, and so on were introduced.

When, in December 1982, a small child died of an affliction similar to that observed after a severe immune compromise as a result of a blood transfusion, it became clear that a transmissible infectious agent caused the disease (Porter, 1997a). In May 1983, researchers at Pasteur Institute, France, reported isolating a virus that they claimed is most likely the cause of AIDS and named it LAV (lymphadenopathy-associated virus). Soon after, Dr. Robert Gallo of the National Cancer Institute, USA, announced discovering the AIDS-causing virus HTLV-III (human T-cell lymphotropic virus, type 3). The dispute on nomenclature was resolved when the International Committee on the Taxonomy of Viruses named it HIV (Human Immunodeficiency Virus).

Gallo also announced that he had a method of identifying the presence of the virus in patients and predicted that an anti-AIDS vaccine would soon become available. Reliable tests for the virus do exist and are routinely used both for diagnostic and forensic purposes. The anti-

AIDS vaccine is still elusive, perhaps because of the unusual nature of the AIDS-causing virus.

The central point of the presentation of this story here is that the cause of a virtually fatal disease like AIDS was discovered within about ten years after its arrival compared with the more than two thousand years that it took to find the cause of malaria and millions of deaths to find the cause of cholera.

Likewise, the causes of SARS (severe acute respiratory syndrome) that first hit Toronto in 2003 and several influenza episodes (e.g., swine flu) that tend to make annual visits with different features are identified rapidly and possible methods of prevention discovered rather effectively and rapidly.

James Lind, a surgeon on a British ship, discovered in 1757 that citrus fruits prevented scurvy in sailors. Surprisingly, no one followed his advice until Lind's death in 1774. In 1775, however, it dawned upon the royalty to provide a bit of lemon juice to every sailor in the ship. Medical science neglected the significance of these findings of Lind for nearly two hundred years. Scurvy is not the only disease caused by a lack of essential nutrients. Egyptian mummies with rickets had been discovered. Night blindness due to vitamin A deficiency was not uncommon. Yet nothing was done about them in modern medicine until the beginning of the twentieth century.

In the next thirty years, all the vitamins, both fat soluble (A, D, E and K), and water soluble (B and C) were discovered in rapid succession and some like vitamin C even synthesized. Even the three dimensional structure of vitamin B_{12} was discovered by Dorothy Crowfoot Hodgkin (1910-1994) in 1956. Axel Holst (1860-1931) and Theodor Frølich (1870-1947) discovered Vitamin C, which was the molecule in citrus fruit that caused scurvy on Lind's ships, in 1907. It became abundantly clear that food should not only provide calories, salts, and water but other essential ingredients as well. Vitamins A, B, and D were discovered within a period of about twenty years. Elmer Verner McCollum (1879-1967) and Marguerite Davis (1887-1967) discovered Vitamin A in 1913. McCollum and Cornelia Kennedy (1881-1969) discovered vitamin B in 1916; it was soon found that what they had discovered was not a single vitamin but a complex of many such as B_1 (thiamine), B_2 (riboflavin), B_3 (niacinamide), B_5 (pantothenic acid), B_6 (pyridoxine), B_7 (biotin), B_9 (folic acid), and B_{12} (cyanocobalamin). Vitamin D was discovered by Elmer McCollum (1879-1967) and Marguerite Davis (1887-1967) (McCollum and Davis, 1914) and Sir Edward Mellanby (1884-1955) (Mellanby, 1919). Vitamin E was discovered in 1922 and K in 1929. Linus Pauling opined that the vitamins serve more purposes than preventing deficiency diseases and advocates liberal consumption of these molecules for a better health (Pauling, 1987).

Theories of Diseases

The quest for disease genesis has been an important human endeavour since antiquity. In the previous chapters, I have provided an historical account of the proposed theories of diseases. Here I provide a brief summary of the causative factors leading to diseases. I hasten to add that the causative factors are essential for a disease but are not sufficient. For example, the majority of Indians are tuberculin-positive indicating contamination by tuberculosis bacteria but only some of them have the actual disease. This is true for most infections.

As we approached the twentieth century, we know that while Ayurvedic, Greek and Chinese medicine made major advances in disease theories, they are not only insufficient but fundamentally wrong.

Disease is not the result of any imbalance, which is presupposed by Hindu, Chinese and Greek medical pioneers; rather, disease is the cause of the imbalance of any or all bodily functions. On a critical examination, one must reach the conclusion that the Hindu, Chinese, or Greek idea of any imbalance-causing disease is in the realm of spiritualism and not truly materialism because it presupposes that some supernatural force has caused the imbalance.

There cannot be a general theory of diseases because what is common are the effects of the diseases and not their causes. All diseases can be classified into three basic groups, caused by diverse and often unrelated factors.

One group of diseases is caused by environmental invasions, be that physical injury, infestation by microorganism or parasites, or ingestion of poisons or drugs. Trauma, burns, AIDS, pneumonia, tuberculosis, malaria, drug poisoning, and so on belong to this group. Almost all these diseases are curable and most trauma reparable by surgical intervention and antibiotic therapy.

The second group of diseases is due to the inability of the body to maintain homeostasis, either due to genetic factors or inappropriate indulgence. Homeostasis refers to body's ability to maintain physiological equilibrium as elaborated by Walter Cannon (1871-1945) and Claude Bernard. Environmental and genetic factors might underlie diseases like diabetes, hypertension, cancers, Parkinson's disease, Alzheimer, epilepsy, and so on. Much progress has been made in this area as well. However, in most cases, diseases belonging to this group can be controlled but most cannot be cured for the time being. Certain cancers, like testicular cancer, Hodgkin's cancer, prostate cancer and breast cancer are either curable or controllable for a much longer period than was the case in the past.

The third group of diseases is caused by a deficient supply of essential needs of the body, either because of inadequate nutrition, inappropriate living style, or physical damage to an organ. Diseases caused by an the inadequate intake of vitamins or essential metals like iodine, iron or zinc, too little or too much exposure to sunlight, or the destruction of an endocrine organ like thyroid or lungs belong to this category. Scurvy, rickets, iron-deficiency anaemia, iodine-deficiency goitre, etc., also belong to this group and are curable. Deficiency in hormones due to damage or ablation of the appropriate organ is often not curable, but substitution therapy for all of them exists.

Modern medicine has perfected the understanding of the causes of diseases belonging to the first and third category, namely those caused by external factors and those caused by a deficiency of essential foods. It is the second category of diseases, namely those due to a disturbance in homeostatic mechanisms, where it has made great strides but as yet the unequivocal answer has been elusive.

We almost know the cause of cystic fibrosis. We even know the probability of breast cancer on the basis of family history and genetic mapping well enough to advise mastectomy as a prophylactic measure and yet we do not know why two identical siblings living under identical conditions do not die at the same time and do not suffer from the same diseases. Why does an obese person with high cholesterol and a sedentary lifestyle not die at a young age but one without any of these signs and symptoms does? We do not know why some people do and some do not suffer from Alzheimer's at identical ages. Smoking and lungs provide another kind of puzzle; every long-time smoker has compromised lung function; this is understandable and can be explained; but why doesn't every smoker get lung cancer?

Therapeutics

In Chapter 13, I have already indicated the gigantic progress made in therapeutics since the mid-twentieth century.

Discovery of sulphonamides followed by penicillin changed the face of modern medicine; a number of killers could now be controlled.

Highly effective drugs with acceptable toxicity exist for most diseases. Constant efforts are made to improve upon existing therapeutics to the extent that it is sometimes difficult to decide which is the best. Just to illustrate this point, I would refer to two therapeutic approaches, which have been indicated earlier in different contexts.

High blood pressure is a common disease. There was a period when no effort was made to treat it; it was argued that high blood pressure is the body's normal response to something that has gone wrong; in short, high blood pressure is a desired compensatory response. Then it was recognized that a proper control of blood pressure prolongs longevity and reduces debilitating complications like stroke or heart failure. This naturally led to efforts to treat hypertension. The regimen for the treatment of hypertension has also undergone drastic changes in the last sixty years or so. Drugs, like ganglion blocking agents, antagonists of noradrenaline at alpha-receptors, methyldopa, which were used in the 1950s and 1960s, are no longer used to treat high blood pressure. Up until the 1970s, it was argued that only an increase in diastolic pressure is harmful, and one should not worry about the systolic pressure. Then it was realized that while this is true up to about fifty years of age, abnormality in systolic pressure is the main problem as we get older. The treatment of hypertension has become individualized rather than population based. The desired upper and lower limits of blood pressure have undergone revision just in the last twenty years or so.

Heart failure is another area. More than two hundred years ago in 1785, William Withering published his report on the effectiveness of foxglove (containing digitalis) on heart failure. Digitalis remained the primary drug for heart failure almost until the end of 1975 when its limitations were realized. Satisfactory treatment of heart failure is still evasive, but digitalis is no longer the primary drug. Instead, other drugs, including many used to treat hypertension, are used; and intensive research is on at many centres to find a more suitable therapy.

Supportive Therapy

Modern medicine has almost perfected this art. The majority of serious emergency cases are not rescued by drugs but by other measures starting with the first aid by ambulance operators to careful care by the nursing staff assisted by the availability of gadgets within a hospital setting for maintaining respiration, circulation, and nutrition. Many diseases, like diabetes, ultimately kill by causing kidney failure. Modern medicine has perfected dialysis techniques, administered at home (peritoneal dialysis) or in a hospital setting (hemodialysis); these procedures can restore near-normal life for quite sometime.

Often, emergency services are successful in resuscitating stopped heart or terminating fatal ventricular fibrillations. We often hear of stories when someone with stroke, completely unconscious, unable to perform any function, has been kept alive for months by supportive therapy. With existing laws in most countries of the world, the physician makes the decision to keep the patient alive. It is not their prerogative to decide that death is a preferred option. The ethics of all this is an important subject, but beyond the scope of this book. Indeed, these developments have resulted in a new controversy – when is a person really dead?

Maintaining body fluid balance by infusion of an appropriate solution or blood, if needed, has been of great benefit in saving lives.

Prophylaxis

Prophylaxis is a very common practice. Its use is not limited to physicians' advice. Every mother tells her child what to eat and what not to, and her pregnant daughter or daughter-in-law what to do and what not to do. Not smoking or quitting smoking is a prophylactic measure. Obviously, prophylaxis is not a treatment of a disease but a measure to prevent diseases, especially those that are more likely to be encountered during life. Indeed prophylaxis was the pivotal aspect of ancient medicine.

In most developed countries, there is a specific season when people rush to get anti-flu vaccine. Also, in developed countries and urban areas in many developing countries, a child begins life with DPT (against diphtheria, pertussis-whooping cough, and tetanus), and in some countries, against polio as well. More recently anti-HPV (human papilloma virus) vaccine has been introduced as a measure against cervical cancer.

Vaccines against many diseases have been developed since Edward Jenner developed the anti-smallpox vaccine in 1796. Louis Pasteur developed the anti-anthrax and anti-rabies vaccine in 1881-1882, and Jonas Salk (1914-1995) advanced medicine by introducing anti-polio vaccine in 1952.

The benefits of these discoveries are immense and so common that their significance is not noted with the admiration they deserve.

Ever since the recognition of a virus as the cause of AIDS, much effort has been poured into discovering an anti-AIDS vaccine. Herbert W. Virgin and Bruce D. Walker (2010) describe the status of this effort in the journal *Nature*; I quote below a part of their summary:

> Developing a human immunodeficiency virus (HIV) vaccine is critical to end the global acquired immunodeficiency syndrome (AIDS) epidemic, but many question whether this goal is achievable.
>
> Natural immunity is not protective, and despite immunogenicity of HIV vaccine candidates, human trials have exclusively yielded disappointing results. Nevertheless, there is an indication that success may be possible, but this will be dependent on understanding the antiviral immune response in unprecedented depth to identify and engineer the types of immunity required.

Generally, drugs are taken as a prophylactic measure on the advice of physicians. Here the issue is not as clear-cut. I pointed this out while referring to the wide use of oestrogens against possible miscarriage or tamoxifen against breast cancer.

The most common prophylactic measure at this time is prescribing lipid-lowering drugs against cardiovascular morbidity and mortality (see Pahan, 2006). These drugs belong to several groups, the most commonly used are statins (atorvastatin or Lipitor, simvastatin or Zocor, lovastatin or Mevacor, pravastatin or Pravachol, rosuvastatin or Crestor) and fibrates. Statins inhibit cholesterol synthesis as well as produce many other effects by complex mechanisms. Fibrates inhibit cholesterol absorption and decrease fatty acids and triglycerides but perhaps produce other effects as well. Numerous publications for and against this practice exist and there seems no unequivocal answer.

Lipid-lowering drugs are recommended on the basis of a statistically significant decrease in mortality and morbidity in a population, who are more likely to develop atherosclerosis because of certain risk factors such as diabetes. Clearly, all people who take lipid-lowering drugs would not develop symptomatic atherosclerosis had they not taken the medication. This means that the drug has been consumed by a subset of the population who did not need it. This is in contrast to therapeutic drugs that are individualized and administered to treat existing diseases. In the case of the therapeutic use of drugs, its desirability and appropriateness can be satisfactorily ascertained by taking a balance between toxic and therapeutic effect. No such method of assessing the desirability of consuming lipid-lowering drugs exists. The toxicity of lipid-lowering drugs is claimed to be minor (see Pahan, 2006) though contrary opinions also exist. Are lipid-lowering drugs as safe and effective as toothpaste, fluoridinated water, or iodized salt? Are lipid-lowering drugs like polio vaccine? If not, then medical science must be obligated to identify better markers for identifying people who need lipid-lowering drugs than the currently used risk factors.

The story of rather common use of SSRIs (selective serotonin reuptake inhibitor) to treat what is diagnosed by self or the physician as depression is another area charged with controversy, which is highlighted in the book *Let Them Eat PROZAC* (Healy, 2004). The same, or nearly the same, can be said about autism, which is diagnosed and treated more often than it should be.

Surgery and Dentistry

Twenty-seven hundred years ago, the Indian surgeon Susruta proclaimed that surgery is curative. Since then, the art of surgery has made great strides especially since the discovery, first of general anaesthetics and then of muscle relaxants. Highly sophisticated tools for surgery have been developed. The method of training a skilled surgeon is simpler than training a skilled physician because it is fundamentally based on apprenticeship. From opening of clogged arteries to replacement of whole organs and fixing detached retina has become possible, so much so that it is only in this area that modern medicine is not challenged by any other school of medicine.

Likewise, the art of dentistry has advanced enough to promise teeth are for lifetime, if not your own then implanted ones. While by no means undermining the benefits to health offered by surgery and dentistry, it must be recognized that art supersedes science in these areas, and advances owe a great deal to advances in other fields primarily physics, chemistry, electronics and mechanics.

Thanks to bypass surgery in which patients' good artery (most commonly mammary artery) is used to replace portions of diseased coronary artery or angioplasty in which a catheter is inserted into the coronary artery to dilate it, patients with coronary artery atherosclerosis can resume almost normal physical activity and for a long life.

The heart can get diseased beyond recovery. Either the patient should be left to die or given a good heart. In the most publicized surgical feat in the history of the world, Dr. Christiaan Barnard (1922-2001) replaced the heart of the patient Louis Washkansky on December 3, 1967, with the heart of the female Denise Darvall, who was killed the day before in a road accident. Washkansky survived for only nineteen days. The second heart transplant was done on January 2, 1968. The recipient was Philip Blaiberg, a white South African, and the donor was a coloured man named Clive Haupt; Blaiberg survived for nineteen months. The third heart recipient was a black woman, Dorothy Fisher, who lived for twelve years (Gonzalez-Crussi, 2009).

Many doctors were opposed to apartheid. Dr. Barnard not only trespassed religious and gender barriers, he was also the first to dismantle apartheid, twenty-six years before Nelson Mandela, its arch enemy, and F. W. de Klerk, its chief custodian, reached an agreement for which they received the 1993 Nobel Peace Prize. The increasing duration of the survival of heart transplant patients as of other organ transplant patients is an achievement, not so much of better surgery alone but also of the availability of better drugs to control infection and prevent transplant rejection, cyclosporine being the chief one.

Normally, the heart beats regularly once per second or a bit faster or slower, but regularly nonetheless. But heart can also start beating irregularly; this irregularity is often confined to the atria, which has the potential of increasing ventricular beats to great discomfort to the patient. As well, when the atria are fibrillating, they lose their power to contract and blood sits inside and can form clots, which can leave the atria and block some vital artery. Medical science has some system to correct the irregularity and prevent blood clotting. This kind of arrhythmia can also affect the ventricle, which is quite serious, and fibrillation of the ventricle means death. Modern medicine has developed techniques to defibrillate the heart and even restart a heart that had stopped beating.

Obstetrics

Pregnancy is a physiological state. Most pregnancies are normal, uneventful, and the baby can be delivered by a midwife or in a hospital setting. However, complications specific to pregnancy do occur. Ectopic pregnancy in which the foetus is anchored to parts other than the uterus such as the fallopian tube used to be a very serious complication. Aside from ectopic pregnancy, three major complications of pregnancy are diabetes, hypertension, and infection; these were killers.

Considerable progress has been made in all these areas. In most urban centres, the progression of pregnancy is routinely monitored, and most complications can be detected early and managed appropriately. Ectopic pregnancy is detected and surgically managed. So is diabetes, whether already existing before pregnancy or induced by pregnancy; it is adequately monitored and controlled. The lungs of the foetus of a diabetic mother do not mature properly and are deficient in a substance called surfactant. Surfactant is a substance that affects surface tension of the lung tissue, ensuring easy inflation during breathing. Inadequate surfactant makes breathing very difficult because inhaled air is not at sufficient pressure to cause inflation of the lungs. Surfactant synthesis can be stimulated by glucocorticoids (e.g., dexamethasone). In the past, preeclampsia, which is characterized by abrupt rise in blood pressure and can be associated with seizures, used to be fatal in a great majority of cases. Protocol to control the onset of preeclampsia has also been developed. Most infections can also be avoided and controlled. These developments, along with awareness of the need for asepsis, have greatly reduced infant and maternal mortality.

However, medical advances can also create new problems. A case in point is premature delivery. Every effort is made to prevent premature delivery as long as possible. In the past, deliveries before thirty-six weeks were often associated with non-survival of the baby. Neonatology has sufficiently advanced so that even twenty-sixth – to twenty-seventh-week babies survive. However, very premature babies tend to develop complications that could include patent ductus arteriosus, which does not allow venous blood to go to lungs as was the case during intrauterine life, cerebral haemorrhage with attendant complications, retinopathy of prematurity, and so on (Stephens and Vohr, 2009; Stoll et al., 2010). Although these continue to remain a challenging therapeutic problem, the area is under intensive investigation at many centres including by a team led by my colleague Dr. Sylvain Chemtob at the Ste Justine Hospital, Montreal, Canada (Varvarigou et al., 1996; Kooli et al., 2008; Sapieha et al., 2008).

Prognosis

Prognosis implies projection of the course of a disease in response to or in the absence of therapy. The very reason for instituting therapy for any disease is to alter its course in favour of the host. This requires a grasp of the pathology of the disease, the potential of therapy and appropriate advice on life style. Physicians and surgeons are not soothsayers, but very close to it, when it comes to forecasting about the course of many diseases. This reflects advances in clinical medicine.

Basic Medical Science

From the time when Susruta showed that the skin from the arm could be used to repair a severed nose in the sixth century BC to the time of deciphering the double helix structure of DNA in the 1950s[3] biological science has accomplished a lot. Erwin Schrodinger's hope that there ought to be no major distinction between physics, chemistry, and biology[4] is being steadily realized. Indeed, advances in medical practice are only a small fraction of this monumental progress in biology. Here I will simply highlight significant advances in medical science; some of these have been translated into applied medicine, but most not as yet, just as is the case with physics and chemistry.

Neurology

Ages passed before we found out that consciousness is a function of the brain and not the heart, though as a respect to the tradition, we still think that the seat of love and hate, generosity and stinginess, kindness and cruelty is a function of the heart (Gonzalez-Crussi, 2009). It is the brain that performs all these functions, but it is the heart that gets the credit.

The brain is the most complex organ and performs two different sets of functions. One set comprises basic functions like control of respiration, activities of the autonomic nervous system, homeostasis like hormonal secretion, and so on. These functions are controlled by parts of the brain like the hypothalamus and midbrain; neuroscientists have worked out fairly well the physiology of these areas of the brain.

The second set of functions include cognition and interpretation and the responses to these; it is the most complex field of study especially because the investigator and the subject of investigation are the same. When the physiology of cognition is understood or even approximately understood, we could declare that Buddha's postulate of self-realization has reached its pinnacle.

Cognition

If one were to grade functions of the brain in order of complexity, cognition would be on the top of the list. Cognition is linked to the creation of the new to the ultimate flight of imagination and analytical power, which distinguishes Einstein from commoners, mathematicians from machinists, astronomers from astrologers, and *Homo sapiens* from the rest of life forms. Extensive researches in the twentieth century have solved much of the physiology of the first set of functions, that is, the basic functions of the brain. The second set of functions, namely cognition and analytical function, has occupied the imagination of philosophers to neuroscientists.

What is cognition? Has it evolved too since the birth of *Homo sapiens*? Is it related to the emergence of language as an organ (Anderson and Lightfoot, 2000; Chomsky, 1995)? All these are puzzling questions needing an answer, and I think the answer will be found.

Aristotle analyzed the views of his predecessors Pythagoras, Democritus, Plato, and Hippocrates. Aristotle (see Barnes, 1984) considered that the "primary form of sense is touch" and opined as follows:

> Generally, about all perceptions, we can say that a sense is what has the power of receiving into itself the sensible forms of things without the matter, in the way in which a piece of wax takes on the impress of a signet-ring without the iron or gold; what produces the impression is a signet of bronze or gold, but not qua bronze or gold: in a similar way the sense is affected by what is coloured or flavoured or sounding not insofar as each is what it is, but insofar as it is of such and such a sort and according to its form.

Almost two thousand years later, René Descartes, usually considered the founder of modern philosophy and otherwise dismissive of Aristotle, appears to echo Aristotle by coincidence or design when he asks us in *Rules for the Direction of the Mind* (about 1628) to imagine that:

> ...although it is by an action (more precisely, by a local movement) that we apply our external senses to objects, nevertheless, insofar as they are parts of the body, they really sense only passively, like a wax which receives its configuration from the seal. And do not think this is a simple analogy; the real modification of the external configuration of the sensing body, by the object, should be pictured in exactly the same way as the modification, by the seal, of the superficial configuration of the wax. (Morris, 1969)

Immanuel Kant says (1781), "Human reason has this particular fate that in one species of its knowledge it is burdened by questions which, as prescribed by the very nature of reason itself, it is not able to ignore, but which, as transcending all its powers, it is unable to answer." Kant has pinpointed the problem and no wonder mind and nature have occupied the attention of mathematicians and physicists as well. The selected writings of Hermann Weyl – who, according to Einstein, was "one of the greatest mathematicians of the first half of the twentieth century ...on philosophy, mathematics and physics" – have been titled *Mind and Nature* (Weyl, 2009). Physicist Erwin Schrodinger (1967) says, "The world is a construct of our sensation, perceptions, memories. It is convenient to regard it as existing objectively on its own. But it certainly does not become manifest by its mere existence."

In recent years, the availability of advanced technologies in the form of PET (positron emission topography), MEG (magneto encephalogram), MRI (magnetic resonance imaging), and so on has enabled neuroscientists to probe into the mechanism of cognition. PET is the first major technical advance over radiogram (x-rays). It is a versatile and expensive instrument and operative at a limited number of centres. The internationally recognized Montreal Neurological Institute, of which noted neurosurgeon Wilder Graves Penfield (1891-1976) was once the director, had acquired PET quite early. One of the earliest investigators to use PET was the young brilliant scientist Justine Sergent (1952-1994). She was using PET to study how the brain responds to human behaviour, for example, upon exposure to music. For reasons never fully explained, the administration created conditions so she could not pursue her research. Having failed to reverse this restriction on her research, the sole passion of this young woman, she and her husband Yves Sergent committed suicide on April 12, 1994. The administration might have won a victory but science lost; one would never know – how much? It seems pushing someone to the brink, especially an innocent hardworking woman, is not a criminal offense; at best, it leads to an inconclusive inquiry as happened in the case of Justine Sergent.

Regeneration and Transmitters

The Spanish neuroscientist Santiago Ramón Y Cajal (1852-1934) used the staining technique of Camillo Golgi (1843-1926) to demonstrate that the brain is not one lump of tissue but consists of millions of neurons connected with each other; he also provided evidence of neuronal regeneration after injury, usually thought to be impossible. The discovery was profound enough for the Nobel Committee to honour both Cajal and Golgi with the Nobel Prize in medicine in 1906. Once it became known that these multiple neurons communicate with each other to make the brain do what it does, researchers mapped out which part of the brain does what and how one neuron communicates with another.

Given the fact that the brain practically modulates all functions of the body by one mechanism or another, researches in the twentieth century allocated various bodily functions to specific brain regions with the cerebral cortex recognized as the one performing the most complex task, which is known as mind or consciousness or intelligence, etc.

Starting with the mid-twentieth century, evidence started accumulating that neurons in the brain communicate with each other by means of chemicals very much like they do in peripheral tissues.

Chemicals like acetylcholine, noradrenaline, dopamine, glycine, *gama*-amino butyric acid (GABA), glutamate, serotonin, and so on were shown to convey information from one neuron to another by exciting or inhibiting them or altering ion (sodium, potassium) channels; they also play a role in drug effects.

Brain Receptors

An important but less recognized contribution was made by McGill University pharmacologists Kenneth Ivan Melville (1902-1975), my doctorate supervisor, and his graduate student Norman Share; they reported (Share and Melville, 1963) that the receptors for noradrenaline, which were already known to be present in peripheral tissues, are also present in the brain. This opened a new field. Since receptors for morphine, acetylcholine, noradrenaline, dopamine, serotonin, glutamate, GABA, and other molecules have been identified in the brain. This knowledge is exploited to explore drugs modifying functions of the brain, which I narrated in Chapter 13.

Neuroplasticity

In a way neuroplasticity is related to cognition and is a challenging field. We know that the visual cortex perceives "what we see," just as sound is processed by the auditory cortex. But are these and other functions of the brain absolutely fixed or there is some flexibility? Massachusetts Institute of Technology (MIT) Professor Mriganka Sur tested this possibility using newborn ferrets; his group of researchers used a surgical technique to induce retinal cells to travel to auditory nuclei instead of their normal destination, the visual cortex. In these ferrets, the auditory nuclei responded to visual signals and auditory cells developed the characteristics of visual cells (Sur et al., 1988). In other words, the part of the brain that normally hears can be made to see. These observations of Sur and his co-workers have implications wider than vision; they demonstrate that environmental factors can qualitatively modify functions and clearly obliterate the distinction between nature and nurture. McGill University researchers (Weaver et al., 2004) have recently shown how maternal behaviour toward the newborn can have a genetic imprint. Vilayanur S. Ramachandran and his group at the Center for Brain and Cognition, University of California, have been studying phantom pain; their research also provides strong evidence in support of the plasticity of the brain.

These three observations – nerve regeneration, neuroplasticity at the highest level of the brain, and specific receptors and transmitters – have opened new possibilities of immense clinical benefits, which have only partially been realized.

Pain

Pain is the most common symptom and the very first recognition of a disease. All kinds of diseases, which may have nothing in common, can produce pain; trauma does it, so does the myocardial ischemia, a stone in the kidney or gall bladder and an infection of the appendix.

There is even such a thing as phantom pain experienced by a limb, which no longer exists. Whatever be the cause of pain, it is ultimately recognized by the brain; not only that, the brain also pinpoints the site of the pain. Pain is a unique pathology. It is physiology because it is needed for survival. It is pathology after it has served its purposes of warning the host. It is no wonder that a study of the pathophysiology of pain has been and remains a subject of intensive investigation.

The philosopher René Descartes did many things. He developed a philosophical system that combined imagination and science. He dealt with pain as well. However, compelled by his outlook of looking at mind and body as unrelated entities, his theory about pain does not conform to scientific data. Melzack and Wall (1965) proposed what was a major breakthrough on the mechanism of pain that they designated as "the gate-control theory of pain."

Accidental loss of a limb in encounters with wild animals or tribal wars must surely have been routine in antiquity. If the person survived, she or he would have complained of feeling pain in the non-existing leg or arm. The healers of that in turn would have concluded that either the patient had been bewitched or had become mad. It is only when soldiers of modern wars, and in large numbers, began complaining of pain in a non-existing organ did neuroscientists realize that the pain is real and called it phantom pain.

The first to document phantom pain in detail was the sixteenth century French barber-surgeon Ambroise Paré (1510-1590) (Keil, 1990). Obviously, Paré could not elaborate on the mechanisms of phantom pain. Since that time, many researchers have studied the pathophysiology of phantom pain. Ramachandran and Hirstein (1998),[5] leading researchers in this area, are of the opinion that the severed limb is represented in the brain; this not only explains the mechanism of the phantom pain but also supports the idea of plasticity of the brain throughout life.

Cardiology

Blaise Pascal (1623-1662) was a great French mathematician and physicist and, as was customary, a philosopher as well. Even biologists have heard his name though they, as in my case, do not know what are the problems that Pascal solved. But like many great men, Pascal also created a problem when he said "the heart has its reason which reason knows nothing about." This is most likely untrue, but difficult to disprove. But let us assume that Pascal was wrong in this case and the heart has no reason; rather, like a robot, it pumps oxygenated blood to the rest of the body and oxygen-poor blood to the lungs for recharging from day one to the last day of life while sparing the lungs during intrauterine life.

Death is difficult to define; for that reason, it was declared to have arrived when the heart stopped beating and could not be resuscitated. With the technique of heart transplant, the brain has taken the place of the heart, and the law will probably hold on to this definition until brain transplant becomes a reality. With so many attributes, the question of what the heart really does remained a mystery for much of human history.

Taking on the many leads from his predecessors, notably from the eleventh-century Persian physician Avicenna (Ibn Sina), William Harvey solved a social and physiological problem. Harvey mapped the physiology of blood circulation in the seventeenth century. However, even Harvey thought that the heart had many functions and was the "foundation of life." Since then, notably, starting with Ernst Henry Starling (1866-1927) who elaborated on the mechanisms of capillary circulation and the relationship between the heart size and force of contraction, much progress has been made in the physiology and pathology of the heart. We know the electrophysiological basis of heart irregularities (arrhythmias), the reasons for angina (chest pain arising from ischemia of the heart), the relationship between blood pressure and heart function and size, coronary artery circulation, and all the diseases that are due to the malfunctioning of any cardiac function. The heart could also be considered an endocrine organ since it produces the diuretic hormone, atrial natriuretic factor (De Bold, 1981).

With all the knowledge about the heart, it still remains the single most important determinant of life and death. Material prosperity has expanded the domain of the heart from the affluent West to countries like India and Pakistan as the major killer. Therapeutics has not kept pace.

Bacterial and Viral Infections

Many diseases caused by micro-organisms, like the tuberculosis (Johnston, 1993), are very old. Robert Koch proved the bacterial basis of tuberculosis in 1882, a year before he identified *Vibrio cholera Pacini 1854.*[6] Since the time of Ross and Koch, the cause and the mode of transmission of practically every disease – bacterial, viral, or parasitic – has been identified. Modern medicine could declare victory on all infective disease if it were not for the emergence of multidrug-resistant bacteria and relatively toxic drug regimen against AIDS; however, these are not insurmountable problems. In the meantime, a certain creed of sociologists (Nettleton, 2006) have discovered that the "Germ theory" of Pasteur, Koch and Ross, a landmark in the history of medicine, as a proof of reductionism in science.

Parasitic Infection

Parasitic infections are mainly problems of tropical countries. The interest of scientists in parasitic diseases was primarily to solve the problem faced by colonial expansion and the fact that the South of the United States has features of a tropical country. A side effect of colonialism, fortunately a desirable one, was the intensive effort to identify the cause of parasitic diseases and find a treatment. I have previously described the story of malaria. Actually, the life cycle of other parasites is also very complex, and a lot of imagination and research was needed to find that out.

Take the case of hookworm disease; it is caused by an infestation by the parasite hookworms, *Ancylstoma duodenale* (most common in India) and *Necator americanus* (common in the Americas). Hookworms anchor in the intestine and suck sufficient blood to cause iron-deficiency anaemia that can be severe enough to incapacitate the victim to bed, incapable of physical activity and often enough with a bulging abdomen due to oedema. During my medical school days (1950-1955) in the North Indian city of Lucknow, almost all cases of anaemia were due to hookworm disease, and the severe ones had to be admitted into the hospital for treatment. I will not go into the fascinating history of how the cause of transmission and the pathology of hookworm disease were discovered since the first identification of the parasite in 1838 by the Italian physician Angelo Dubini (1813-1902). I would just describe the life cycle of the *A. duodenale* in the Indian setting and leave it to the imagination of the reader to wonder how the whole thing was worked out.

A vast majority of rural Indians defecate in the field. According to a report by Stephanie Noel in the Toronto Globe and Mail of March 12, 2012, even today there are more cell phones than toilets in India. Many Indians, especially rural women, did not use any shoes until recently. As they walked in the field for work, or to defecate, their feet came in contact with larvae of parasites in faeces. Larvae entered through the skin, mainly through the toenail bed, and were carried to the lungs through the venous blood. During a cough or the equivalent, they were deposited in the oral cavity and then found their way into the oesophagus and the gut. Some, not destroyed by the stomach acid, would reach the small intestine and anchor themselves to the intestinal mucosa and start nourishing themselves on the blood of their host. When fully grown, they may be approximately one centimetre long and may live for one to five years. The adult female may produce thousands of eggs per day and eventually enough to deplete the host of blood. They are passed in the stool from where they find new customers. Wearing shoes is the greatest prophylactic measure; treatment had changed from the very toxic carbon tetrachloride in the 1950s to less toxic bephenium hydroxynphthoate in 1970s to even less toxic albendazole in the 2000s.

Malaria

Like tuberculosis, malaria is also a very old problem (Dunn, 1993). From antiquity, people recognized the similarities in signs and symptoms of cases of malaria or tuberculosis. However, not until Alphonse Laveran in Algeria and Ronald Ross in India discovered *Plasmodium* and the role played by *Anopheles* mosquito between 1880-1887 did we have a clear understanding of malaria.

In Chapter 3, I have mentioned the scientific and political dimensions of malaria and the problem of resistance to chloroquine. I am reintroducing this subject because of a very recent development, which, if successful, might make malaria a disease of the past like smallpox and plague. The Toronto-based *Globe and Mail* (July 16, 2010) highlighted an article "Genetically Altered Mosquito May Spell End of Malaria" on page 3. The *Globe and Mail* news was based on an article by a team of researchers led by Michael A. Riehle of the Department of Entomology,

University of Arizona, published in *Public Library of Science Pathogens* (Corby-Harris et al., 2010). I was surprised that the paper was not published in *Nature* or *Science*, the two top science journals. I contacted the senior author Dr. Riehle and asked him why they had not got the article published in *Nature* or *Science*. I was happy to know that they did try both journals but were disappointed that the editors of these journals did not find the findings of sufficient interest. In my opinion, the story reveals the lack of a broad vision on the part of the editors of *Nature* and *Science;* they are techno-centric and tend to find transgenic mice more fascinating than tinier mosquitos and can be oblivious to the significance of certain researches. But this is beside the point. The point is that Riehle's team is tackling one of the greatest scourges in human history by trying to make mosquitos incapable of transmitting malaria.

Plasmodium, which is the source of malaria, absolutely needs two hosts – mosquitos and humans. What Dr. Riehle and his colleagues have done is to generate mosquitos that no longer allow parasite development and render plasmodium ineffective. Of course, this is only a beginning. Their mosquitos are still in a confined laboratory. How to release them to ultimately replace all mosquitos of the world by their type is the next problem. And when they do so, would there be unforeseen consequences? Nonetheless, it is a monumental discovery.

Immunology

Advances in the field of immunology have been spectacular as well. The immune system is the body's own mechanism for dealing with infections. Phagocytes, granulocytes, leucocytes, lymphocytes, and the thymus are organs like all other organs – and better ones at that – because they protect the body from a host of infections. Even before the specific roles of the immune system were recognized, vaccinations were introduced as a therapeutic measure, starting with the anti-smallpox vaccine. Babies are protected because they have received protective mechanisms from the mother while still in the womb.

As early as 1890, Robert Koch thought that tuberculin could cure tuberculosis; it did not cure tuberculosis, but the reaction to tuberculin opened up an understanding of the phenomenon of allergy, and it was developed as a diagnostic test later on. In tuberculosis-prone countries like India, a positive tuberculin test has little meaning, but a negative one conclusively rules out the presence of hidden tuberculosis. Perhaps for all these reasons, none of which were known before 1778, the year of Voltaire's death, Voltaire announced, "The art of medicine consists of amusing the patient while nature cures the disease" (quoted by Hager, 2006).[7]

A significant advance in the field of immunology was the development of the hybridoma technique for generating monoclonal antibodies by César Milstein (1927-2002), Georges Jean Franz Kohler (1946-1995) and Niels K. Jerne (1911-1994); all three won the 1984 Nobel Prize in medicine.

The deadly human immunodeficiency virus would possibly have been quite innocuous on its own if it did not suppress the body's immune system. It is not a wild conjecture that the exploitation of knowledge about the immune system might prove to be the therapeutics of the future. If AIDS and malaria could be eliminated like smallpox and plague, it would not be because of drugs better than the ones we have but because immunologists and biochemists would have solved the problem of anti-AIDS and anti-malaria vaccines.

Artificial Cells

Thomas Ming Swi Chang, an undergraduate student at McGill University, Canada, in the 1950s, felt inspired by the entrepreneurship of his grandfather in China and wanted, as many young idealists do, to apply "basic research to medical treatment." He started with artificial red blood cells with semi-permeable microcapsules containing functional haemoglobin, inside and reported his results with haemoglobin first in 1957 followed by a publication in the prestigious journal *Science* (Chang, 1964). Chang's imaginative findings have now metamorphosed into a big field concerned with delivery and removal of molecules by artificial cells into and out of the body (Chang, 2007).

Unsuspected Effects of Molecules

Matt Ridley (1999) conjectured that chromosomes have personalities; perhaps they do. But chromosomes contain too many DNAs and too much proteins. It is natural for them to have personalities. What is even more significant is that drugs – which are not a package of many things, like chromosomes, but single entities – too have personalities, both open and hidden. We know drugs by their open personalities; we come to know other features of their personalities bit by bit, but we can never be sure that we know everything about them. In a certain way, the question of knowledge about drugs can be conceived as the general question of knowledge described by physics Nobel laureate Werner Heisenberg (1901-1976), the founder of quantum mechanics:

> The philosophic thesis that all knowledge is ultimately founded in experience has in the end led to a postulate concerning the logical clarification of any statement about nature ...The words "position" and "velocity" of an electron, for instance, seemed perfectly well defined ...But actually they were not well defined, as is seen from the relations of uncertainty ...This shows that we can never know before hand which limitation will be put on the applicability of certain concepts by the extension of our knowledge into the remote parts of nature, into which we can only penetrate with the most elaborate tools. (Heisenberg, 2007)

I could randomly select many drugs to illustrate my point, but I am choosing vitamin D (vitamin D_3 and vitamin D_2) because of its clinical significance (Hollick, 2007; White, 2008). Since Sun is the centre of our solar system and sunshine makes the skin manufacture vitamin D, it can be assumed that vitamin D has existed ever since Darwin's species came into being. The healing effect of sunshine has been known since antiquity, but it was left to McCollum (1879-1967) and Mellanby to figure out that what prevents rickets is not sunshine but vitamin D (McCollum and Davis, 1914; Mellanby, 1919). In subsequent years, it became clear that vitamin D is not only a vitamin but also a hormone with an aptitude for nuclear receptors like other steroids (oestrogen, progesterone, cortisol) and a drug with both therapeutic and toxic effects.

The active form of vitamin D, 1,25-dihydroxyvitamin D, is generated by enzymatic activity, mainly in the liver and kidneys; it has many effects in addition to increasing the absorption of calcium to make bones; it modulates the immune system, suppresses infection, possibly prevents heart failure and cancer and much more (Hollick, 2007; White, 2008). Vitamin D is not a prescription drug. An enthusiastic consumption of vitamin D can lead to a deposition of calcium in soft tissue and may even cause skin cancer like what is known with too much sunlight. Vitamin D is made from cholesterol; if cholesterol-lowering drugs (Pahan, 2006) produce vitamin D deficiency, their use might be helping the heart by one mechanism and harming it by another.

Not to be left behind, vitamin A, a sister molecule of vitamin D, also present in milk but not as stable, decided to reveal its many features. If too little vitamin D can cause rickets or osteoporosis, too little vitamin A can cause night blindness or skin problems. In many other ways, it is similar to vitamin D, but in some way, it is very different from it.

Regeneration of tissues is a well-known phenomenon. In certain animals, like lizards and frogs, if a limb is severed, it grows back. According to the generally accepted law of regeneration, if an organ is amputated, it will grow back in time, but only the portion that was amputated.

The Indian biologist Iqbal Niazi – who did his PhD at McGill University in the early the 1960s and accepted an academic position at Jaipur, India, known for its royal palaces and not science – observed that vitamin A can lead to the formation of the entire limb from the point of amputation, not just the severed portion (Niazi and Saxena, 1968, 1978; Niazi et al., 1985); this defied the then-existing law of generation and could only happen if the genes for the limb formation are present in the entire limb and can be activated by vitamin A. These startling data of Niazi and Saxena published in less known journals by India-based scientists did not catch the attention of researchers until Professor Malcolm Maden of King's College, London, took note of it (Maden, 1982) and a group of Indian biologists published confirmatory data in *Nature* (Mohanty-Hejmadi et al., 1992). The vitamin A-induced mis-regulation of mice limb development observed by McGill University researchers (Galdones and Hales, 2008) is indeed an extension of the original data of Niazi et al. (1968, 1978, 1985). I have been trying to persuade my associates to test the effect of vitamin A on neuronal regeneration in Alzheimer's, but without any success.

The story of vitamin C is similar to that of vitamins D and A. Unlike vitamins A and D, vitamin C is water-soluble. Linus Pauling was an accomplished scientist (Paradowski, 1983; Herman and Munro, 1996), who, though a chemist, contributed to clinical medicine more than any other single individual I can think of. Pauling was a socially conscious scientist and a pacifist (Pauling, 1983). Aside from path-breaking discoveries about chemical bond, sickle-cell anaemia, and the structure of a number of molecules, and coming close to deciphering the helical structure of DNA, Pauling's insight into the chemistry of vitamin C and a vitamin C-promotional letter from biochemist Irwin Stone (1907-1984) led him to propose its use against the common cold (Pauling, 1971) and cancer (Pauling, 1976). His conjecture on orthomolecular psychiatry relies on creating inside the body a new balance of normally present endogenous molecules (Pauling, 1968). Pauling also proposed a general theory on the mechanism of action of general anaesthetics (Pauling, 1961). Tom Hager (1998) provided an excellent summary of the achievements of the many-faceted Linus Pauling.

Being a chemist and well-versed in quantum physics, Pauling could deduce that vitamin C acted as an antioxidant. Because of his radical political views, Linus Pauling not only earned the wrath of the US administration, to the extent of being denied a passport for a while, but of many run-of-the-mill scientists who claimed to be averse to politics while steadfastly holding on to their conservatism. Linus Pauling's conjecture about vitamin C and an orthomolecular approach toward psychiatry is somewhat forgotten, without being seriously examined. Surprisingly, the role of oxidants and antioxidants is a big puzzle in health and disease including in cancer and in birth defects, but most researchers in this area are unaware of the fact that the initiator of this area was Linus Pauling. What especially concerns us here is that vitamin C is more than a vitamin, and the reason we are aware of this is the work of Linus Carl Pauling.

New Uses of Old Drugs

There are many examples of drugs finding new uses; here I describe just a few of them.

The exact cause of cancer is still not known. It was generally thought in the 1950s and 1960s that most cancers are caused by viruses. This encouraged scientists to synthesize antiviral drugs. The American scientist Jerome Horwitz synthesized azidothymidine (AZT, Zidovudine) in 1964 as a potential anticancer drug. AZT proved of little value against tumours in mice. AZT was sidelined until AIDS appeared on the scene, which is caused by a retrovirus. Suddenly, AZT came into prominence in the treatment of AIDS and made a fortune for Burrows-Welcome, which holds the patent on AZT.

Arsenic is a well-known molecule. It has been used to cure and kill since ancient times. After the discovery of penicillin, the use of arsenic in the treatment of syphilis was abandoned, and it became pure poison. But as I mentioned before, one can never know everything about drugs and chemicals. Recent reports suggest that arsenic may be a miracle drug against certain forms of leukaemia (Chou and Dang, 2004).

Thalidomide, which produced fetal abnormality found a place in the treatment of leprosy.

Science and Society

In general, scientists live in their exclusive world from which the general public is excluded. Pythagoras had a strict rule of secrecy for his school, and one of the pupils was drowned because he violated that rule of secrecy. This was fortunately replaced by a trend of public discourse about scientific findings. Many discoveries were publicly announced. Darwin's book on evolution was intended as much for the public as for biologists. In the twentieth century, however, science became largely confined to the laboratories, as far away from the public as possible. Findings were published in scientific journals exclusively for scientists. Scientists were no longer involved in creating a culture of science.

It is redeeming to note that modern science, including medical science, is beginning to recognize the significance of interaction between scientists and the general public; and important media, both print and television, are beginning to highlight scientific discoveries in open channels. On the other hand, modern scientific research has become very technical and most of the publications in prestigious journals like *Nature* and *Science* are incomprehensible even to scientists in different fields. The cautious note by Yves Quéré (2010) that "academics must engage with society" is a welcome development. Hopefully, all major journals will find a way of communicating to the public at large a culture of science and public awareness about scientific medicine.

Conclusion

Scientists – be they physicists, chemists, biologists, or just physicians – have made great strides in the task allotted to them by history. It took almost two hundred thousand years to find out that consciousness is a function of the brain and not the heart, but it took less than fifty years from the discovery of the double-helical structure of DNA to the introduction of stem cell in therapeutics. The achievements of modern medicine are monumental, but challenges still remain, even in common ailments like diabetes and hypertension. Each advance is met with new challenges, like effective chemotherapy is met with resistance by stubborn micro-organisms. There is, however, reason to hope that all diseases can be conquered; at some stage we can all echo the 1963 optimism of Martin Luther King (1929-1968): "I [we] have a dream!"

Notes

1. From *Ancient Society* by Lewis Henry Morgan (1818-1881), first published in 1877; the First Meridian Printing in 1963 (page 3). Morgan was an American anthropologist of eminence. He was appalled by white oppression of native Americans. He did an in-depth study of the Iroquois Indians and was adopted as a citizen by the Iroquois Confederation. Morgan's book is the basis of Friedrich Engels's *The Origin of the Family, Private Property and the State,* first printed by Progress Publishers, Moscow, in 1948. Both Engels and his associate, Karl Marx, expressed their great admiration for the scholarly and analytical achievement of Morgan.

2. Einstein, A. *Ideas and Opinions* (New York: Crown Publishers [1954] (1985), 336-337.

3. James Dewey Watson, Frances Compton Crick, and Maurice Hugh Wilkins won the Nobel Prize in medicine and physiology in 1962 for discovering the double helix structure of DNA. Elizabeth Blackburn, Carol W. Greider, and Jack W. Szostak won the 2009 Nobel Prize in medicine and physiology for the discovery of how chromosomes are protected by telomeres.

4. Erwin Schrodinger in *What is Life?* (Cambridge: Cambridge University Press, 1944).

5. The article is based on the Donald Olding Hebb (1904-1985) lecture at McGill University in 1997 given by Ramachandran. D. O. Hebb was an influential psychologist of the twentieth century. He was professor of psychology at McGill University, Montreal, from 1848 to 1859, vice dean from 1964 to 1966, and chancellor from 1970 to 1974.

6. The formal name *Vibrio cholerae Pacini 1854* was given in 1965; the term *Pacini* was added to credit Filippo Pacini (1812-1883), who was the first to identify the bacteria in 1854; Robert Koch was not aware of this discovery. Italian scientists made a number of significant discoveries in the area of tropical medicine. Angelo Dubini (1813-1902) had discovered hookworms, and Giovanni Batista Grassi had independently discovered malaria parasite in 1889. This is because Italy, of all European countries, is prone to tropical diseases, but since it was not a major colonial power, the contributions of Italian scientists did not often get them appropriate recognition.

7. Thomas Hager's book *The Demon Under the Microscope* (New York: Harmony Books, 2006) is a fascinating story of the life of Gerhard Domagk, whose discovery of sulphonamide, the first antibiotic, is mentioned in Chapter 13. Most of Domagk's research was done in the years preceding and during the ascendency of Nazism, which Domagk did not admire.

References

Anderson, S. R. and Lightfoot, D. W. "The Human Language Faculty as an Organ," *Annual Review of Physiology*, 62 (2000): 697-722.

Barnes, J. Ed. *The Complete Works Aristotle: The Revised Oxford Translation*, V. I. (Princeton: Princeton University Press, 1984), 674.

Chang, T. M. S. "Semipermeable Microcapsules," *Science* 146 (1964) 524-525.

——. *Artificial Cells* (Singapore: World Scientific Publishing, 2007).

Chomsky, N. "Language and Nature," *Mind*, 104: (1995): 1-69.

Chou, W-C., and Dang, C. V. "Acute Promyelocytic Leukemia: Recent Advances in Therapy and Molecular Basis of Response to Arsenic Therapies," *Current Opinion in Hematology* 12 (2004): 1-6.

Corby-Harris, V., Drexler, A., de Jong, L. W. et al. "Activation of *AKT* Signaling Reduces the Prevalence and Intensity of Malaria Parasite Infection and Lifespan in *Anopheles stephensi* Mosquitoes," *Public Library of Science Pathogens (PLoS Pathogens)* 6 (2010): 1-10.

De Bold, A. J., Borenstein, H. B., Veress, A. T., and Sonnenberg, H. "A Rapid and Potent Natriuretic Response to Intravenous Injection of Atrial Myocardial Extract in Rats," *Life Sciences* 28 (1981): 89-94.

Dunn, F. L. "Malaria," In *The Cambridge World History of Human Disease*, edited by K. F. Kiple (Cambridge: Cambridge University Press, 1993), 855-862.

Galdones, E. and Hales, B. F. "Retinoic Acid Receptor Gamma-Induced Misregulation of Chondrogenesis in the Murine Limb Bud *In Vitro*," *Toxicological Sciences* 106 (2008): 223-232.

Gonzalez-Crussi, F. *Carrying the Heart: Exploring the Worlds within Us* (New York: Kaplan 2009).

Groopman, J. *How Doctors Think* (New York: Houghton Mifflin, 2007).

Hager, T. *Linus Pauling and the Chemistry of Life* (New York: Oxford University Press, 1998).

——. *The Demon under the Microscope: From Battlefield Hospitals to Nazi Labs, One Doctor's Heroic Search for the World's First Miracle Drug* (New York: Harmony Books, 2006), 11.

Healy, D. *Let Them Eat PROZAC: The Unhealthy Relationship between the Pharmaceutical Industry and Depression* (New York: New York University Press, 2004).

Heisenberg, W. *Physics and Philosophy: The Revolution in Modern Science* [1962] (New York: Harperperennial, 2007), 59-60.

Herman, Z. S. and Munro, D. B. *Publications of Linus Pauling.* (Palo Alto: The Linus Pauling Institute of Science and Medicine, 1996).

Hollick, M. F. "Vitamin D Deficiency," *New England Journal of Medicine* 357 (2007): 266-281.

Illich, I. *Limits to Medicine. Medical Nemesis: The Expropriation of Health* [1976] (New York: Penguin Books, 1977).

Johnston, W. D. "Tuberculosis," In *The Cambridge World History of Human Disease*, Ed. K. F. Kiple (Cambridge: Cambridge University Press, 1993): 1059-1068.

Kant, E. *Critique of Pure Reason* (1781). Trans. Norman Kemp Smith (New York: ST Martin's Press, 1965), 7.

Keil, G. "Sogenannte Erstbeschreibung des Phantomschmerzes von Ambroise Paré," *Fortschritte der Medizin.* 108 (1990): 62-66.

Kooli, A., Kermorvant-Duchemin, E., Sennlaub, F., et al. Trans. Arachidonic Acids Induce Heme Oxygenase-Dependent Vasorelaxation of Cerebral Microvasculature. *Free Radical Biology & Medicine*, 44 (2008): 815-825.

Maden, M. "Vitamin A and Pattern Formation in the Regenerating Limb", *Nature* 295 (1982): 672-675.

McCollum, E. V. and Davis, M. "Observations on the Isolation of the Substance in Butter Fat which Exerts a Stimulating Effect on Growth," *Journal of Biological Chemistry* 19 (1914): 245-250.

Mellanby, E. "An Experimental Investigation on Rickets," *Lancet* 196 (1919): 407-412.

Melzack, R. and Wall, P. D. "Pain Mechanisms: A New Theory," *Science* 150 (1965): 973-978.

Mohanty-Hejmadi, P., Dutta, S. K., and Mahapatra, P. "Limbs Generated at Site of Tail Amputation in Marbled Balloon Frog after Vitamin A Treatment," *Nature* 355 (1992): 352-353.

Morris, J. "Pattern Recognition in Descartes' Automata," *ISIS* 60 (1969): 451-460.

Nettleton, S. *The Sociology of Health and Illness* (Cambridge: Polity Press, 2006).

Niazi, I. A. and Saxena, S. "Inhibitory and Modifying Influences of Excess of Vitamin A on Tail Regeneration in *Bufo* Tadpoles," *Experientia* 24 (1968): 852-853.

——. "Abnormal Hind Limb Regeneration in Tadpoles of the Toad, *Bufo andersoni*, Exposed to Excess Vitamin A," *Folia Biologica [Krakow]* 26 (1978): 3-11.

Niazi, I. A., Pescitelli, M. J., and Stocum, D. L. "Stage-Dependent Effects of Retinoic Acid on Regenerating Urodele Limbs," *Roux's Archives of Developmental Biology* 194 (1985): 355-363.

Pahan, K. "Lipid-Lowering Drugs," *Cellular and Molecular Life Sciences* 63 (2006) 1165-1178.

Paradowski, R. J. "About the Author (Linus Pauling)". In *No More War* by Linus Pauling [1958] (New York: Dodd, Mead & Co. 1983).

Pauling, L. *No More War* [1958] (New York: Dodd Mead, 1983).

——, "A Molecular Theory of General Anesthesia," *Science* 134 (1961): 15-21.

——, "Orthomolecular Psychiatry: Varying Concentrations of Substances Normally Present in Human Body may Control Mental Disease," *Science* 160 (1968): 265-271.

——, *Vitamin C and the Common Cold* (New York: Bantam Books, 1971).

——, *How to Live Longer and Feel Better* (New York: Avon Books, 1987).

——, "Vitamin C and Cancer," *National Academy of Preventive Medicine Journal* 1 (1976): 6-10.

Porter, R. *The Greatest Benefit to Mankind: A Medical History of Humanity* (New York: W. W. Norton, 1997).

Ibid., 1997a. 494-495.

Quéré, Y. "Academies Must Engage with Society," *Nature* 465 (2010): 1009.

Ramachandran, V. S. and Hirstein, W. "The Perception of Phantom Limbs. The D.O, Hebb Lecture," *Brain* 121 (1998): 1603-1630.

Ridley, M. *Genome: The Autobiography of a Species in 23 Chapters* (New Delhi: Harper-Collins, 1999), 3.

Sapieha P., Sirinyan M., Hamel D. et al. "The Succinate Receptor GPR91 in Neurons Plays a Major Role in Retinal Angiogenesis," *Nature Medicine*, 14: 1067-1076, 2008.

Schrödinger, E. *What is Life? With Mind and Matter and Autobiographical Sketches.* (Cambridge: Cambridge University Press [Combined Reprint] 1967), 93.

Share, N. N. and Melville, K. I. "Centrally Mediated Sympathetic Cardiovascular Responses Induced by Intraventricular Norepinephrine," *Journal of Pharmacology and Experimental Therapeutics* 141 (1963): 15-21.

Stephens, B. E. and Vohr, B. R. "Neurodevelopmental Outcome of the Premature Infant," *Pediatric Clinics of North America* 56 (2009): 631-46.

Stoll, B. J., Hansen, N. I., Bell, E. F. et al. "Neonatal Outcomes of Extremely Preterm Infants from the NICHD Neonatal Research Network," *Pediatrics 126* (2010):443-56.

Sur, M., Garraghty, P. E., and Roe, A. W. "Experimentally Induced Visual Projections into Auditory Thalamus and Cortex," *Science* 242 (1988): 1437-1441.

Varvarigou A., Bardin C. L., Beharry K., Chemtob, S., Papageorgiou, A., and Aranda, J. V. "Early Ibuprofen Administration to Prevent Patent Ductus Arteriosus in Premature Newborn Infants." *Journal of American Medical Association 275(1*996): 539-44.

Virgin, H. W. and Walker, B. D. "Immunology and the Elusive AIDS Vaccine," *Nature* 464 (2010): 224-231.

Warner, J. H. "The History of Science and the Science of Medicine," *OSIRIS* 10 (1995): 164-193.

Weaver, I. C. G., Cervoni, N., Champagne, F. A. et al. "Epigenetic Programming by Maternal Behavior," *Nature Neuroscience* 7 (2004): 847-854.

Weyl, H. *Mind and Matter: Selected Writings on Philosophy, Mathematics, and Physics* [with an Introduction by Peter Pesic] (Princeton: Princeton University Press, 2009).

White, J. H. "Vitamin D Signaling, Infectious Diseases, and Regulation of Innate Immunity," *Infection and Immunity* 76 (2008) 3837-3843.

CHAPTER 15

Medical Ethics and Medical Science

Parpalaid: *You may think me too much of a stickler for ethical standards, but doesn't your method subordinate the interest of the patient just a bit to that of doctor?*

Knock: *Dr. Parpalaid, you're forgetting that there is an interest which is greater than either.*

Parpalaid: *What?*

Knock: *The interest of medicine. I serve that interest and that alone … You've given me a township inhabited by several thousand neutral individuals, individuals without direction. My function is to direct them, to lead them into a life of medicine. I put them to bed and see what can be made of them: tuberculosis, neurasthenia, arteriosclerosis, whatever you like, but* **something** [emphasis in the original], *for God's sake. Nothing gets on my nerves like that indeterminate nonentity called a healthy man.*

Jules Romains[1]

In actuality, the Hippocratic Oath, whether in its original or revised form, is like other declarations of moral principles; it is no stronger than the will of the people to respect and uphold it. The Declaration of Independence proclaimed that liberty is an inalienable human right; this did not prevent Americans from holding the Negro in bondage. Similarly, the Hippocratic Oath proclaims that the physician's primary loyalty is to the patient; this did not prevent physicians from betraying this loyalty – to the Church in the Middle Ages, and to the State in the modern world.

Thomas S. Szasz[2]

Introduction

In social relationships, people generally know what is ethical and what is not. However, professions like medicine have their specialized ethics. From the books on medical ethics, I infer that authors – both individuals as well as British and American medical associations – think of medical ethics in relation to the law of the land, religion, training of medical personnel, euthanasia, care of the elderly, right to abortion, professionalism, clinical trials, and so on. Questions of ethics are designed to gain public respectability for the profession.

Jonsen (2000) dealt with the historical account of medical ethics from Hellenic and Roman medicine to modern times. The books *Bioethics: An Anthology* edited by Kuhse and Singer (2006) and *Doing Right: A Practical Guide for Medical Trainees and Physicians* by Hébert (2009) deal with practically every technical aspect of medical ethics. Indeed there are almost 100 books on medical ethics.

The book *Let Them Eat PROZAC* by David Healy (2004) is not specifically on medical ethics, and yet, by dealing with the mania of mass consumption of the antidepressant drug Prozac, the book elegantly exposes ethical issues involving societal pressure, the interests of major pharmaceutical industries, and of physicians who function as intermediaries between the drug industry and the population.

I am not intending to narrate all the technical dimensions of medical ethics; rather, I dwell on social, political and monetary factors that determine the attitude of physicians toward ethics and of the population towards the medical profession.

Questions of medical ethics fall into two different domains. One deals with the intervention by the state or physicians in alleviating the clearly identifiable suffering of the patient. Denial of medical assistance in such cases, for whatever reason, is clearly a violation of medical ethics. The second category falls in the philosophical domain (Culver and Gert, 1982); this second category concerns conduct under political pressure or inclination.

Social and Political Role of Doctors

Indeed, much of the criticism of modern medicine is based on the role played by the medical profession (Rosen 1968; Szasz, 1961,1971; Ehrenreich. and English, 1973; Waitzkin and Waterman, 1974; Illich, 1976; Brown, 1979); these authors are not critical of medical science.

The professional organizations of physicists, chemists, mathematicians, historians, philosophers, et cetera, are primarily or exclusively concerned with their specific disciplines. On the other hand, the organizations of physicians and surgeons defend the monetary, professional and legal interests of their members as well as of the profession; they influence government policies toward health care, prevent encroachment of their profession, both on rational and irrational grounds; they decide upon the number of doctors a country can or should have, and so on. In recent years, for example, medical associations have played a crucial role in determining the rights of immigrant physicians to practice their profession in the West.

The American Medical Association (AMA) played an important role in preventing health reforms introduced in the 1940s by President Franklin Delano Roosevelt (1882-1945), Lyndon Baines Johnson (1908-1973), and Senator Hillary Clinton during Bill Clinton's presidency. Although each time the AMA claimed that its position is determined by a consideration of the greater good of patients, it was clearly determined by the monetary interests of the profession. However, public pressure for some kind of health-care system, inspired by the successes of their Canadian neighbours, forced the AMA to support the health-care reforms introduced by President Obama in 2009-2010.

In Canada, an attempt to introduce universal health care was first made in the 1930s by Norman Bethune, albeit without success. Ultimately, Saskatchewan's premier, Thomas (Tommy) Clement Douglas (1904-1986), implemented it in 1962 in his state; it met fierce opposition from the medical profession, including a strike by the doctors. On Tommy Douglas's persuasion, the Canadian prime minister, Lester B. Pearson (1897-1972), who won the 1957 Nobel Peace Prize for defusing the Suez crisis, introduced universal health care in all of Canada in

1966. This measure too was opposed by the medical profession, but not as vigorously as the one in Saskatchewan.

Public support for the Canadian Health Care Plan was formally expressed when Tommy Douglas was voted as the Greatest Canadian of All Times in a poll conducted by the Canadian Broadcasting Corporation in 2004. The opposition of Canadian physicians to the health-care plan in contrast to public support is an indication of divergent views on ethics by doctors and the public.

Gender bias is universal although in the last twenty-five years or so, there has been much progress in removing at least the most blatant methods of discrimination against women. However, there are still fewer women in science than there should be (Williams and Ceci, 2007, Editorial, 2010). Gender bias is a cultural expression of social evolution. Feudal order and religious beliefs play a major role in perpetuating discrimination against women and are often able to recruit even the support of women.

A very grotesque expression of this, which directly concerns the medical profession, is the preference of the family for a male child. With the availability of ultrasound, the termination of pregnancy if the foetus is female has reached epidemic proportions. During the last decade of the twentieth century, female infanticide accounted for a staggering ten million in India (Jha et al., 2006), which could not happen without the active involvement of medical professionals.

The physiology of males and females is different and so are the consequences of disease. Most researchers in medicine pay little attention to the effect of sex in their data, and no journal or funding agency insists that all researches must address the issue of gender as a variable. So when we read that a certain drug is a better antidepressant than another, we do not know if the statement applies to both males and females or just to males or to females. A recent article in *Nature* (Editorial, 2010) and other articles (Baylis, 2010; Kim et al., 2010; Zucker and Beery, 2010) have reassuringly raised some of these issues.

Ethics of Confidentiality and Secrecy

Confidentiality about a patient is treated as a valued ethical principle of medicine. The doctor is not expected to divulge information about a patient even in a court of law unless specifically commanded by the judge to do so. Thomas S. Szasz (1971) eloquently discussed this subject and extensively quotes Donald Gould (1919-2002) in connection with this subject matter.

Donald Gould was a physiologist who taught at medical schools in England, Hong Kong, and Singapore. He gave up physiology to serve as editor of prestigious medical magazines like *World Medicine, Medical News,* and *New Scientist* and he was also a regular correspondent for *New Statesman*; additionly, he served as the chairman of Medical Journalists Association (Richmond, 2002).

Gould (1967) expressed his views on the physicians' privilege of confidentiality in an article appropriately titled "To Hell with Medical Secrecy!" The title says it all and Szasz (1971a) quotes him as follows: "We do not argue that a more or less adequate statement of our financial affairs should not be made available at regular intervals to the inspector of taxes. Why then should we jibe at the idea that a full, accurate, and regular account of our physical (and, indeed, mental) state should be rendered to some central authority?"

Szasz (1971a) himself adds, "Like the zealous inquisitor intoxicated with the glory of God and the supreme good of man's salvation, for whom personal liberty was a subsidiary value (if not a positive evil) – so the zealous medical collectivist, intoxicated with the glory of science and the supreme good of man's health (bodily and mental, of course), regards personal liberty as a subsidiary value (if not a positive evil)."

The 383-page book *The Manufacture of Madness* by Szasz (1971) is a fascinating, if a depressing, story of the role of the medical profession, particularly in relation to its handling of mental illnesses. The magnitude of this problem must have been big enough to have occupied the attention of other authors as well (Rosen, 1968; Hoenig and Hamilton, 1969; Parry-Jones, 1972; Jonsen, 2000). I discussed the role played by psychopharmacology in Chapter 13; the benefits delivered by psychoactive drugs is a minor affair compared with the role played by the medical profession and the state in condemning people to mental asylums and declaring them unfit for the society.

Juridical Role of Doctors

Doctors are often called to verify if a mother is fit to raise her children, if a prisoner should be granted parole, if a person is fit to drive a vehicle, and a host of other things. Doctors' dictum in these matters carries undue weight although their competence in these matters can rarely be verified. Couldn't a doctor be as much at fault in such cases as they are sometimes known to be in diagnostics (cancer cases) and forensic testimonies? Doctors are products of society like everyone else, and there is no reason to assume they are always above personal, religious and moral prejudices.

One of the most difficult problems that doctors face is to arrive at a decision to save or not save the life of a terminally ill patient in agony, unable to eat and breathe and kept alive by mechanically supporting nutrition and respiration and preventing infection using multiple drugs. A great deal has been written on this subject, and an article by Udawadia (2009) discusses this issue with reference to different socio-cultural contexts. There are no clear guidelines in such cases and Hospital Ethics' Committees, which by now exist in almost all major hospitals, often make the decisions.

Nobody likes to die in a hospital. Everyone prefers to die at home. And yet, at least in developed countries like Canada, most people die in a hospital, at much cost to the healthcare system and much agony to the dying person. In most cases, it is possible to provide the necessary support and let the person die at home in comfortable surroundings.

In her book *First, Do No Harm*, Lisa Belkin (1994) gives a moving account of real stories of patients in a major hospital in Houston, Texas, whose ultimate fates reveal the compassion of the nursing staff, the matter-of-fact and yet ethically sound attention of the doctors, the factors that lead the ethics' committee to terminate the life-support system of helpless patients and of the financial consideration of the hospital.

In many countries, formal laws exist that are used to punish sex workers, drug addicts, homosexuals, and a host of other practices, which includes the right to abortion. Doctors abide by this because abortion is illegal. Doctors can also dare to violate this law against abortion openly because they feel, and according to feminist movement correctly so, that women must have the final choice. The doctor who took this challenge to its limits in Canada, until the Supreme Court ruled in 1988 that denying abortion was against the Charter of Rights, was Henry Morgantaler.

Henry Morgantaler's whole life is nothing but a struggle to survive – and to survive with dignity and defy whatever comes in the way of the rights of women. He was born in Poland in 1923. His father, being Jewish, was killed by the Gestapo. Henry Morgantaler is a survivor of the notorious Auschwitz and other incarcerations rescued by the US Army in 1945. He migrated to the United States and then to Canada, and completed his MD from the Université de Montréal in 1953.

He practiced medicine in a poor locality in Montreal and performed abortions, which were then illegal except in cases where pregnancy threatened the life of the mother, as determined by a committee of experts. He was arrested and jailed in Montreal. His clinic in Toronto was firebombed, and he himself was attacked. However, he never succumbed to the laws of the land or threat by male chauvinist bigots.

The story of Morgantaler shows that ethics is only compatible with fundamental human rights, but might be at odds with the law of the land.

More recently, a controversial issue centres around the disease multiple sclerosis (MS). It is widely assumed that it is an autoimmune disease. More recently, the Italian neurologist Dr. Parlo Zamboni has claimed that MS is caused by blocked blood vessels to the brain; he claims that angioplasty, as in the case of coronary artery disease, can relieve the patient of debilitating symptoms. As is usually the case, many neuroscientists, most importantly from the United States, say more research is needed before angioplasty can be considered a treatment for MS. A recent report in the Canadian newspaper *Globe and Mail* (April 29, 2010) says that a patient Paulette O'Leary went from her home in Toronto to Pennsylvania to be operated by doctor Joseph Bonn, who was very confident that his surgery would alleviate the MS symptoms of O'Leary. However, just as the operation was to begin the lawyer for the hospital ordered a cancellation of the operation on her and many other patients who had been booked for the same surgery. The patient's husband is a doctor and health-care researcher, and he took his wife for the surgery. In the meantime, Paulette O'Leary is considering going to Bulgaria to get her operation for less money.

The question is this: is it ethical to deny a possible treatment for a debilitating disease like MS? Would insulin have been allowed to treat diabetes and penicillin to treat infection if the current laws existed in the 1920s and 1940s? I think that law firms should be barred by law from handling medical cases, which should be left only to the jurisdiction of medical associations. The lawyers only increase the cost of therapies.

The rider that more research is needed before a certain treatment can be given or a certain medical procedure can be used has no objective criteria. There are many patients of MS in the United States. What would more research constitute has not been spelled out by the US medical profession. There are animal models of MS. The MS specialists in the United States could have ascertained by non-invasive procedures if indeed blood supply to the brain is compromised in cases of MS. It would seem to me that what is not discovered in the United States is considered by the US establishment to be suspect. Metformin, which had been in use in Europe for several years to manage type-2 diabetes, was not approved in the United States until just a few years ago. Perhaps the Zamboni method has to wait; in the meantime, however, American and Canadian patients are flocking to Bulgaria to go through the Zamboni treatment.

Interaction with Patients

The demoralising experiences of the patients with health services and, on the other hand, advertisements of medical benefits from other schools of medicine is the major factor determining a patient's choice between modern and alternative medicine. The vast majority of the population lives in countries where universal health care does not exist; this includes populous countries like India. Primary health-care facilities are free, but a good number of doctors either do not pay reasonable attention to patients unless they are paid, legally or otherwise, and patients somehow appear to be convinced that proper care will not be available unless the doctor is paid.

According to Groopman (2007), the thinking process of many doctors is stereotypical, such that they do not pay sufficient attention to what the patient is saying and ultimately reach an erroneous diagnosis. He describes many cases. The very first case is of a young woman reduced to around 40 kg over a fifteen-year period of consulting numerous doctors and ingesting three thousand calories a day. To most doctors, she fitted the description of being a neurotic. She finally and fortunately reached one Dr. Myron Falchuk in Boston who cared to patiently listen to her and thought of all possibilities outside the standard algorithm. By endoscopy, he discovered that the patient had celiac disease, an autoimmune disease, essentially allergy to gluten, the source of her problem of malabsorption and weight loss. Groopman (2007) provides many case histories of diagnostic errors resulting from stereotypical attitudes by doctors and their reluctance to properly heed the information provided by their patient.

Why are not all drugs freely available, as alcohol is? The medical profession does not allow the pharmacist to dispense drugs deemed prescription drugs. For a long period of time, midwives were not allowed to deliver babies. Most educated patients know a lot about their own diseases and appropriate therapeutics. The regulations on the availability of prescription drugs ensures the mediating role of a doctor, never without cost to someone.

In summary, monetary consideration and relative inaccessibility of medical assistance compels patients to seek alternative therapy. Of course, there are other reasons for the popularity of other schools of medicine, which I wish to discuss in the final Chapter 17 entitled "Survival of the Fit and the Unfit."

Pharmaceuticals, Patent Laws, and Clinical Trials

In earlier times, say before 1960, new drugs were introduced by university researchers. This is no longer true. In the United States, for example, the Food and Drug Administration (FDA) and the Department of Health, Education, and Welfare rigidly control the development and evaluation of new drugs. Regulations instituted by the Drug Amendments Act of 1962 require proof of both efficacy and safety. Earlier regulations only required test of safety and not efficacy. In the case of new molecules, efficacy and safety can only be tested by clinical trials, which are too costly to be undertaken by individual researchers or small laboratories. Clinical trials are undertaken by giant pharmaceutical companies and require the recruitment of physicians and human volunteers. Physicians are paid and volunteers are usually offered free drugs and monitoring and sometimes money as well.

The logistics of clinical trials and the potential of legal complications are such that the majority of clinical trials comprise several phases and are usually done in developing countries. India is a preferred country because it is bestowed with technical competence and with subjects willing to volunteer. Paradoxically, India, an example of a dismal health-care system, is a haven both for clinical trials and organ transplants (Srinivasan, 2009). What is relevant is the ethics of these clinical trials. Starting with the clinical trials of high oestrogen dose oral contraceptives, which were mainly done on Puerto Rican women, several reports have appeared of biased reporting by physicians because of the pressure of pharmaceutical industries. Obviously, controversial trials such as testing the efficacy of sterilization by the introduction of the irritant quinacrine into fallopian tubes were conducted in India, Bangladesh, Vietnam, and some Latin American countries and not in North America and Europe; these trials were unethical by any standards of judgment (Mulay, 1997).

Organ Transplants

The story of organ transplant is even more grotesque than that of clinical trials. Kidney transplant is a big business in India (Amaloraparvanathan, 2007) and the subject of the book *Kidneys for Sale* by Mark J. Cherry (2005). In all cases, the beneficiaries are the rich, mostly Americans, because getting donors is more difficult in the USA than in developing countries. Popular media sometimes reports how an American tourist of modest means went to India to get a heart transplant for less than US $40,000; with this money, he had a new heart as well as a visit to the Taj Mahal. Various people are involved in illegal and unethical acquisition of organs; but ultimately, a reasonably trained surgeon, a hospital or equivalent setting, and a set of nursing staff are essential components of this transaction. It is true that a healthy individual can lead a normal life with one kidney, and so donating the other one to someone is by itself not unethical. Indeed, in some cases, it can be the most precious gift one can give to dear ones. However, removing a kidney from a prisoner or a poor person for a small sum is a test of ethics and lots of doctors have failed.

Doctors and Wars

Doctors could be accessory to the war or just function as doctors. Both aspects are described below.

Doctors as Heroes

By its very nature, wars against another country or civil wars result in deaths and injuries of soldiers and civilians. Doctors tend to these injuries at great risk to themselves. During the Spanish Civil War (1936-1939), Canadian doctor Norman Bethune worked day and night from 1936 to 1937 performing sometimes more than one hundred operations a day; out of necessity, he introduced the first mobile blood transfusion. Between 1938 and 1939, Bethune worked with the Chinese Communist Party resisting Japanese aggression. He treated injured Japanese soldiers as well. Bethune trained other doctors and nurses. While with the Eighth Route Army of the Chinese Communist Party, Bethune developed sepsis by accidental injury during surgery and died on November 12, 1939. He is revered in China more than in Canada.

French doctors in Biafra started Medecins Sans Frontiéres (MSF) in 1971. It was a period of civil war when Biafra was fighting to separate from Nigeria. The sacrifice of doctors and their relentless efforts lead to the formation of the international body Doctors Without Borders as its English counterpart is called. MSF was awarded the 1999 Nobel Peace Prize. The hard work and sacrifice of these doctors and volunteers and the risks they take is exemplary. There are heroic stories of other doctors as well. In earthquakes such as in Haiti, during the tsunami in East Asia and India, and during the Bhopal industrial disaster, it was volunteer doctors who carried the heaviest burden. A recent survey reveals how a number of doctors opt to go to rural areas in Chhattisgarh (Sheikh et al., 2010), a poor province of India and centre of violent activities by Indian Maoists.

Mother Teresa (Agnes Gonxhe Bojaxhiu: 1910-1997) was not a doctor but she did what doctors should have done for the poor and helpless. Albert Schweitzer (1875-1965) trained himself in medicine so that he could help the needy (Brabazon, 1975).

Doctors as Assassins

Doctors can also descend to the lowest level possible under certain situations, such as during the rise of German and Japanese fascism, which goes on to show that doctors are more likely to side with the establishment than scientists of other disciplines.

In Nazi Germany, doctors identified and engineered the death of thousands of persons declared unfit for the 'superior race' even before the sword descended on homosexuals, Gypsies, communists, and millions of Jews (Grodin, 1992). We must thank our fortune that Plato, Michelangelo (1475-1564), and Leonardo da Vinci (1452-1519) – who, according to Sigmund Freud, were homosexuals – did not live in Adolf Hitler's (1889-1945) Germany or Benito Mussolini's (1883-1945) Italy.

Sadly, however, even in the citadel of democracy, that is England, its prudishness could not tolerate even Oscar Wilde (1854-1900) a hundred years ago (Ellman, 1988) and Alan Mathison Turing (1912-1954) in modern times (Hodges, 1992; Singh, 1999), the two geniuses driven to death in their forties.[3]

Proctor (1992) describes the horrific role played by doctors, which I quote in some detail below:

> In 1929 a number of physicians formed the National Socialist Physicians' League to ...purify the German Medical community of "Jewish Bolshevism." By Jan 1933 (before the rise of Hitler to power, 3000 doctors (6% of total) had joined the League. By 1942, more than 38,000 doctors had joined the Nazi Party representing about half of all doctors in the country. The discipline of racial hygiene (Rassenhygiene) was founded by Alfred Ploetz (1860-1940) and Wilhelm Schallmayer (1857-1919); medical scientists

were the ones who invented racial hygiene. Major expansion came before Hitler came to power.

Three laws were passed: the Sterilization Law, the Nuremberg Law and the euthanasia operation. Approximately 350,000 to 400,000 people were sterilized for conditions including feeblemindedness, schizophrenia, manic depression, epilepsy, Huntington's chorea, genetic blindness, deafness and "severe alcoholism." Some German doctors argued that this was not enough, 10-15 % should be sterilized. Nonsurgical sterilization by injecting supercooled carbon dioxide was used. In 1943, Carl Clauberg (1898-1957) announced to Heinrich Himmler (1900-1945) he could sterilize 1,000 women per day. Sterilization methods were initially devised in the US and used on 15,000 individuals. "In fact, Nazi physicians on more than one occasion argued that the German racial policies were relatively 'liberal' compared with the treatment of blacks in the United States."

By August 1941, when the first phase of euthanasia plan was brought to a close, more than 70,000 patients from German mental hospitals had been killed in an operation which provided rehearsal for the subsequent destruction of Jews, homosexuals, communists, Gypsies, and prisoners of war.

Physicians forced people to drink sea water to find out how long a man might survive without fresh water. At Dachau, Russian prisoners of war were immersed in icy water to see how long a pilot might survive when shot down over the English Channel and to find out what kind of protective gear or re-warming technique were most effective. Prisoners were placed in vacuum chambers to find out how the human body responds when pilots were forced to bail out at high altitudes.

At Fort Ney, near Strasbourg, 52 prisoners were exposed to phosgene gas in 1943 and 1944 to test possible antidotes; at Auschwitz, physicians experimented with new ways to sterilize or castrate people as part of the plan to repopulate Eastern Europe with Germans. Physicians performed limb and bone transplants (on persons with no medical need) and, in at least one instance, injected prisoners' eye with dyes to see if eye colour could be permanently changed. At Buchenwald, Gerhard Rose (1886-1992) infected prisoners with spotted fever to test experimental vaccines against the disease; at Dachau, Ernst Grawitz (1899-1945) infected prisoners with a broad range of pathogens to test homeopathic preparations.

Contrary to postwar apologies, doctors were never forced to perform such experiments. Physicians volunteered – and in several cases, Nazi officials actually had to restrain overzealous physicians . . .

> How and why physicians were able to engage in these medical crimes and atrocities? How could men and women sworn to the Hippocratic oath, trained as professionals in the world's most advanced scientific culture, come to commit crimes that even today stand as exemplars of evil?

In the documentary *An Indian Story,* the director Tapan Bose shows pictures of prisoners having been blinded by doctors with intraocular injection of acids, ostensibly to prevent them from committing crimes in the future. During the 2002 anti-Muslim riots in the Gujarat state of India, some Hindu doctors refused to treat injured Muslims even in hospital settings. It is likely that some doctors in other countries also placed their social prejudice and monetary interest above medical ethics.

Iserson (2002) documents cases where doctors acted as serial killers; however, I think these are deranged individuals who happen to be doctors and their cases do not constitute questions of ethics but rather a malaise.

The book *Molecules for Murder* by John Emsley (2008) is a masterly narration of many cases of homicide using chemicals such as ricin, hyoscine or scopolamine, atropine, diamorphine or diacetylmorphine or heroin, adrenaline, chloroform, carbon monoxide, cyanide, the weed killer paraquat and radioactive polonium. However, only two of these killers were doctors; Dr. Hawley Harvey Crippen (1862-1910) killed his wife with hyoscine so he could marry his mistress; Dr. Harold Frederick Shipman (1946-2004) killed an elderly woman suffering from emphysema with heroin. Digitalis, a molecule that has been used by doctors to commit homicide because it would kill by ventricular fibrillation is hard to identify at autopsy.

Medical Education

In the beginning doctors were trained as apprentices by watching their masters and assisting them where they could. But the situation has changed in a fundamental way. A medical degree is one of the most sought after university qualifications. It brings fame and money and allows the recipient to claim that he/she is doing it for neither of these but rather to serve humanity. The competition for admissions to medical schools is tough and the cost of medical education is high, although medicine is not intellectually as demanding as mathematics or physics, or even some disciplines in humanities such as economics or philosophy. Medical professional organizations limit the number of doctors that a country produces and it is usually less than that needed by society. In the United States (now in countries like India as well) a medical graduate incurs a large debt before graduation; because it is a safe investment, lending institutions are always available. What is generally not realized is that ultimately all education is subsidized by the entire population; if it were not so the cost would me much higher than it is – indeed in the absence of a social contribution, institutions of learning would not have come into existence. Notwithstanding these considerations, a doctor feels entitled to high earnings to make up for the debt incurred during education, several years of training and the high cost of insurance; the latter is the contribution of law firms which function like extortion factories. These different considerations are the principal determinants of medical ethics and not the Hippocratic oath.

The Push to Prescribe

The Push to Prescribe is the title of a book by Ford and Saibil (2009); these authors are primarily concerned with over medication of women, who are about one-half of the world's population at any time. They menstruate, bear children, go through menopause, and have to look better than they are; for all these there are drugs and surgery. However, these do not constitute a sufficient number of consumers and more have to be found. What could be easier than to identify a need for psychotropic drugs. It is estimated that "five psychotropic drugs (three SSRIs [selective serotonin reuptake inhibitor] and two antipsychotics) appear on the list of top twenty drug sellers of 2002" with a total sale of over $11 billion (Duncan et al., 2004). The result is not cure but an increase in mental illnesses (Whitaker, 2010). This is a huge topic. All I can add is that societal pressures, physicians' enthusiasm and giant pharmaceuticals have all joined hands to make humanity depend upon drugs just as they do upon food.

Scientific Research and Ethics

Biological and epidemiological research does not fall in the exclusive domain of physicians; indeed, a rather small percentage of practicing physicians are involved in clinical or experimental research. I mentioned their role in clinical trials. But ethical questions also concern basic laboratory research in areas clearly relevant to patient care. This point can be made by numerous examples that could include not giving due credit to the actual researcher as was the case in the discovery of the structure of DNA, misrepresentation of data, suppression of unpleasant data not to the liking of the sponsoring pharmaceutical, and so on.

Here I illustrate my point through the story of HeLa cells, how they came to exist, from whom these cells were derived and who did and did not benefit from the discovery of these cells. Rebecca Skloot in the book *The Immortal Life of Henrietta Lacks* [1920-1951] (Skloot, 2010)tells the story of HeLa cells with the tenderness it deserves. HeLa cells are immortalized human carcinoma cells; they might well be the most important tools in biological research so far; "they helped with some of the most important advances in medicine: the polio vaccine, chemotherapy, cloning, gene mapping, in vitro fertilization" (Skloot, 2010a).

HeLa cells are named using the first two letters of the donor Henrietta Lacks. She was a black woman who made a living growing tobacco where a generation ago her family worked as slaves. She diagnosed herself with something abnormal in her womb by the age of twenty-nine, just before her fifth pregnancy. A few months after the birth of her fifth child, on February 5, 1951, her doctor noted the result of a biopsy report – an aggressive cervical cancer. She was to be subjected to radium therapy. During the insertion of the radium pellet, a portion of her cancerous cervix was removed; this was the beginning of HeLa cells reproducing every twenty-four hours ever since when in culture.

Skloot writes,

> If you could pile all HeLa cells ever grown onto a scale, they'd weigh more than 50 million metric tons – an inconceivable number, given that an individual cell weighs almost nothing. Another scientist calculated that if you could lay all HeLa cells ever grown end-to-end, they'd wrap around

> the Earth at least three times, spanning more than 350 million feet. In her prime, Henrietta herself stood only a bit over five feet tall. (Skloot, 2010a)

Although the doctor of the Johns Hopkins Hospital, who excised the cervical piece had only research interest in mind, the piece of cervix was nevertheless removed without consent. The ultimate beneficiaries of this theft were not Henrietta and her family but others.

This book by Skloot is also an eye-opener about the state of health care in the United States until the 1950s. By the prevailing law of the land, all patients were not equal. A coloured person could not have access to all hospitals. Even at Johns Hopkins, which did treat black people, beds and operating facilities were separate from those reserved for white patients. This is almost like what had been the fate of the Dalits (untouchable caste) in India.

Conclusion

Medical ethics, like the ethics of all other professions, is determined by numerous social, political and monetary considerations. In no way is a doctor different from other professionals. The conscientiousness of doctors is determined by the prevailing socio-cultural milieu of the society in which they function and that differs widely as does the ethics of individual doctors.

Notes

1. Jules Romains (1885-1972) in *Knock* (1923) (New York: Barron's Educational Series 1962), 59-60. The play was made into a film in 1951, directed by Guy Lefranc. Knock was a self-made doctor without a formal degree. This is how he learned medicine (in Knock's words): "I had a passion for medical and pharmaceutical advertisements and for reading the Directions for Using on the bottles and pill boxes my parents brought. At the age of nine I had learned by heart a number of speeches on the faulty elimination of the constipated . . ." (Act 1, p.13). Knock's first assignment as a doctor was on a ship bound for India with thirty-five people including the crew; when asked how many patients he had, Knock said thirty-five. This portion is also quoted in *The Manufacture of Madness* by Thomas S. Szasz (London: Routledge & Kegan Paul, 1971), 207.

2. Thomas S. Szasz in *The Manufacture of Madness* (London: Routledge & Kegan Paul, 1971), 219. The reference to "revised form" is to the modification adopted at the Geneva Convention of 1949, which incorporated provisions against any discrimination

based on nationality, religion, race, gender, and political opinion.

3. Oscar Wilde was imprisoned in England for sodomy and wandered in Europe after his release; he died penniless in Paris (*Oscar Wilde: A Biography* by R. Ellman, New York: Penguin, 1988). Alan Turing opted for female hormonal treatment instead of prison as a punishment for his homosexuality; he committed suicide in 1954. For details on Turin's life and his historic contribution to the development of computer science and his other scientific feats, see *Alan Turing: the Enigma* by Andrew Hodges (London: Vintage Books, 1992), *The Code Book* by Simon Singh (New York: Anchor Books, 1999) and the Special Issue of *Nature* (Volume 482, February 23, 2012) on the 100th anniversary of his birth. Both Wilde and Turin, driven to their deaths in their forties, were a great loss to the world of literature and science. It is heartening to know that both are being honoured now and that a Turing Award, (an award equivalent to a Nobel Prize in computer science) has been instituted by the Association of Computing Machinery.

References

Amaloraparvanathan, J. "Kidneys for Sale," *Economic and Political Weekly*, Mumbai, April 14, 2007: 1332-1333.

Baylis, F. "Pregnant Women Deserve Better," *Nature* 465 (2010): 689-690.

Belkin, L. *First, Do No Harm* (New York: Ballantine Books, 1994).

Brabazon, J. *Albert Schweitzer: A Biography* (New York: G.P. Putnam's Sons, 1975).

Brown, E. R. *Rockefeller Medicine Men: Medicine and Capitalism in America* (Berkley: University of California Press, 1979).

Cherry, M. J. *Kidneys for Sale by Owner: Human Organ, Transplantation, and the Market.* Washington, DC: Georgetown University Press, 2005).

Culver, C. M. and Gert, B. *Philosophy in Medicine: Conceptual and Ethical Issues in Medicine and Psychiatry* (New York: Oxford University Press, 1982).

Duncan, B. L., Miller, S. D. and Sparks, J. A. *The Heroic Client: A Revolutionary Way to Improve Effectiveness through Client-Directed Outcome-Informed Therapy* (San Francisco: Jossey-Bass, 2004), 164.

Editorial. "Putting Gender on the Agenda," *Nature* 465 (2010): 665.

Ehrenreich, B. and English, D. *Witches, Midwives, and Nurses: A History of Women Healers* (Old Westbury, NY: The Feminist Press, 1973).

Ellman, R. *Oscar Wilde: A Biography* (New York: Penguin, 1988).

Emsley, J. *Molecules of Murder: Criminal Molecules and Classic Cases* (Cambridge: The

Royal Society of Chemistry, 2008).

Ford, A. R. and Saibil, D. (Ed.). *The Push to Prescribe: Women & Canadian Drug Policy* (Toronto: Women's Press, 2009).

Gould, D. "To Hell with Medical Secrecy!" *New Statesman*, May 3, 1967 (quoted from Szasz, 1971, 210-214).

Grodin, *The Nazi Doctors and the Nuremberg Code* (Oxford: Oxford University Press, 1992), 17-31.

Groopman, J. *How Doctors Think* (New York: Houghton Mifflin Company, 2007), 15-16.

Healy, D. *Let Them Eat PROZAC: The Unhealthy Relationship Between the Pharmaceutical Industry and Depression* (New York: New York University Press, 2004).

Hebert, P. C. *Doing Right: A Practical Guide for Medical Trainees and Physicians* (2009).

Hodges, A. *Alan Turing: The Enigma* (London: Vintage Books, 1992).

Hoenig, J. and Hamilton, M. W. *The De-segregation of the Mentally Ill* (London: Routledge & Kegan Paul, 1969).

Illich, I. *Limits to Medicine. Medical Nemesis: The Expropriation of Health* (New York: Penguin, 1976).

Iserson, K. V. *Demon Doctors: Physicians as Serial Killer* (Tucson: Galen Press, 2002).

Jha, P., Kumar, R., Vasa, P., Dhingra, N., Thiruchelvam, D., Moineddin, R. "Low Male-to-Female Sex Ratio in Children Born in India: National Survey of 1.1 Million Households," *Lancet* 367 (2006): 211-218.

Jonsen, A. R. *A Short History of Medical Ethics* (New York: Oxford University Press, 2000).

Kim, A. M., Tingen, C. M. and Woodruff, T. K. "Sex Bias in Trials and Treatment Must End," *Nature* 465 (2010): 688-689.

Kuhse, H. and Singer, P. Ed. *Bioethics: An Anthology* (New York: Wiley-Blackwell, 2006).

Mulay, S. "Quinacrine Sterilization: Unethical Trials," *Economic and Political Weekly*, Mumbai, India 32 (1997): 877-879.

Parry-Jones, W. L. *The Trade in Lunacy: A Study of Private Madhouses in England in the Eighteenth and Nineteenth Century* (London: Routledge & Kegan Paul, 1972).

Proctor, R. N. "Nazi Doctors, Racial Medicine, and Human Experimentation." In G. J. Annas and Michael A. Grodin *The Nazi Doctors and the Nuremberg Code: Human Rights in Human Experimentation* (Oxford: Oxford University Press, 1992).

Richmond, C. "Donald Gould," *The Independent*, March 4, 2002.

Rosen, G. *Madness in Society: Chapters in Historical Sociology of Mental Illness* (Chicago: Chicago University Press, 1968).

Sheikh, K. Sundararaman, T., Jain, K. et al. "Why Some Doctors Serve in Rural Areas: A Qualitative Assessment from Chhattisgarh State." (*http://www.phfi.org/downloads/pdf/Report_WhyDoctorsStay.pdf*) 2010.

Singh, S. *The Code Book: The Science of Secrecy from Ancient Egypt to Quantum Cryptography* (New York: Anchor Books, 1999), 165-189.

Skloot, R. *The Immortal Life of Henrietta Lacks* (New York: Crown Publishers, 2010).

Ibid., 2010a. 2.

Srinivasan, S. "The Clinical Trials Scenario in India," *Economic and Political Weekly*, Mumbai (August 29, 2009), 29-33.

Szasz, T. S. *The Myth of Mental Illness* (New York: Hoeber-Harper, 1961).

——. *The Manufacture of Madness* (London: Routledge & Kegan Paul, 1971).

——. 1971a. 210-214.

Udawadia, F. E. *The Forgotten Art of Healing and Other Essays* (New Delhi: Oxford University Press, 2009), 32-58.

Waitzkin, H. B. and Waterman, B. *The Exploitation of Illness in Capitalist Society* (Indianapolis: Bobbs-Merrill, 1974).

Whitaker, R. *Anatomy of an Epidemic: Magic Bullets, Psychiatric Drugs, and the Astonishing Rise of Mental Illness in America* (New York: Crown Publishers, 2010).

Williams, W. M. and Ceci, S. J. "Introduction: Striving for Perspective in the Debate on Women in Science." In *Why Aren't More Women in Science?* Ed.

Zucker, I. and Beery, A. "Males Still Dominate Animal Studies," *Nature* 465 (2010): 690.

CHAPTER 16

The Sun Rises in the West

When I first formed the idea, about 1938, of writing a systematic, objective and authoritative treatise on the history of science, scientific thought, technology and medicine in the Chinese culture-area, I regarded the essential problem as that of why modern science had not developed in Chinese civilisation (or Indian or Islamic) but only in that of Europe. Nevertheless, as they say in sunny France, "Attention! Un train peut cacher un autre!" [Attention! One train may hide another!]

Joseph Needham[1]

The centralization of capital is essential to the existence of capital as an independent power. The destructive influence of that centralization upon the markets of the world does but reveal, in the most gigantic dimensions, the inherent organic laws of political economy now at work in every civilized town. The bourgeois period of history has to create the material basis of the new world – on the one hand, the universal intercourse founded upon the mutual dependency of mankind, and the means of that intercourse; on the other hand, the development of the productive power of man and the transformation of material production into scientific domination of natural agencies. Bourgeois industry and commerce create these material conditions of a new world in the same way as geological revolutions have created the surface of the earth.

Karl Marx[2]

Introduction

"What do these things have in common? Fireworks, wood-block printing, canal lock-gates, kites, the wheelbarrow, chain suspension bridges and the magnetic compass. The answer is that they were all invented in China . . ." This is how the British Broadcasting Corporation (BBC) provided the background to the Joseph Needham question on October 16, 2006.

Joseph Needham was a distinguished biologist at Cambridge University, England. His treatise on China is unique. I am not aware of any comparable book on Indian and Egyptian science and civilization. Needham's pioneering work has been compared with Sir George Frazer's *The Golden Bough* (Frazer, 1922) and Arnold Toynbee's *A Study of History* (Toynbee, 1946, 1957). In this chapter, I am re-examining the broader implications of the Needham question and have attempted to provide an answer.

What Needham asked was not exactly what the BBC said. Even if it is in passing, Needham does extend the question also to Indian and Islamic civilization and does not limit it to China as the BBC did.

In reality, the Needham question is as follows: why were China, India, Persia, and Egypt – which were pioneers in medicine, philosophy, mathematics and astronomy, among other things – so far behind Europe?

Other commentators (Said, 1978; Frank, 1998) have also wondered on this matter in a similar vein. Toynbee (1946a) qualifies western supremacy when he writes, "While the economic and political maps have now been Westernized, the cultural map remains substantially what it was before our Western Society started on its career of economic and political conquest."

Needham went on to answer his own question; he says (Needham 2004), "The answer to all such questions lies, I now believe, primarily in the social, intellectual and economic structure of different civilizations." This is true. However, Needham's answer is evasive; it can easily be paraphrased as a question – why did the social, intellectual and economic structures of China, India, and the Islamic world differ from that of Europe? Critics of the West (Said, 1978; Frank, 1998) describe the expression of the Western bias in historiography but do not provide the reasons for the stalemate in the East. The only one I am aware of who does attempt to answer this question with regard to the Mughal period in India is the Indian historian Irfan Habib (1995).

The Coming of Age of Europe

The ascendency of Europe and of its extended arm America is relatively recent in the long history of civilization. According to political economist Andre Gunder Frank, even England, more developed than Germany and France and of course all other European countries, was not much ahead of India until the eighteenth century; Frank (1998a) says:

> Europe was certainly not central to the world economy before 1800. Europe was not hegemonic structurally, nor functionally, nor in terms of economic weight, or of production, technology or productivity, nor in per capita consumption nor in any way in its development of allegedly more "advanced" "capitalist" institutions. In no way were the sixteenth-century Portugal, the seventeenth-century Netherlands, or eighteenth-century Britain "hegemonic" in world economic terms. Nor in political ones. None of the above! In all these respects, the economics of Asia were far more "advanced," and its Chinese Ming/Qing, Indian Mughal, and even Persian Safavid and Turkish Ottoman empires carried much greater political and even military weight than any or all of Europe.

Consequently, the Needham quiz really refers to Europe from the eighteenth century on and not from an earlier period. This might be because the contribution of Europe to science, as well as to politics and economics (Toynbee, 1946a) was spectacular between the eighteenth and early twentieth century. Europe in this period produced such greats as Isaac Newton, Charles Darwin, James Clerk Maxwell, Joseph John Thomson (1856-1940), Max Karl, Ernst Ludwig Planck (1858-1947), Marie Curie, Ernest Rutherford (1871-1937), Albert Einstein, Niels Henrik David Bohr (1885-1972), Enrico Fermi (1901-1954), and many others. The American contribution, undoubtedly significant, cannot be detached from its European parentage; the Indian contribution by Raman, Satyen Bose, and Jagdish Chandra Bose is the product of colonization rather than indigenous. In any case, the world would be as primitive today as it was during the Middle Ages were it not for the Industrial Revolution, which produced these great figures, and which occurred in England and Europe but not in China, India and Egypt.

The rapid advances in science in the West essentially coincide with the birth of capitalism and the Industrial Revolution. The characteristics of capitalist production as distinct from the feudal mode of production, the source of capital and the part played by labour, machines, and commerce have been extensively and critically examined by Adam Smith (1776), Karl Marx (1867, 1885, 1894),[3] and many others.

Even critics of capitalism like Karl Marx would not dispute that it propelled science to new heights although opinions on the functions of science under capitalism differ (Bernal, 1939; Lewontin, 1991; Hobsbawm, 1975, 1977, 1994, 1995). So the real question is not why science blossomed in Europe, but rather, why did the Industrial Revolution begin in Europe and not in the East?

I would attempt to answer this. However, it is basically a question of political economy, which I know little of. Even Karl Marx of the nineteenth century or Eric Hobsbawm of the twentieth century describe the consequences of the Industrial Revolution and of the stalemate in India but do not specifically tell why this happened in England and not in India. Edward Said (1978) and Andre Gunder Frank (1998) lament the Western bias in historiography but do not answer why Asia was left behind.

The Obligatory Relationship between Capitalism and Natural Sciences

According to Karl Marx, the source of capital is labour and the means of production operated by labour; an essential feature of capital is to expand (Marx, 1867, 1885, 1894). This can be done by intensifying the exploitation of labour and improvement in the means of production. However, there is a physical limit to the exploitation of labour. On the other hand, there is no limit to renovations in the means of production. The survival of scientists depends upon innovations and not upon reproducing what already exists. Once they have created a new product, they can also create a market when a market does not really exist, such as in armaments. So the expansion of commerce is integral to the capitalist mode of production. A glaring testimony to this is provided by the relative scarcity of goods and services in the seventy years of the existence of the Soviet Union and the emergence of China as a world economic power in just the last thirty years, during which it parted from the Soviet model of socialism.

Three different factors, each a product of the capitalist mode of production, operate concomitantly to propel scientific advances. The first is societal need for the new; unprecedented advances in telecommunications are an example. Two, the unforeseen inquisitiveness made possible by rapid scientific advances; exploration of what lies beyond our planetary system is an example. Three, the demand for an answer to the mysteries of life, its origin, its functioning in health and disease, its interaction with the changing environment and the consequences of this interaction.

Bass (1992) writes, "It has been said of modern science that whereas the first half of the twentieth century belonged to physics, the second half belongs to biology." This is because for its own advance, biology requires tools, which must be provided by physics and chemistry. Indeed, major advances in biology have occurred since the beginning of the second half of the twentieth century. In general, advances in biology and medical science follow and do not precede advances in the natural sciences.

Why the Stalemate in India and China?

India, as a geographical entity, is ancient, but it begins to shape as a nation state only late during the Mughal period, particularly during the rule of Akbar the Great (1543-1605); a number of books deal with this period, but the ones most relevant to capitalist development are the writings of Karl Marx (see Husain et al., 2006) and Irfan Habib (1995). Marx characterized the mode of production in pre-British India as consisting of two elements – the village community and oriental despotism (Husain et al., 2006a) and attributed to British colonialism the role of acting as an unconscious tool of transforming India. Irfan Habib (1995) noted:

> In so far as capital, confined practically to the sphere of commerce, had failed to develop any independent basis for itself, its fortunes would lie with the Mughal ruling class, and, after its collapse, with such other classes as imitated or inherited the methods and institutions of that class. Denied during the eighteenth century, the large market that it had been provided with by the Mughal Empire, merchant capital had no choice but to atrophy. With this receded into the background those prominent economic land-

marks, which in the better days of the Mughal Empire might have been mistaken for capitalist features.

There must be socio-political reasons why Egypt, India, and China could not come out of feudalism. I think the reason lies, in part, with the rivers Nile, Ganges, and Yangtze, the providers of health and wealth in these three great civilizations of the past. True, there were shortages of the means of sustenance in the lands of these great rivers but they were never without a hope and never without a promise for the future. This led to strengthening feudalism with no compelling need to shatter it. India too had a shipping industry (Habib, 1995) but had no need to conquer territories, which European vassals found essential, and considered conquest as their natural right. Neither India nor China sought outside outlets.

In contrast, Europe was warring to establish nation states; boundaries were changing in search of something more promising, but most of all, to find a solution to impending shortage in their means of livelihood. The dismantling of feudalism at home, and the acquisition of land, countries, and continents in distant places, changed Europe first and eventually, the world. The steam engines of England and newly found America with no history of feudalism ushered an era which delivered more than anticipated. Toynbee (1946b) might have been correct when he wrote that the greater the hurdles, the greater the ushering in of initiatives to overcome them.

The American case in many ways is unique and revealing. It was the first country to break away from a colonial power (Britain) in 1776; by the end of World War II in 1945, that is in less than two hundred years, it emerged not only as the leading world power but also a leader in scientific and technological fields. To some extent science developed in America because it could draw talented immigrants from Europe; but the indigenous contribution of America in advancing science cannot be ignored; moreover, talented scientists would not have migrated to America unless it offered more than was possible in Europe either in the form of conducive culture for research or the requisite facilities or both.

It also follows that societies that did not make a breakthrough in the means of production also did not advance scientific achievements beyond what they had already made. This is one of the reasons why Ayurveda and yin-yang did not evolve into modern medicine.

Democracy, Secularism, and Science

The capitalist mode of production not only acts as an impetus for science and for innovation, it also necessitates a democratic culture far greater than that under feudalism, religious states, and socialist systems as witnessed to date. Democracy, freedom of the press, and a free atmosphere for research and academic pursuit is a desirable, perhaps necessary, requirement for the advance of science. The capitalist mode of production as we know of provided all that and hence science flourished in the West.

In recent years, three modes of production have been witnessed – feudal, capitalist, and the Soviet model of socialism. As I mentioned before, feudalism neither creates the necessity for science nor provides the necessary culture for its advance.

Although Marx envisioned the unfettered advance of science under socialism, his ideas have been distorted beyond recognition. How science would progress under Marx's socialism, therefore, is hypothetical. Of the major social orders that we know of, capitalism has provided the greatest impetus to science. The socialist order, as it was practiced in the former Soviet Union and Eastern Europe or as it is now practiced in Cuba, made significant advances in public health and health delivery and in armament and space technology rather than in the basic sciences and in medical science.

Conclusion

Joseph Needham posed the question of why science grew in the West and not in China, India, and the Islamic world. He was correct in his supposition that it was due to differences in social structure and culture. I have concluded that for a variety of reasons, the ascendency of science in the West is a consequence of the factors that propelled the Industrial Revolution and the capitalist mode of production in the West but not in India, China, and the Islamic world. The economic order is rapidly changing and one can anticipate a period in the near future where science will become universal and no longer confined to any specific region.

Regarding the developments in India, Marx observed (1853):

> The Indians will not reap the fruits of the new elements of society scattered among them by the British bourgeoisie, till in Great Britain itself the now ruling classes shall have been supplanted by the industrial proletariat, or till the Hindoos themselves shall have grown strong enough to throw off the English yoke altogether. At all events, we may safely expect to see, at a more or less remote period, the regeneration of that great and interesting country, whose general natives are, to use the expression of Prince Soltyko,[4] even in the most inferior classes, "plus fins et plus adroits que les Italiens,"[5] whose submission even counterbalanced by a certain calm nobility, who, notwithstanding their natural langor have astonished the British officers by their bravery, whose country has been the source of our languages, our religion, and who represent the type of the ancient German in the Jat, and the type of the ancient Greek in the Brahmin.

The first part of Marx's prediction – that is, the overthrow of the bourgeoisie by the proletariat – has not been achieved, and one cannot anticipate it being achieved anytime soon, if ever, but the second part of his prediction, that is Indians overthrowing British rule, did occur in 1947, and its consequences are being realized, primarily under a capitalist system.

Notes

1. Joseph Needham was a brilliant biochemist and a sinologist. His interest in China was triggered by the presence in his laboratory in Cambridge of three visiting Chinese scientists, notably Lu Gwei-Djen (1904-1991), whom he married in 1989 two years after his first wife, Dorothy Needham (1896-1987), died. The quote is from: Needham, J. *Science and Civilisation in China, VII, Part 2* (Cambridge: Cambridge University Press, 2004), 1.

2. Karl Marx. "Future Results of British Rule in India," *New York Daily Tribune*, August 8, 1853 (London, July 22, 1853). From *Karl Marx on India*, ed. I. Husain, I. Ḥabib and P. Patnaik (New Delhi: Tulika Books, 2006), 50.

3. Karl Marx's *Capital* consists of three volumes; volume 1 (1867), was published by Marx; Volume 2 (1885) and Volume 3 (1894) were edited by F. Engels and published posthumously.

4. Prince Alexei Dimitrievich Soltykoff (1806-1859) was a Russian traveller, writer and painter, who travelled in India, between 1841-1843 and 1845-1846 (Husain et al., 2006).

5. More subtle and adroit than the Italians.

References

Bass, L. "Schrödinger: A Philosopher in Planck's Chair," *British Journal of Philosophy of Science* 43 (1992): 111-127.

Bernal, J. D. *The Social Function of Science* (London: George Routledge & Sons, 1939).

Frank, A. G. *ReOrient: Global Economy in the Asian Age* (Berkeley: University of California Press, 1998).

Ibid., 1998a. 5.

Frazer, J. G. *The Golden Bough: A Study in Magic and Religion* (New York: Simon & Schuster, 1922).

Habib, I. *Essays in Indian History: Towards a Marxist Perception* (New Delhi: Tulika Books, 1995), 232.

Hobsbawm, E. J. *The Age of Capital 1848-1875* [1975] (London: Abacus.1975).

——. *The Age of Revolution 1789-1848* (1962) (London: Abacus, 1977).

——. *The Age of Empire 1875-1914* (1987) (London: Abacus.1994).

——. *The Age of Extremes 1914-1991* (1994) (London: Abacus.1995).

Husain, I., Habib, I. and Patnaik, P. *Karl Marx on India* (New Delhi: Tulika Books, 2006).

Ibid., 2006a. xxxi.

Lewontin, R. C. *Biology as Ideology* (New York: Harper Perennial, 1991).

Marx, K. "The Future Results of British Rule in India," *New York Tribune*, August 8, 1853 (London, Friday, July 22, 1853), From *Karl Marx on India*. Ed. Husain, I., Habib, I. and Patnaik, P. (New Delhi: Tulika Books, 2006), 49-50.

——. *Capital: A Critique of Political Economy, Volume 1.* [1867]: *The Process of Production of Capital.* Translated from the Original German by Samuel Moore and Edward Aveling, Edited by F. Engels, Online Version: Marx/Engels Archive (marxist.org) 1995.

——. *Capital: A Critique of Political Economy, Vol. II* [1885]: *The Process of Circulation of Capital.* Edited and translated by F. Engels (Chicago: Charles H. Kerr and Co., 1909).

——. *Capital: A Critique of Political Economy, Vol. III.* [1894]: *The Process of Capitalist Production as a Whole.* Translated by David Fernbach. London: Penguin Books, 1991.

Needham, J. *Science and Civilisation in China, VII, Part 2* (Cambridge: Cambridge University Press, 2004), 1.

Said. E. W. *Orientalism* (New York: Vintage Books, 1978).

Smith, A. *The Wealth of Nations* [1776] (New York: Bantam Classics, 2003).

Toynbee, A. J. *A Study of History.* Abridgement of Vols. I-VI by D. C. Somervell (New York: Oxford University Press, 1946).

Ibid., 1946a. 36.

Ibid., 1946b. 187-243.

——. *A Study of History.* Abridgement of Vols. VII-X by D. C. Somervell, New York: Oxford University Press, 1957.

CHAPTER 17

Survival of the Fit and the Unfit Medicines

The Collective principle asserts that ...no society can legitimately call itself civilised if a sick person is denied medical aid because of lack of means.

Aneurin Bevan[1]

The trumpet of a prophecy! O, Wind,
If Winter comes, can Spring be far behind?

Percy Bysshe Shelley[2]

Introduction

In the preceding pages, I have attempted to present the strength and weaknesses of all the major schools of medicine (Ayurveda, Chinese, homeopathy, modern medicine). I have come to the conclusion that the popularity of alternative medicine is not based on its strength; rather, it is based partly on the lacunae in modern medical science, but mainly because of poor health-care systems in most countries of the world.

The socio-political factors that gave rise to different schools of medicine from witchcraft to homeopathy do not exist now in any significant way, but their effects do. Scientific advances are not accompanied by scientific culture, which is a prerequisite for the overwhelming dominance of science over myths. Even in the twenty-first century, more people believe in creationism than in Darwin's theory of evolution. Mooney and Kirshenbaum (2009) paint an alarming picture of scientific illiteracy in the United States, which perhaps can be extended to the whole world. Hence the unfit and the fit in medicine exist because modern medicine has not solved all problems of health and disease, and governments have not ensured universal health care.

Modern Medicine Versus Other Schools of Medicine

Modern medicine is the most rational evolution of witchcraft. However, at each critical stage of the evolution of medicine, vestiges of the old continued either in their original shape such as the case with Hindu medicine or as a new aberration such as homeopathy.

Despite all advances in medicine, however, rational and effective treatment of many diseases is still illusive. Ordinarily, a false promise to cure a disease is unethical as is the case with any other social interaction. Modern medicine accepts its therapeutic limitations. On the other hand, nothing is considered beyond the means of alternative medicine. Other schools of medicine give hope where modern medicine has conceded defeat.

Spurious assertion has become popular that the difference between modern medicine and other schools of medicine is the use of synthetic versus natural products. While this is clearly not true, it has a profound effect. Iatrogenic diseases, irrational therapy by physicians of modern medicine, and the culture of "what is natural is better" has created a place for other schools of medicine. The time is not yet ripe to expect the demise of alternative medicine. Rather, it is still a time when all healing practices – the unfit and the fit – are bound to exist for some time.

Modern medicine, like any other science, can never be perfected. However, human desire to get rid of any unpleasant physical experience is universal.

While writing a manuscript to tell his children "the entire story of the Crows from A to Z," Canadian biologist William Rowan (1891-1957) pointed out that "in Science there is no Z. Nothing in Science ever reaches finality . . ."[3] (Ainley, 1993). This is true for modern medicine in contrast to other schools of medicine, which started and ended with Z.

In this concluding chapter, I do not wish to deal with other schools of medicine. Rather, I will point to the salient weaknesses of health-care systems that allow their survival. By and large, other schools of medicine succeed when they treat self-limiting diseases. Modern medicine accumulates discredit because it cannot treat all maladies; cancer is an example.

The 1978 Declaration of Alma-Ata on Primary Health Care

The International Conference on Primary Health Care, held at Alma-Ata, in the Kazakh Republic of the former Soviet Union during September 6-12, 1978, called for urgent action by all governments and health institutions to protect and promote the health of all people of the world. The Alma-Ata declaration had a broad vision of health and declared that health – which is a complete state of physical, mental, and social well-being and not merely the absence of disease or infirmity – is a fundamental human right and that the attainment of the highest possible level of health is a most important worldwide social goal. It called upon all governments to formulate national policies, strategies, and plans of action to launch and sustain primary health care as part of a comprehensive national health system and in coordination with other sectors. The Alma-Ata declaration projected an acceptable level of health for all people of the world by the year 2000. That was a decade ago. Things have not changed much. Indeed, in many parts of the world, health care has taken a downward dive.

Hurdles against Health Care

I think that poor health care in most parts of the world is not due to scanty resources but rather reflects the failures of governments. I will attempt to illustrate this by briefly presenting the state of health care in three countries – the United States, the richest country of the world, India, the second most populous country of the world and on a path of aggressive development, and Cuba, a rather poor country neighbouring the US and facing a US embargo ever since Fidel Castro came to power in 1959.

There are two types of hurdles against universal health care. The first, where therapy is not presently available, and the second, where it is, but not made available to the needy.

The Non-availability of Therapy

This is a very minor problem in the overall context of health care. Although all diseases cannot be cured, almost all can be managed reasonably well with available drugs, technology, and a support system.

The Availability of Therapy

This second hurdle is where modern medicine does possess effective therapy but its delivery is faulty for a number of reasons. It is here that the comparison among the United States, India, and Cuba becomes meaningful, which is briefly presented below.

The Case of the USA

The pre-colonial America was a "healthy land of bracing air, clean water and acres of fertile soil" (Fee, 1994). America was conquered by small pox which eliminated 50 to 90 percent of native Americans in some areas (Duffy, 1953) and was developed by slave labour. Such a beginning is incompatible with public health, which hardly occupied any important place until the beginning of the twentieth century (Fee, 1994). Even in the beginning of the twenty-first century the difference in the healthcare available to the rich and poor is enormous. The sorry state of health care in the United States has been pointed out by numerous scholars (Brown, 1979; Illich, 1976; Konner, 1994; Rosen, 1968; Szasz, 1971; Waitzkin and Waterman, 1974; Whitaker, 2010).

On the other hand, the contribution of the United States to medical science is second to none. Its health institutions are equipped with the most sophisticated diagnostic and therapeutic gadgets and available to those who can afford them. The Food and Drug Administration (FDA) is always on the alert to ensure drugs meet the toughest tests of efficacy and safety. The United States continues to innovate its medical curriculum in the hope of producing quality doctors.

And yet, from the point of view of public good, the US health-care system would rate poorly, in comparison to many other developed countries, including Canada and a poor country like Cuba. The state of healthcare available to a substantial number of Americans is described by Konner (1994) as follows:

> I believe that America will move toward, and eventually attain, a single-payer system for the delivery of health care. What counts most in the meantime are not niceties of ideology, nor even our agreed-upon abstract ethical principles, but faces: the faces of the uninsured, sitting in pain hour after hour in emergency-ward waiting rooms not far from where we sit; of parents who worked and paid their premiums for years but have been dropped from coverage because their child has become chronically ill; of women who cannot afford routine gynaecological care; of men denied insurance because they are florists and hairdressers; of middle-class families who must spend their entire life savings before they can qualify for the assistance of their community when faced with a catastrophic illness.

Health is designated a private matter and therefore outside the domain of the state. State intervention is shunned. Moreover, the cost of medical education is needlessly high, which is followed by the absurdly high cost of insurance; the doctor must recover this cost through patient care, which many patients cannot afford. Preventive measures are not fully utilized. The culture of what is natural is superior is very high in the USA and well off Americans more than any one else feel entitled to the best in the world. United States is a thriving ground for other schools of medicine.

The Case of India

Health care in India is perhaps the worst of all countries with a comparable economy.

According to the Indian Planning Commission, India is short of 600,000 trained physicians. Standard medical schools are fewer than needed and spurious private, money-minting medical schools of the poorest quality possible, have mushroomed.

Approximately 70 percent of Indians live in rural areas; the shortage of doctors in general, and in rural areas in particular, has become a fertile ground for quackery and alternative medicine. India spends exorbitant amounts to produce doctors of Ayurvedic medicine and supports Ayurvedic and Unani-tibb hospitals, which serve no purpose because all emergency cases reaching these hospitals are referred to hospitals of modern medicine. A Committee set up in 1943 under the chairmanship of Sir Joseph Bhore (1878-1960) had recommended against producing doctors of Ayurveda and Unani-tibb but India gained independence in

1947 and did not abide by Bhore Committee directives (Gautham and Shyamprasad, 2009).

Nationalism in India also meant revivalism; instead of modernizing medical education, reducing the number of years required to train a doctor from five to four or even less, preventing excessively high failure rates, emphasis was laid on reviving indigenous medical systems. Indeed, China, poorer and less industrialized than India at the time of liberation in 1949, has solved much of its health problems as noted by a delegation of visiting American scientists (Science for the People, 1974).

Aside from acute shortage of doctors, the other problem faced by the Indian population is the cost of medical care. Many poor families incur debt to have their children treated by qualified doctors. They borrow money from loan sharks sometimes at 100 to 200 percent interest, which pushes them into perpetual servitude.

The Case of Cuba

In contrast to the United States and India, a poor country like Cuba produces enough doctors to be able to send to other countries during emergencies. A doctor is in charge of the health of a designated population; at least one doctor and one nurse must reside in their constituency, and they must make sure that no pregnant woman loses her baby; and if they feel that they cannot manage it, they transfer her to major hospital facilities. Since the real cost of treatment is not very high, no sick person suffers more than absolutely necessary because of the lack of availability of a healer or drugs. Homeopathy still exists in Cuba, but its scope is limited. By all known standards of healthcare, Cuba is easily on the top, even better than China, with a similar economic and political system.

Projection into the Future

There are two important functions of medical science. One is to solve the problems of human biology and the second is to cure all diseases without producing new ones. This is not a simple assignment, but it is achievable. Sufficient advances have already taken place in medical science to allow speculation that all aspects of human physiology will eventually be known. However, from a practical point of view, it is not the science of medicine but rather its application that will determine its place in society. The following points, in my view, are key to establishing the supremacy of scientific medicine over non-scientific approaches.

Primary Health Care

Universally available health care is, by far, the most important determinant of the future of medicine; it is not organ transplant, not our ability to save a twenty-four-week-old preemie, and not to prolong the life – rather the agony – of a terminally ill patient. Priority in medicine must be proportional to the prevalence of a disease. Primary health care must reach to the farthest corner within a country and around the world. This, in my opinion, is achievable within existing world resources and the resources of each and every country.

Alleviation of Poverty

Poverty is incompatible with a healthy body (Kawachi et al., 1999). Just as the community of nations recognizes the necessity of intervening in national disasters and genocides anywhere in the world, so also it should be recognized that poverty is simultaneously a national and international problem. Substantial evidence exists that poverty is directly related to illness.

It is important to note that while primary health care is universally accessible in some countries, no country in the world has been able to abolish poverty, India being at the bottom of the ladder; in many advanced countries like the United States, Canada, Australia, and New Zealand, poverty is linked to racial bias; the victims are primarily indigenous people, and in the case of the United States, poverty is conspicuous among indigenous Americans, African-Americans and Hispanics.

Disease Prevention

In purely economic terms, it is a lot cheaper to prevent diseases than to treat them. The experience of smallpox, plague, cholera and polio clearly reveals the virtues of preventive measures. In the US setting, the care of just a few patients with polio would have amounted to the total cost of all vaccinations. However, disease prevention requires simultaneous alleviation of poverty, provision of clean water, and education. In some cases, disease prevention may entail early diagnosis, such as tuberculosis or complicated pregnancies.

Control over Pharmaceuticals

Major pharmaceuticals function like any other enterprise. Many drugs for the same illness are just like soaps, doing the same thing at different costs. Governments should find some system of determining the cost of drugs and shortening patent time in order to promote generic drugs.

Universal Access to Abortion

A majority of maternal deaths are caused by complications resulting from illegal abortions carried out under unhygienic conditions by unqualified persons. Pregnancy outside marriage is treated worse than a crime, forcing young women to seek help in secrecy. Abortion is still illegal in many countries. Even in countries where abortion is legal, such as India, the social stigma against pregnancy of an unmarried girl or woman is so powerful that they seek secret abortions by quacks. Provision can be made and should be made to facilitate free and secret abortion within modern medical facilities.

Health for All

Finally, the emphasis of the health-care system must shift from taking care of the sick to ensuring health for all. In a highly developed system, the physician is custodian of the health and not only a caretaker of disease.

The Fit and the Unfit

At some stage, I considered using the terms "fit, fittest, and unfit." The term "fittest" was to be borrowed from Darwin, who borrowed it from Herbert Spencer (1820-1903), who too had conceived of the evolution of species before Darwin although his treatise *The Principles of Biology* is dated December 5, 1868 (Spencer, [1868] 2009), nine years after Darwin's *The Origin of Species* (Darwin, [1859] 1999). I must assume that Darwin used the term *fittest* in a metaphorical way rather than in a mechanistic sense. Obviously, *fittest* cannot be defined; it would reduce the number of species to fewer and fewer than there are and put an end to the very process of evolution. Likewise, the fittest in medicine does not yet exist and is unlikely to ever exist because no one can ever say that the ultimate therapy for any ailment has already been discovered and no further research is needed. For this reason, I have limited myself to the use of the terms, "fit" and "unfit." As long as the convincingly best therapy for an ailment has not been discovered, there will always be a room for the unfit. Homeopathy, Ayurveda, Chinese medicine, and chiropractic will be with us for a long time; so far, they have only accepted defeat when it comes to medical emergencies.

Notes

1. Aneurin Bevan (1897-1960) was the minister of health (1945-1951) after his Labour Party came to power in UK after World War II. Bevan's "National Health Services Act of 1946" was the beginning of the universal health care outside the Socialist block. The quote is from Bevan, A. *In Place of Fear* (New York: Simon Schuster, 1952), 110.

2. Percy Bysshe Shelley (1792-1822) was a charismatic British poet who got expelled from Oxford University after only five months for publishing a pamphlet "The Necessity of Atheism." At the time of his death, he was living in Italy. He was drowned in 1822 in the Bay of Spezia, when his boat caught a sudden violent storm. The quote is from his poem "Ode to the West Wind."

3. The quote is from a manuscript written by William Rowan for his children and, according to biographer Marianne Gosztonyi (1993), is preserved in the archives of the University of Alberta.

References

Ainley, M. G. *Restless Energy: A Biography of William Rowan 1891-1957* (Montreal: Vehicule Press, 1993), 184.

Brown, E. R. *Rockefeller Medicine Men: Medicine and Capitalism in America* (Berkley: University of California Press, 1979).

Darwin, C. *The Origin of Species* (New York: Bantam Books, [1859] 1999).

Duffy, J. *Epidemics in Colonial America* (Baton Rouge, La: Louisiana State University Press, 1953).

Fee, E. "Public Health and the State: The United States". In *The History of Public Health and the Modern State*. Ed. Dorothy Porter (Amsterdam: Editions Rodopi B.V. 1994), 224-275.

Gautham, M. and Shyamprasad, K. M. "Needed: 'Basic' Doctors of Modern Medicine," *The Hindu* (Indian Daily) November 5, 2009.

Illich, I. *Limits to Medicine. Medical Nemesis: The Expropriation of Health* (New York: Penguin, 1976).

Kawachi, I., Kennedy, B. and Wilkinson, R.G. Ed. *The Society and Population Health Reader: Income inequality and Health* (New York: New Press, 1999).

Konner, M. *Medicine at the Crossroads* (New York: Vintage Books, 1994), 252.

Mooney, C. and Kirshenbaum, S. *Unscientific America: How Scientific Illiteracy Threatens Our Future* (New York: Basic Books, 2009).

Rosen, G. *Madness in Society: Chapters in the Historical Sociology of Mental Illness* (Chicago: University of Chicago Press, 1968).

Science for the People. *China: Science Walks on Two Legs* (New York: Avon, 1974).

Spencer, H. *Principles of Biology* V. 1. and 2 [1864] (Danvers, MA: General Books, 2009).

Szasz, T. S. *The Manufacture of Madness* (London: Routledge & Kegan Paul, 1971).

Waitzkin, H. B. and Waterman, B. *The Exploitation of Illness in Capitalist Society* (Indianapolis: Bobbs-Merrill, 1974).

Whitaker, R. *Anatomy of an Epidemic: Magic Bullets, Psychiatric Drugs, and the Astonishing Rise of Mental Illness in America* (New York: Crown Publishers, 2010).

APPENDIX I

Natural Drugs

A partial list of natural drugs currently in use by modern medicine for therapy or as research tool. Ayurveda and Chinese medicine most likely possess many more drugs but they are yet not listed here.

Acacia: Gummy exudation from many plants of the family *Fabaceae*. High molecular weight substances once used as a diuretic, like glucose and sucrose. Acacia plants contain many pharmacologically active chemicals.

Adrenaline: Present mainly in adrenal gland but has been synthesized. Used to treat anaphylaxis and asthma.

Aldosterone: Principal hormone-maintaining sodium and potassium balance. Antagonists of aldosterone, like spironolactone, are used as diuretics.

Aloe: Laxative.

Aminoglycosides: A group of antibiotics (streptomycin, gentamycin, tobramycin) produced by soil actinomycetes and can also be synthesized.

Angiotensin: Both I and II are present in the body, and their antagonists are used in heart failure and hypertension.

Antibiotics: Most antibiotics naturally exist in moulds although synthetic ones are more practical. Some are mentioned below.

Antidiuretic hormone (vasopressin): Diabetes insipidus, characterized by too much water loss through urine (this is distinct from diabetes mellitus, which is a disturbance in sugar metabolism).

Antimony: Antimony salts against leishmaniasis caused by protozoa; one form of the disease is *Kala-azar* (black fever).

Arecoline: Present in betel nuts (*Arecca catechu*). It is used to cause euphoria in South Asia but has no clinical use.

Arsenic: Against certain leukemia and sleeping sickness (trypanosomiasis).

Artemisinin: Derived from Chinese weed Qing hao (*Artimisia annua*); anti-malaria drug effective against chloroquine-resistant malaria.

Ascorbic acid (vitamin C): Citrus fruits, with many uses, prevent scurvy.

Aspirin: Modified from salicin present in willow bark; analgesic, antirheumatic, and antithrombotic.

Atropine: From *Atropa belladonna*; suppresses excessive secretion such as during dentistry and anaesthesia and exposure to war gases. Also used against asthma like conditions.

Azelaic acid: Naturally occurring dicarbolic acid. Used against acne and pigmentary disorders.

Berberine: Extracts of families of Ranuculaceae and Berberidadaceae; effective against bacterial diarrhea and cholera.

Bismuth: Against diarrhea and gastric irritation.

Blood: Matching human blood is commonly used to replace blood loss.

Botulinum toxin (BOTOX): Toxin from anaerobic bacterium *Clostridium botulinum*, used to treat strabismus, facial wrinkles and many other conditions.

Bran: Bran, like other bulk-forming food (fruits, vegetables), an anticonstipation agent.

Bungarotoxin: Toxic constituent of cobra venom used as research tool.

Caffeine: Present in tea and coffee. Respiratory stimulant for preterm babies.

Camptothecin: Derived from Chinese tree *Camptotheca acuminate*; natural and modified form against different kinds of cancer.

Cannabis (hashish, marihuana, bhang): Derived from hemp plants (*Cannabis sativa*). Used to treat nausea and vomiting and analgesic; also a drug of abuse because of its mood altering action.

Cascara: Derived from the bark of buckthorn tree and acts as a laxative.

Castor oil: Derived from the bean of castor plant *Ricinus communis*. It contains toxic ricin and a triglycerides, the latter are laxatives.

Charcoal: Used to neutralize orally ingested poisons, often in activated form.

Chaulmoogra oil: Obtained from trees of the *Flacourtaceae*, used to treat leprosy.

Cocaine: From coca shrub *Erythroxylon coca*; first local anaesthetic and a drug of abuse.

Codeine: Derived from poppy (*Papaver* somniferum); used against pain and cough.

Colchicine: Derived from the corn and seeds of the plant meadow saffron (*Colchicum autumnale*); effective against acute gout.

Colistin: A polymixin antibiotic produced by *Bacillus colistinus* reserved for topical application to avoid renal toxicity.

Conotoxin: Poison present in the venom of the marine cone snail; used as a research tool to study ion channels and the acetylcholine receptors.

Corticosteroids: Cortisol is the normal human glucocorticoids; synthetic substitutes of cortisol are more frequently used than cortisol in diseases involving inflammation and many other anomalies.

Curare: The South American arrow poison; its main constituent, d-tubocurarine, was the first muscle relaxant during surgery.

Dicumarol (bishydroxycoumarin): Derived from spoiled sweet clover of the *Melilotus* family. Like heparin, it prevents clotting. A synthetic congener warfarin is more commonly used than dicumarol to prevent blood clotting and also as rat poison.

Digitalis glycosides: Present in many plants and toad skin; individual glycosides described below.

Digitalis (digoxin): Present in *Digitalis lanata*. Primary drug against heart failure until late 1960s but used less commonly now. Also effective against certain type of cardiac arrhythmias.

Digitalis (digitoxin): Present in *Digitalis purpurea*. Same use as digoxin.

Ergot alkaloids: Produced by fungus *Claviceps purpurea*. Ergotamine is used against migraine and ergonovine occasionally to produce postpartum uterine contraction.

Estrogens. *See Oestrogens*

Ethanol (alcohol): Topical antiseptic at high concentrations; wine reputed to protect against cardiac diseases. Chronic use associated with liver toxicity and foetal alcohol syndrome.

Ferrous salts (iron): To treat iron deficiency anaemia.

Folic acid: Essential vitamin derived from fruits and vegetables; deficiency can cause neural tube defects and inadequate blood formation.

Green fluorescent protein: Isolated from jellyfish and used as a biosensor (research tool) to monitor movement of particles inside cells. The 2008 chemistry Nobel Prize was awarded for this discovery.

Glucose: Essential nutrient.

Glycerin: Laxative and diuretic.

Gold: Used against rheumatoid arthritis not responsive to conventional therapy.

Helium: Used in pulmonary function tests and in pulmonary obstruction.

Heparin: Present in human and animal tissues. Usually extracted from porcine intestine or bovine lungs; prevents blood clotting.

Heroin: Not natural but can be easily made from morphine. Drug of abuse but is a potent analgesic.

Histamine: Present in venoms, bacteria, plants, and animals tissues; some use in diagnosis of bronchial hyperactivity. Antagonists of histamine are more commonly used.

Huperzine A: Derived from club moss *Huperzia serrata*. Used to enhance memory in Alzheimer's disease and also as a memory booster.

Insulin: Bovine or porcine pancreas for any type of diabetes.

Interferons: Natural or synthetic, used against certain viral infections and Kaposi's sarcoma.

Iodine: Essential for the synthesis of thyroid hormone, prophylaxis against thyroid deficiency.

Lithium: Bipolar disorders.

Lobeline: Derived from certain tobacco (*Lobelia inflate*). Previously used as expectorant and anti-asthmatic drugs but now used as a research tool to stimulate carotid body.

Lovastatin: Derived from mold (*Penicillium citrinum*). One of the group of statins used to lower cholesterol.

Lysergic acid diethylamide (LSD): Synthesized from lysergic acid, which is present in fungus that grow on rye. Hallucinogenic and not a therapeutic agent.

Magnesium: Against cardiac irregularity, magnesium salts as antacids and laxatives, and in toxemia of pregnancy.

Mannitol: Used to prevent cerebral edema; in lead poisoning and to prevent kidney failure.

Mercury: In the past used as a diuretic.

Morphine: Poppy (*Papaver* somniferum) contain morphine, codeine and papaverine. Morphine and codeine are used against pain, diarrhea and cough. Heroin is acetyl morphine and synthesized.

Muscarine: Derived from mushrooms, a source of poisoning.

Nicotine: Derived from leaves of tobacco, *Nicotiana tabacum*; cause of addiction to smoking. Use associated with decrease in Parkinson's disease.

Nitric oxide: First discovered in inner lining of blood vessels and now known to be active ingredient of many drugs including nitroglycerin used to control cardiac pain. Used to treat pulmonary hypertension in children.

Oestrogens: Natural female hormone; multiple uses.

Ouabain: Derived from *Strophanthus gratus*. Like digitalis mentioned above.

Papaverine: Derived from poppy (*Papaver* somniferum). Not analgesic, not addictive. Of little use but can suppress intestinal colic.

Physostigmine: Derived from Calabar beans (*Physostigma venenosum*). Used against glaucoma; in the past used as an antidote against atropine but no more used for this purpose.

Pilocarpine: Like arecoline and muscarine but derived from shrubs of the genus *Pilocarpus*. Used to prevent dryness of eyes. Potentially can be used in all conditions requiring cholinergic simulation.

Predates sildenafil (Viagra) against erectile dysfunction.

Plasma: Free blood cells and used for fluid replacement. Platinum: Platinum containing compounds (e.g., cisplatin) are used in cancer chemotherapy.

Podophyllin: Derived from plant *Podyphyllum peltatum*, applied topically for anogenital warts.

Polymixin: An antibiotic produced by various strains of *Bacillus polymyxa*; used mainly topically in view of serious renal toxicity.

Progesterone: Naturally occurring hormone but also synthesized. Many uses including in oral contraceptives.

Prostaglandins: Derived from arachidonic acid, present in diet. First identified in human semen.

Psoralens: Present in many plants including limes, lemons, and figs. Photosenistive and act like ultraviolet waves.

Pyridoxine (Vitamin B6): Source same as other water soluble vitamins; useful against certain forms of anaemia.

Quinidine: It is derived from Peruvian bark, is an isomer of antimalarial drug quinine, and is used to treat certain type of irregularity of heartbeat.

Quinine: It is derived from Peruvian bark and remained the main drug against malaria for thousands of years and is still used.

Reserpine: Derived from Rauwolfia serpentina. Occasionally used to treat hypertension.

Retinoids: Include all natural compounds with vitamin A-like activity.

Salicin: Present in willow bark; its antipyretic and antirheumatic activity was improved by modifying it into aspirin and salicylate.

Scopolamine: From *Hyoscyamus niger*; like atropine and also hallucinogenic. Used as preanaesthetic medication.

Senna: Plants containing laxative property.

Serotonin (5-hydroxytryptamine): Present in many tissues; many mood changing drugs act by modifying its concentration or action.

Sodium chloride (common salt): Constituent of all fluid replacement therapy.

Streptomycin: Produced by *Streptomyces griseus* was the second antibiotic after penicillin but now has been replaced by other less toxic antibiotics.

Strychnine: Derived from the seeds of Indian plant *Nux vomica*; antagonizes glycine receptor and used as a research tool.

Sulfur: Against certain skin disorders.

Taxanes: Paclitaxel isolated from the bark of Western yew tree effective against certain cancers.

Testosterone: Major male hormone; natural or modified testosterone can be used as substitution therapy. Consumption of many animal parts as a part of folk medicine is based on the assumption of deriving testosterone-like chemicals.

Tetrodotoxin: Poison present in puffer fish; an important research tool to block nerve conduction.

Thebaine: Present along with morphine in poppy but does not have analgesic activity.

Theobromine: Present along with caffeine in tea leaves, *Thea sinensis*, but does not possess caffeine-like activity.

Theophylline: Present in coffee and tea, is often modified to aminophylline. Useful in the treatment of asthma.

Thyroxin: Thyroid hormone used in substitution therapy.

Trabectedin: First isolated from sea squirt, *Ecteinascidia turbinate*. Approved form used for the treatment of soft tissue tumors, like ovarian tumor.

Tryptophan: Present in foods and can be converted into serotonin (5-hydroxy-typtamine).

Ultraviolet: In combination with naturally occurring psoralens, used in the treatment of vitiligo (loss of skin pigments), psoriasis, and cutaneous lymphoma.

Urea: End product of protein metabolism excreted in urine and the first organic compound synthesized from inorganic reagents. Diuretic, used in kidney failure.

Vancomycin: An antibiotic produced by *Streptococcus orientalis*.

Vasopressin: A pituitary hormone used to treat paralysis of intestine and diabetes insipidus (excess of water loss distinct from the commonly known diabetes associated with abnormal glucose metabolism. Usually, a synthetically modified vasopressin, which is more stable, is used.

Veratrum alkaloids: A family of chemically related substances obtained from liliaceous plants of the suborder *Melanthaceae*. Used in certain cases of hypertension but mainly as research tool.

Vinca alkaloids: Vinblastine, vincristine, vinleurosine and vinrosidine are derived from Madagascar periwinkle plant *Catharanthus roseus*. Used to treat certain types of cancer (leukemia, lymphoma and some solid tumours).

Water: Essential body constituent.

Yohimbine: An alkaloid derived from West African tree, Yohimbéhé. At one time promoted as an aphrodisiac but currently used as a research tool.

Ziconotide: Isolated from the venom of marine cone snail. Used to treat chronic pain resulting from spinal cord injury and research tool.

Zinc: Zinc oxide is used as a sunscreen against UVA.

Subject Index

Other Titles from Three Essays

Aijaz Ahmad, *On Communalism and Globalisation: Offensives of the Far Right*

Amar Farooqi, *Opium City: The Making of Early Victorian Bombay*

Angana Chatterji, *Violent Gods: Hindu Nationalism in India's Present – Narratives from Orissa*

Antoinette Burton, *Brown Over Black: Race and the Politics of Postcolonial Citation*

Archana Prasad, *Against Ecological Romanticism: Verrier Elwin and the Making of an Anti-Modern Tribal Identity*

AR Vasavi, *Shadow Space: Suicides and the Predicament of Rural India*

Arup Banerji, *Old Routes: North Indian Nomads and Bankers in Afghan, Uzbek and Russian Lands*

Ashraf Aziz, *Light of the Universe: Essays on Hindustani Film Music*

Badri Raina, *The Underside of Things: India and the World – A Citizen's Miscellany*

Barbara Harriss-White, *India's Market Society: Three Essays in Political Economy*

Biswamoy Pati, *Identity, Hegemony, Resistance: Towards a Social History of Conversions in Orissa, 1800-2000*

Brinda Karat, *Survival and Emancipation: Notes from Indian Women's Struggles*

Colin Leys, *Total Capitalism: Market Politics, Market State*

Deepa Ganesh, *A Life in Three Octaves: Gangubai Hangal and Her Times*

Eduardo Galeano, *Open Veins of Latin America: Five Centuries of the Pillage of a Continent*

Harsh Mander, *A Fractured Freedom: Chronicles of India's Margins, 2004–2011*

Jackie Assayag and Véronique Bénéï (eds.), *Re-mapping Knowledge: The Making of South Asian Studies in India, Europe and America, 19th-20th centuries*

John S Saul, *Development After Globalisation: Theory and Practice for an Embattled South in a New Imperial Age*

John S Saul, *Decolonisation and Empire: Contesting the Rhetoric and Practice of Resubordination in Southern Africa and Beyond*

John S Saul, *Liberation Lite: The Roots of Recolonisation in Southern Africa*

KN Panikkar, *An Agenda for Cultural Action and Other Essays*

KN Panikkar, *History as a Site of Struggle: Collected Essays on History, Politics and Culture*

Kristoffel Lieten, *Views on Development: The Local and the Global in India and Pakistan*

Meera Nanda, *Breaking the Spell of Dharma and Other Essays*

Meera Nanda, *The Wrongs of the Religious Right: Reflections on Science, Secularism and Hindutva*

Madhu Trivedi, *The Emergence of the Hindustani Tradition: Music, Dance and Drama in North India, 13th to 19th Centuries*

Meeto (Kamaljit Bhasin-Malik), *In the Making: Identity Formation in South Asia*

Mukul Dube, *The Path of the Parivar: Articles on Gujarat and Hindutva*

Nasreen Ahmed, *Muslim Leadership and Women's Education: Uttar Pradesh, 1886-1947*

Omar Khalidi, *Khaki and Ethnic Violence in India: Army, Police and Paramilitary Forces during Communal Riots*

Omar Khalidi, *Muslims in Indian Economy*

Paul R Brass, *Forms of Collective Violence: Riots, Pogroms, and Genocide in Modern India*

Patricia Jeffery and Roger Jeffery, *Confronting Saffron Demography: Religion, Fertility, and Women's Status in India*

Perry Anderson, *The Indian Ideology.*

Pritam Singh, *Economy, Culture and Human Rights: Turbulence in Punjab, India and Beyond*

Radhika Desai, *Slouching Towards Ayodhya: From Congress to Hindutva in Indian Politics*

Rajesh Sharma, *In/disciplines: Notes on Culture, Politics and Education*

Ralph Russell, *Findings, Keepings: The Autobiography of Ralph Russell, Early Years, 1918-1945*

Ralph Russell, *Losses Gains: The Autobiography of Ralph Russell, Middle Years, 1945-1958*

RK Jain, *Indian Transmigrants: Malaysian and Comparative Essays*

Romila Thapar, *The Aryan: Recasting Constructs*

S. Irfan Habib, *To Make the Deaf Hear: Ideology and Programme of Bhagat Singh and His Comrades*

Shereen Ratnagar, *The Other Indians: Essays on Pastoralists and Pre-Historic Tribal People*

Shubh Mathur, *The Everyday Life of Hindu Nationalism: An Ethnographic Account*

Subhash Gatade, *The Saffron Condition: Politics of Repression and Exclusion in Neoliberal India*

Sunil Kumar, *The Present in Delhi's Pasts: Five Essays*

Sunil Kumar (ed.), *Demolishing Myths or Mosques and Temples: Readings on History and Temple Desecration in Medieval India*

Utsa Patnaik, *The Republic of Hunger and Other Essays*

Vasudha Dalmia, *Orienting India: European Knowledge Formation in the Eighteenth and Nineteenth Centuries*

Vijay Prashad, *The American Scheme: Three Essays*

Vina Mazumdar, *The Mind and the Medium: Explorations in the Evolution of British Imperial Policy in India*

Zaheer Baber, *Secularism, Communalism and the Intellectuals*